Series editor
Daniel Horton-Szar
BSc (Hons) MBBS (Hons)
Kent & Canterbury Hospital
Canterbury
Kent

Faculty advisor
Simon S Cross
MB BS BSc MD MRCPath
Senior Lecturer in
Pathology and Honorary
Consultant
Histopathologist
University of Sheffield
Medical School

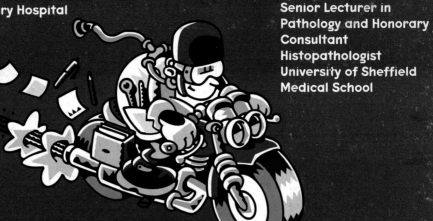

Pathology

Bethan Goodman Jones
BSc (Hons) PhD
University of Sheffield Medical
School
Sheffield

M Mosby

London • Philadelphia
St Louis • Sydney • Tokyo

Editor	Louise Crowe
Development Editor	Filipa Maia
Project Managers	Adèle Collins
	Ian MacQuarrie
Designer	Greg Smith
Layout	Rob Curran
Illustration Management	Danny Pyne
Illustrators	Deborah Gyan
	Amanda Williams
	Jeremy Theobald
	Milvia Romici
	Sue Tyler
	Robin Dean
	Matthew McClements
Cover Design	Greg Smith
Production	Andrea Ford
Index	Janine Ross

ISBN 0 7234 3142 6

020219

Published by Mosby, an imprint of Mosby International Ltd, Lynton House, 7–12 Tavistock Square, London WC1H 9LB, UK.

Printed by GraphyCems, Navarra, Spain, 1998.
Text set in Crash Course—VAG Light; captions in Crash Course—VAG Thin.

Cataloguing in Publication Data
A catalogue record for this book is available from the British Library.

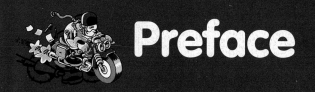

Preface

Sifting through large volumes of pathology and wading through pages of irrelevant data can be a daunting task for many medical students, particularly when time is limited and exams are looming on the horizon. Yet, a basic knowledge of pathology is essential towards an understanding of not only how different diseases arise, but also their clinical effects, outcomes and treatments.

In this book, we have tried to present clinically relevant pathology in a way that is concise and to the point, yet contains sufficient factual detail to satisfy examination requirements. From past experience, we have found that being able to visualise a process is key to understanding. With this in mind, an abundance of illustrations have been included throughout the text to enhance the understanding of the more difficult concepts, and to highlight key features of the more important diseases. We hope this works for you, too.

Bethan Goodman Jones

Pathology lies at the core of medical practice. Without knowledge of the pathology of a disease it is difficult to predict what features might be present in a patient with the disease and diagnosis may be problematic. Treatment must also be related to pathology; a tumour that is known to metastasise early in its development is not going to be cured by local surgical excision—it requires systemic therapy. Unlike treatments, the principles of pathology remain relatively constant, so the student who learns pathology well will benefit from a long-term payoff.

This book covers the whole spectrum of human pathology with a great emphasis on instructive diagrams and summary tables that give a succinct overview of the subject. The author has a background in cell biology as well as studying medicine, so there is good integration between the basic clinical sciences and clinical pathology. The text includes all recent developments in pathology such as acquired immunodeficiency syndrome, inherited cancer syndromes and molecular biology of tumours.

Dr Simon S Cross
Faculty Advisor

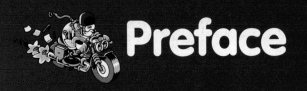# Preface

OK, no-one ever said medicine was going to be easy, but the thing is, there are very few parts of this enormous subject that are actually difficult to understand. The problem for most of us is the sheer volume of information that must be absorbed before each round of exams. It's not fun when time is getting short and you realize that: a) you really should have done a bit more work by now; and b) there are large gaps in your lecture notes that you meant to copy up but never quite got round to.

This series has been designed and written by senior medical students and doctors with recent experience of basic medical science exams. We've brought together all the information you need into compact, manageable volumes that integrate basic science with clinical skills. There is a consistent structure and layout across the series, and every title is checked for accuracy by senior faculty members from medical schools across the UK.

I hope this book makes things a little easier!

Danny Horton-Szar
Series Editor (Basic Medical Sciences)

Acknowledgements

I would like to thank all those who helped to produce this book, in particular Dr Simon Cross for useful suggestions and sneak previews of pathology lecture outlines.

Contents

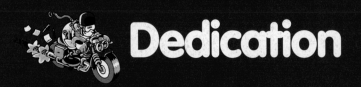

Dedication

To my Father

who would have enjoyed seeing

the completed version of this book

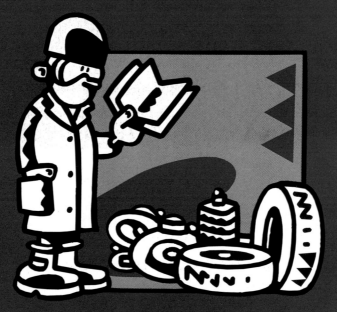

PRINCIPLES OF PATHOLOGY

DISEASE

Disease can be defined as any condition that limits life in either its power, enjoyment or duration.

PATHOLOGY

Pathology is the scientific study of disease. It is concerned with the causes and effects of disease, and the functional and structural changes that occur during the course of a disease.

These changes range from alterations at the molecular level, to the clinical manifestations of the disease at the level of the individual.

Understanding the processes of disease is essential for accurate recognition, diagnosis and treatment of disorders.

Divisions of pathology

Pathology is traditionally subdivided into five main disciplines according to how it is practised within hospitals. The divisions are:

- Histopathology—the study of histological abnormalities of diseased cells and tissues.
- Haematology—the study of primary diseases of the blood, and the secondary effects of other diseases on the blood.
- Chemical pathology—the study of biochemical abnormalities associated with disease.
- Microbiology—the study of infectious diseases and the organisms that cause them.
- Immunopathology—the study of diseases through analysis of immune function.

The 'surgical sieve' approach to pathology

The causes of disease are numerous and diverse, therefore it is useful to classify these causes according to a 'surgical sieve' approach. The cause of any disease can be classified into at least one of the following categories.

Congenital

Congenital causes can be either genetic or non-genetic.

Acquired

Acquired causes can be any of the following:

- Trauma.
- Infections and infestations.
- Neoplasms.
- Circulatory disturbances.
- Immunological disturbances.
- Degenerative disorders.
- Nutritional deficiency diseases.
- Endocrine disorders.
- Psychosomatic factors.
- Iatrogenic disease.
- Idiopathic disease.

However, many if not most diseases are due to a combination of causes and are therefore said to have multifactorial aetiology.

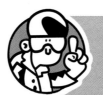

It is useful (and, in examinations, very important!) to have a logical and methodical approach to diseases. See Fig. 1.1 for an outline of a series of characteristics worth applying to any disease.

HOW PATHOLOGY IS COVERED IN THIS BOOK

Part I Principles of pathology

The number of tissue responses that underlie all diseases is limited. These responses are known as basic pathological responses. The first part of this book describes the principles of these.

Part II Systematic pathology

As well as an understanding of the basic pathological responses, it is also necessary to understand how they affect individual tissues and organs. The second part of this book describes the common pathology of the specific diseases as they affect individual organs or organ systems. This approach is termed systematic pathology.

Characteristics worth applying to a disease	
Characteristic	**Explanation**
definition	clear, concise and accurate definition is an essential starting point
epidemiology	incidence/prevalence and variation with age, sex, race and geography
aetiology	the cause of a disease
pathogenesis	the mechanism by which a disease is caused
morphology	morphological, functional and clinical changes which occur during the course of the disease
complications and sequelae	secondary consequences of a disease
treatment	existing treatments, their effectiveness and side effects
prognosis	expected outcome of a disease

- ○ **Define 'disease'.**
- ○ **Define 'pathology'.**
- ○ **What are the divisions of pathology?**
- ○ **What are the different disease categories?**

Fig. 1.1 Characteristics worth applying to any disease. Incidence is the number of new cases of disease occurring in a population of a defined size during a defined period. Prevalence is the number of cases of disease to be found in a defined population at a stated time.

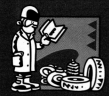

2. Cancer

Definitions

Tumour

A tumour is an abnormal mass of tissue resulting from autonomous disordered growth which persists after the initiating stimulus has been removed. Tumours are:

- Progressive—they are independent of normal growth control and continue to grow regardless of requirements, and in the absence of any external stimuli.
- Purposeless—abnormal mass serves no useful purpose.
- Parasitic—endogenous in origin but draw nourishment from the body while contributing nothing to its function.

All tumours have the suffix '–oma', which means a swelling.

Other definitions are:

- Neoplasm (i.e. new growth)—synonymous with tumour.
- Neoplasia—the process of tumour growth.
- Cancer—a malignant neoplasm (see p. 6).
- Anaplastic neoplasm—a very poorly differentiated neoplasm.

Dysplasia

Dysplasia is the disordered development of cells resulting in an alteration in their size, shape and organisation. It may be reversible but is also known to precede neoplasia. Normal growth, dysplastic growth and neoplastic growth may be viewed as a continuum.

Metaplasia

Metaplasia is the change from one type of differentiated tissue to another, usually in response to an irritating stimulus, e.g. a change from mucus-secreting epithelium to stratified squamous epithelium in the bronchial irritation associated with smoking.

Characteristics of benign versus malignant tumours		
Characteristics	**Benign**	**Malignant**
behaviour • most important feature • invasion • metastases • growth rate	 remains localized no never slow	 spreads yes frequent rapid
microscopic anatomy • cell size and appearance • differentiation (resemblance to normal tissue) • mitoses • nuclear chromatin	 cells of uniform size and appearance good few normal	 cells and nuclei vary in size and shape poor many increased
macroscopic anatomy • direction of growth on skin/mucosal surfaces • ulceration • border	 often exophytic rare circumscribed, often encapsulated	 often endophytic common on skin and mucosal surfaces irregular, ill-defined and non-encapsulated
effects	usually due to compression of normal tissue, e.g. vessels, tubes, nerves, etc., removal alleviates effects	invades and destroys normal tissue removal of tumour does not restore function

Fig. 2.1 Characteristics of benign versus malignant tumours. Note that invasion is the only absolute distinguishing feature between benign and malignant neoplasms.

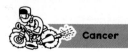

Benign versus malignant

Tumours are classified as either benign or malignant according to their appearance and behaviour (Fig. 2.1).

Nomenclature of tumours

Tumour nomenclature (Fig. 2.2) is based on

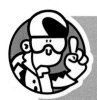

A few simple rules to follow:
- **−oma: suffix for tumours. But there are some non-neoplastic '−omas', e.g. granuloma, tuberculoma and mycetoma.**
- **Carcinomas: malignant tumours of epithelial origin; prefixed by tissue of origin.**
- **−aemia: suffix for neoplastic disorders of the blood (but there is one non-neoplastic '−aemia', i.e. anaemia).**
- **−sarcomas: suffix for malignant tumours of connective tissue origin.**

histogenesis and behaviour. Histogenesis gives information about the type of cell from which the tumour has arisen, while behaviour gives information on whether the cell is benign or malignant.

Classification of carcinomas

Carcinomas can be further categorized according to the extent of their invasion.

Carcinoma *in situ*

This is an epithelial neoplasm which has all the cellular features associated with malignancy but which has not yet invaded through the epithelial basement membrane. The in-situ phase may last for several years before invasion commences.

Intra-epithelial neoplasia

This covers the spectrum of changes short of invasive carcinoma:

1. Mild dysplasia.
2. Moderate dysplasia.
3. Severe dysplasia/Carcinoma *in situ*.

It is usually divided into three categories, e.g. cervical intraepithelial neoplasia: CIN1, CIN2 and CIN3.

Fig. 2.2 Examples of tumour nomenclature. * represents those tumours that are always malignant and do not have benign counterparts.

Examples of tumour nomenclature		
Histological type	**Benign**	**Malignant**
epithelial tumours • glandular • non-glandular, e.g. 　squamous cell 　transitional cell 　basal cell	adenoma papilloma • squamous cell papilloma • transitional cell papilloma • basal cell papilloma	adenocarcinoma carcinoma • squamous cell carcinoma • transitional cell carcinoma • basal cell carcinoma
connective tissue tumours • adipose tissue • cartilage • bone • smooth muscle • voluntary muscle • blood vessels	lipoma chondroma osteoma leiomyoma rhabdomyoma angioma	liposarcoma chondrosarcoma osteosarcoma leiomyosarcoma rhabdomyosarcoma angiosarcoma
haemopoietic tumour	*	leukaemia
lymphoreticular tumour	*	lymphoma
melanocytes	*	malignant melanoma
germinal cell tumour	benign teratoma	malignant teratoma

Invasive carcinoma

This is an epithelial neoplasm which has invaded through basement membrane. The tumour gains access to the vascular supply and lymphatics, and will often metastasise.

Epidemiological aspects of cancer
Cancer in the UK

As a cause of mortality in the UK, cancer is the second biggest killer (after cardiovascular disease). Its incidence (Fig. 2.3) is as follows:

- Almost 1 in 3 of the population will develop cancer during their lifetime.
- Almost 1 in 4 of the population will die of cancer.
- Incidence of cancer deaths increases with increasing age.
- Incidence of cancer varies between males and females.

Cancer worldwide

The incidence of different cancers varies from country to country, and this variation provides clues to the causes of the cancers.

For example, in Japan, gastric carcinoma is 30 times more common than in the UK, whereas pancreatic cancer is much rarer. However, migration of a subset of the Japanese population to different geographical areas (e.g. USA, UK) alters the incidences of these diseases within that population.

These findings suggest that environmental factors (such as diet, occupational, social and geographic) rather than genetic causes account for most of the observed differences between countries.

MOLECULAR BASIS OF CANCER

Oncogenes and tumour suppressor genes
Oncogenes

Oncogenes are genes that are present in normal cells and which encode for proteins involved in growth and differentiation. They include:

- Nuclear binding proteins (e.g. *c-myc*).
- Tyrosine kinase proteins (e.g. *src*).
- Growth factors.

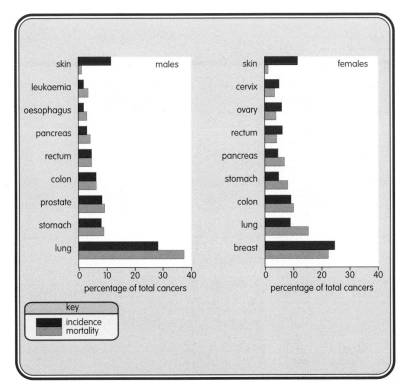

Fig. 2.3 Incidence and mortality of common cancers in men and women in England and Wales. (Adapted from *Textbook of Medicine*, 2nd edn, by Souhami and Moxham, Churchill Livingstone, 1994, p.123.)

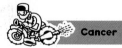
- Receptors for growth factors.
- GTP binding proteins (e.g. *ras*).

In healthy cells, transcription of these genes is tightly controlled as required for cell growth and differentiation.

In neoplastic cells, oncogenes are abnormally expressed leading to uncontrolled autocrine growth of cells whereby the cells drive their own proliferation.

Abnormal expression of oncogenes may occur due to:
- Gene amplification, e.g. due to incorporation of viral oncogene (*v-onc*) into genome.
- Increased gene transcription (due to mutation of controlling gene).
- Increased activity of protein (due to mutation of oncogene).

Tumour suppressor genes

Tumour suppressor genes (e.g. p53 and Rb1) encode proteins that prevent or suppress the growth of tumours by repairing damaged DNA (Fig. 2.4) or by initiating apoptosis if there is extensive cell damage.

Loss of function of tumour suppressor genes (TSGs) or their protein products can result in uncontrolled

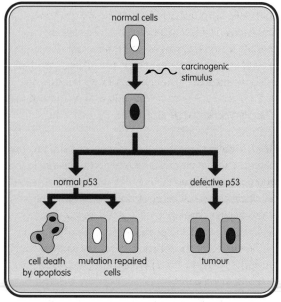

Fig. 2.4 Role of p53 in cells with damaged DNA. (Adapted from JCE Underwood, General and Systematic Pathology 2nd edn, Churchill Livingstone, p.279.)

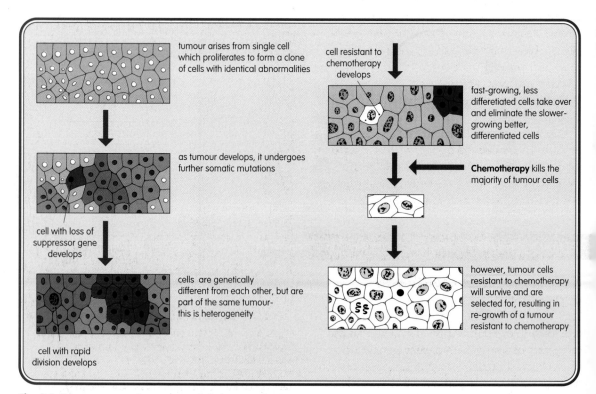

Fig. 2.5 Tumour progression and genetic heterogeneity.

neoplastic cell growth. TSGs can lose their normal function by a variety of mechanisms:
- Mutations (hereditary or acquired).
- Binding of normal TSG protein to proteins encoded by viral genes, e.g. human papilloma virus proteins.
- Complexing of normal TSG protein to mutant TSG protein in heterozygous cells.

Apoptosis

Apoptosis (programmed cell death) is a process whereby a single cell initiates its own death. This type of cell death can be either physiological (e.g. during embryological development) or pathological (e.g. when DNA of cell has sustained injury).

The advantage of pathological apoptosis is that the mutated cell is destroyed before it can perpetuate itself thus preventing potential tumour formation. Some tumour suppressor genes, e.g. p53, can initiate apoptosis in the mutated cell (see Fig. 2.4).

Multistage model of tumour progression

Tumours arise from single cells, which proliferate to form a clone of cells with identical abnormalities. As tumours develop, they undergo further somatic mutations which cause abnormalities in other oncogenes and/or tumour suppressor genes. These additional mutations result in cells which are genetically different from each other but which are part of the same tumour—this is heterogeneity.

Fast-growing, less-differentiated cells take over and eliminate the slower-growing, better-differentiated cells.

Chemotherapy will kill the majority of tumour cells. However, tumour cells that are resistant to chemotherapy will survive and be selected for (due to ablation of competing, non-resistant cells), resulting in the regrowth of a tumour resistant to chemotherapy (Fig. 2.5).

TUMOUR GROWTH

Kinetics of tumour growth and angiogenesis

Tumours cannot grow beyond a few millimetres in diameter without a blood supply. Tumour cells release angiogenic factors which induce vascular proliferation. Eventually, the tumour may outgrow its blood supply, and areas of necrosis may appear, resulting in slower growth (Fig. 2.6).

Mechanisms and pathways of invasion and metastasis

Invasion

Invasion is the only absolute criterion for malignancy. Invading malignant cells have the following properties:
- Abnormal or increased cellular motility—due to loss of contact inhibition.
- Decreased cellular adhesion—due to loss of surface adhesion molecules.
- Increased secretion of proteolytic enzymes, e.g. metalloproteinases.

Metalloproteinases, such as collagenases and gelatinases, are the most important enzymes in neoplastic invasion. These enzymes digest the surrounding connective tissue thus aiding invasion.

Metastasis

Metastasis is the process whereby malignant cells spread from their site of origin—primary tumour—to distant sites forming secondary tumours.

Total mass of secondary tumours usually exceeds that of the primary lesion. Only a proportion of neoplastic cells in a malignant tumour are able to metastasize.

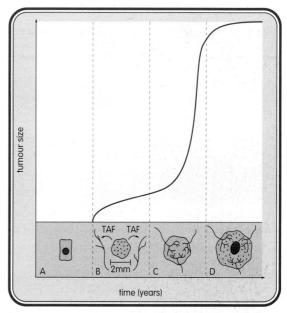

Fig. 2.6 Kinetics of tumour growth and angiogenesis. (A) Transformed cell. (B) Avascular tumour nodule. (C) Vascularized tumour. (D) Vascularized tumour with central necrosis. TAF, tumour angiogenic factors. (Adapted with permission from *General and Systematic Pathology*, 2nd edn, by J.C.E. Underwood, Churchill Livingstone, 1996.)

9

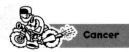

In order to metastasize, neoplastic cells undergo the following sequence of events:

- Detachment of tumour cells from neighbouring cells.
- Invasion of surrounding connective tissue.
- Intravasation into blood/lymphatic vessels.
- Evasion of the host's defence mechanisms.
- Adherence to endothelium at distant site.
- Extravasation of cells from vessel lumen into surrounding tissue.

Following extravasation, the malignant cells proliferate and secrete more angiogenic growth factors for vascularization. Hence a new tumour is formed.

Main routes of metastasis

There are four main routes of metastasis (Fig. 2.7):

- Local invasion—most common pattern of spread of malignant tumours; by direct growth into adjacent tissues.
- Lymphatic spread—forms secondary tumours in lymph nodes.
- Blood-borne spread—cells enter the blood stream and form secondary tumours in organs perfused by blood that has drained from a tumour.
- Transcoelomic spread—in pleural, pericardial and peritoneal cavities.

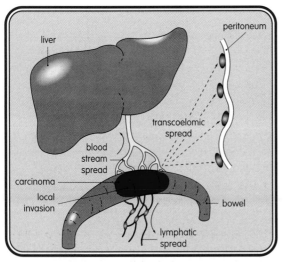

Fig. 2.7 Routes of metastasis exemplified by a carcinoma of the bowel, i.e. via the blood stream, via the lymphatic spread, through peritoneal cavities and via local invasion.

CARCINOGENIC AGENTS

Carcinogens are substances known to cause an increased incidence of cancer.

Carcinogens can exert their effect by either genetic mechanisms (i.e. causing DNA alteration—this is the majority of carcinogens) or epigenetic mechanisms (i.e. acting on the protein product of growth regulating genes).

Chemical carcinogens

Most chemical carcinogens are procarcinogens and require metabolic conversion into active carcinogens (ultimate carcinogens). Some carcinogens act directly to induce cellular damage. Examples of chemical carcinogens are given in Fig. 2.8.

Stages of chemical carcinogenesis

The multistage model of carcinogenesis (Fig. 2.9) is based on observations on the effects of chemical carcinogens on laboratory animals. This model proposes three main stages of carcinogenesis:

Examples of chemical carcinogens	
Chemical compound	**Cancer type**
indirect carcinogens	
polycyclic hydrocarbons • soot [benzo(a)pyrene; dibenzanthracene] • tobacco smoke	skin, colon lung, bladder, oral cavity, larynx, oesophagus
aromatic amines • benzidine, 2-naphthylamine	bladder
nitrosamines • chemotherapeutic agents • cyclophosphamide, chlorambucil, thiotepa, busulphan	oesophagus, stomach leukaemias
vinyl chloride	liver (angiosarcoma)
aflatoxins	liver
unknown mechanisms	
heavy metals • nickel, cadmium, chromium • arsenic	lung skin

Fig. 2.8 Examples of chemical carcinogens.

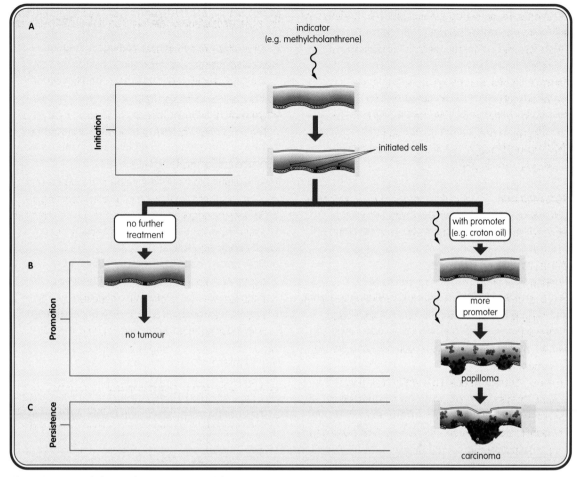

Fig. 2.9 Stages of chemical carcinogenesis. (A) Initiation. (B) Promotion. (C) Persistence.

- Initiation—induction of a genetic alteration in oncogene or tumour suppressor gene.
- Promotion—a stimulus for proliferation of initiated cell; may be an external agent or a further random mutational genetic abnormality.
- Persistence—stage where proliferation of tumour cells becomes autonomous, i.e. it no longer requires the presence of initiators or promoters.

Radiation
Radiation can be:
- Ionizing—natural radiation, therapeutic radiation and nuclear radiation.
- Non-ionizing—ultraviolet (UV) radiation.

Radiation can result in DNA damage in two ways:
- Directly—causing strand breaks, base alterations and cross linking of DNA.
- Indirectly—ionization of H_2O with formation of reactive oxygen free radicals which interact with and damage DNA.

Ultraviolet (UV) radiation
This is associated with many different kinds of skin cancer, particularly:
- Squamous cell carcinoma.
- Basal cell carcinoma.
- Malignant melanoma.

Skin cancer is the most common type of cancer in the UK and USA. It is more common in fair-skinned individuals.

UV light is thought to induce the formation of linkages between pyrimidine bases on DNA molecule. The risk is greatly increased in patients with xeroderma

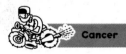
pigmentosum, which is a rare, congenital disease characterised by deficiency of DNA repair enzymes.

Ionizing radiation

X-ray radiation

Radiotherapy can cause cancer as well as curing it! It is associated with radiation-induced malignant neoplasms, usually sarcomas. These tumours occur months or years after radiation therapy, e.g. in the lungs, CNS, bones, kidneys and liver.

Radioisotopes

Radioactive iodine used to treat thyroid disease is associated with increased risk of cancer development 15–25 years post treatment.

Nuclear radiation

Survivors of the Hiroshima and Nagasaki atomic bombs, and of the Chernobyl nuclear power plant accident, have a greatly increased incidence of cancer including leukaemia and carcinoma of breast, lung and thyroid.

DNA repair mechanisms and their failure

DNA is the cellular constituent most sensitive to radiation. Fortunately, cells have DNA repair mechanisms that deal with DNA damage. Repair is usually rapid, but sometimes damage is irreparable and major chromosomal and chromatid alterations occur.

Repair of single-stranded breaks, particularly in rapidly dividing cells, is error prone and introduces single base mutations.

Double-stranded cleavage leads to chromosome breakage, and attempts to repair multiple breaks lead to inappropriate recombination events, e.g. translocation or interstitial deletion.

Viruses

Certain DNA viruses and retroviruses (Fig. 2.10) can cause neoplasia, as follows:

- DNA viruses insert DNA directly into the host genome.
- Retroviruses have reverse transcriptase enzyme to produce DNA copy of viral RNA. DNA copy is then inserted into the host genome.

Mechanism of viral carcinogenesis

Inserted viral genes may be either viral oncogenes (*v-onc*), the expression of which may lead to uncontrolled

_		
Examples of oncogenic human viruses		
Type	**Virus**	**Tumour type**
retroviruses	human T cell leukaemia virus (HTLV)	T cell leukaemia
	human immunodeficiency virus (HIV)	AIDS-related lymphomas
DNA viruses	human papillomavirus	skin papilloma (common wart) cervical carcinoma
	Epstein–Barr virus	carcinoma of the nasopharynx Burkitt's lymphoma
	hepatitis B virus	hepatocellular carcinoma

Fig. 2.10 Examples of oncogenic human viruses.

proliferation, or activators of cellular oncogenes, resulting in overexpression of the cellular oncogene.

active against tumour cells, most tumours are not distinguishable from normal host cells, and are therefore not easily detected by the immune system. The natural history of most cancer cells, if not surgically ablated, is one of relentless progression culminating in death.

HOST DEFENCES AGAINST CANCER

Some tumours are known to stimulate both innate (passive) and adaptive immunological reactions in the host.

Innate immunity
Activation of macrophages and natural killer cells can prevent growth of some tumours *in vitro*. Some tumours activate complement via the alternate pathway.

Adaptive immunity
Humoral
Antibodies may have a protective role, and are more likely to be effective against free cells—e.g. leukaemia or metastasizing tumours—than those in solid lumps.

Cell mediated immunity
Cytotoxic T cells are thought to play a role in tumour regression. Infiltration of the tumour with lymphocytes and macrophages is associated with better prognosis. Reaction is strongest in small tumours and disappears when they enlarge.

Despite many immune mechanisms known to be

- Explain the differences between neoplasia, dysplasia, metaplasia, etc.
- Explain the behavioural and structural differences between malignant and benign tumours.
- How have geographic and environmental factors influenced the prevalence of various types of tumour?
- What are oncogenes and tumour suppressor genes?
- Describe the process of tumour growth, angiogenesis, invasion and metastasis.
- Describe the host defences against cancer.

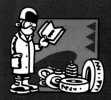

3. Inflammation, Tissue Damage and Repair

INFLAMMATION

Definition
Inflammation is the response of living tissues to cellular injury. It involves both innate and adaptive immune mechanisms.

Purpose
The purpose of inflammation is to localize and eliminate the causative agent, limit tissue injury and restore tissue to normality.

Inflammation can be divided into two types: acute and chronic. These categories are not mutually exclusive as some overlap exists (Fig. 3.1).

Causes of acute inflammation
The causes of acute inflammation are:
- Physical agents—e.g. trauma, heat, cold.
- Chemical substances.
- Microbial infections.
- Immune-mediated hypersensitivity reactions.
- Tissue necrosis, e.g. from ischaemia and anoxia.

Causes of chronic inflammation
Chronic inflammation usually develops as a primary response (chronic *ab initio*) to:

- Micro-organisms resistant to phagocytosis or intracellular cell killing, e.g. tuberculosis (TB), leprosy.
- Foreign bodies—endogenous (bone, adipose tissue, uric acid crystals) or exogenous (silica, suture materials, implanted prostheses).
- Some autoimmune diseases, e.g. Hashimoto's thyroiditis, rheumatoid arthritis, contact hypersensitivity reactions.
- Primary granulomatous diseases—Crohn's disease, sarcoidosis.

Occasionally, chronic inflammation occurs secondary to acute inflammation due to the persistence of the causative agent. Fig. 3.2 shows the sequelae of inflammation.

ACUTE INFLAMMATION

Classical signs of acute inflammation
The classical signs of acute inflammation are:
- Redness (rubor).
- Heat (calor).
- Swelling (tumour).
- Pain (dolor).
- Loss of function (functio laesa).

Comparison of acute and chronic inflammation		
	Acute inflammation	**Chronic inflammation**
response	initial reactions of tissue to injury	persisting reactions of tissue to injury
onset	rapid response	slow response
type of immunity	innate	cell mediated
predominant cell type	neutrophil polymorphs	lymphocytes, plasma cells, macrophages
duration	few hours to few weeks	weeks, months or even years
vascular response	prominent	not very prominent

Fig. 3.1 Comparison of acute and chronic inflammation. Note that the acute and chronic categories are not mutually exclusive.

These classical signs are caused by a rapidly developing vascular response and cellular events characteristic of acute inflammation.

The main function of these events is to bring elements of the immune system to the site of injury.

Vascular response

Widespread vasodilatation (hyperaemia)
Arterioles and precapillary sphincters relax, resulting in increased blood flow and hydrostatic pressure.

Contraction of endothelial cells
The intercellular junctions between endothelial cells widen resulting in:
- Increased fenestrations (i.e. gaps) between endothelial cells.
- Increased permeability of vessels to plasma proteins.

Proteins leak out of the plasma into the interstitial spaces, leading to a decrease in the plasma oncotic pressure.

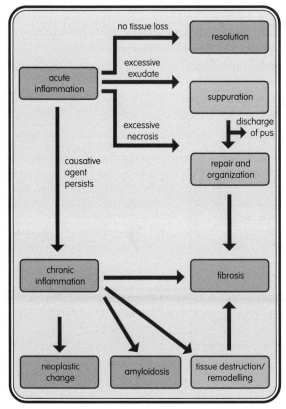

Fig. 3.2 Sequelae of inflammation.

Inflammatory oedema
The combined increase in hydrostatic pressure (from hyperaemia) with the decreased oncotic pressure (from leakage of proteins into interstitial spaces) causes net fluid movement from plasma into tissues; this is inflammatory oedema. As a result, blood viscosity is increased and flow rate is decreased.

Advantages of inflammatory oedema
Fluid increase in tissue dilutes toxins. Protein increase in tissue provides protective antibodies and allows fibrin deposition.

Cellular events
Neutrophil polymorphs pass between endothelial cell junctions and invade damaged tissue to combat the effects of injury.

There are four stages (Fig. 3.3):
1. Margination of neutrophil polymorphs (Fig. 3.4).
2. Adhesion of neutrophil polymorphs ('pavementing')—leukocytes adhere to the vascular endothelium at sites of acute inflammation.
3. Emigration of neutrophil polymorphs—leukocytes pass between the endothelial cell junctions by amoeboid movement through the venule into tissue spaces (diapedesis).
4. Chemotaxis of neutrophil polymorphs—neutrophils are attracted towards, and possibly activated by, chemical substances (chemotaxins) released at sites of tissue injury. These chemotaxins are thought to be leukotrienes, complement components and bacterial products.

Phagocytosis and intracellular killing
At the site of injury, neutrophils and monocytes ingest debris and foreign particles (Fig. 3.5).

Following phagocytosis, leukocytes attempt to destroy phagocytosed material by:
- Discharge of lysosomal enzymes into the phagosome.
- Activation of powerful oxidizing agents, e.g. H_2O_2, oxygen free radicals, acids, etc.

Cytokine release
Neutrophil polymorphs also release further cytokines involved in the following:
- Chemotaxis of more leukocytes.
- Increasing vascular permeability.
- Production of systemic fever (pyrogens).

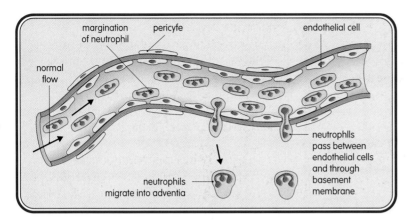

Fig. 3.3 Cellular events in acute inflammation.

Fig. 3.4 Mechanism of margination of neutrophil polymorphs.

Increased plasma viscosity (due to loss of intravascular fluid)	→	Decreased blood flow	→	Cells fall out of axial stream into plasmatic zone (margination)

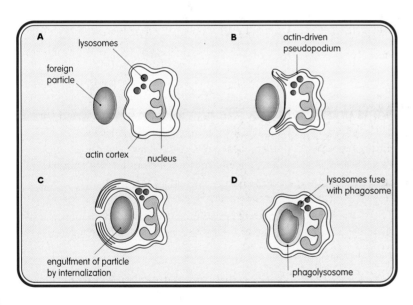

Fig. 3.5 Phagocytosis of foreign particle by leukocyte. (A) Attachment of foreign particle. (B) Pseudopodia engulfing particle. (C) and (D) Incorporation within the cell in a vacuole called a phagosome.

CHEMICAL MEDIATORS OF INFLAMMATION

There are several different inflammatory mediator systems all of which interact together to produce inflammation, but no single chemical mediator can be responsible for any single feature of inflammatory response.

Regulatory mechanisms exist in all mediator systems.

The complement system

This is a cascading sequence of serum proteins, made up of more than 20 proteins; the activated product of one protein activates another (Figs 3.6 and 3.7).

Kinins

Kinins are small vasoactive peptides (about 10 amino acids). Bradykinin is the most well known, and exerts its effects by increasing vascular permeability and producing pain. Both effects are cardinal features of acute inflammation.

The kinin system is activated by activated coagulation factor XII.

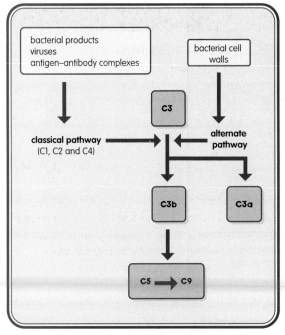

Fig. 3.6 Simplified version of the complement cascade showing how the activated product of one protein activates another.

Arachidonic acid, prostaglandins and leukotrienes

During acute inflammation, the membrane phospholipids of neutrophils and mast cells are metabolized to form prostaglandins and leukotrienes (Fig. 3.8).

The anti-inflammatory action of drugs, e.g. glucocorticoids, aspirin and aspirin-like drugs, is attributable to their ability to inhibit prostaglandin production.

Platelet activation factors

Platelet activation factors are released from mast cells and neutrophils during degranulation. They have the following effects:
- Induce platelet aggregation and degranulation.
- Increase vascular permeability.
- Induce leukocyte adhesion to the endothelium.
- Stimulate synthesis of arachidonic acid derivatives.

Cytokines

Cytokines are a family of chemical messengers released by T lymphocytes and macrophages. They act over short distances (autocrine and/or paracrine) by

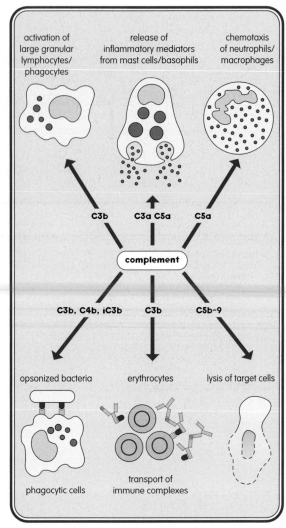

Fig. 3.7 The major functions of the complement system.

binding specific receptors on target cell surfaces. They include:
- Lymphokines—cytokines produced by lymphocytes.
- Monokines—cytokines produced by monocytes/macrophages.
- Interleukins—cytokines which act between leukocytes (more than 15 types).
- Interferons—inhibit replication of viruses within cells and activate macrophages and NK cells.
- Growth factors.
- Tumour necrosis factors—kill tumour cells, but also stimulate adipose and muscle catabolism leading to weight loss.

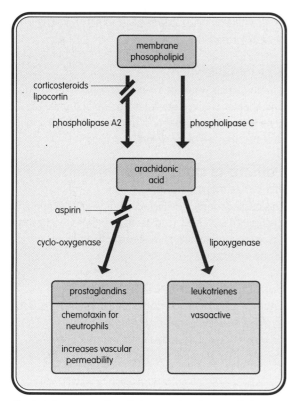

Fig. 3.8 Formation of arachidonic acid and its metabolites.

CHRONIC INFLAMMATION

Mononuclear infiltration and granulation tissue

The cells involved in chronic inflammation are shown in Fig. 3.9. The site of chronic inflammation is dominated by:

- Lymphocytes.
- Plasma cells (for antibody production).
- Macrophages (for phagocytosis). Some macrophages fuse to form multinucleate giant cells.

Damaged tissue is gradually removed by macrophages. It is slowly replaced by granulation tissue, which consists of new capillaries and new connective tissue formed from myofibroblasts (i.e. modified fibroblasts capable of contracting) and the collagen that they secrete.

Wound healing
Healing by first intention
Apposed wound margins are joined by fibrin deposition, which is subsequently replaced by collagen and covered by epidermal growth (Fig. 3.10).

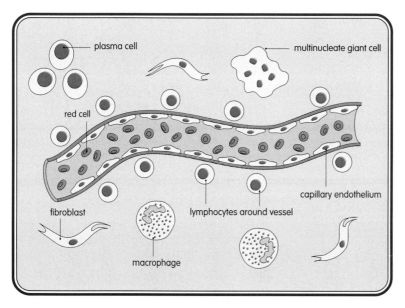

Fig. 3.9 Cells involved in chronic inflammation.

Healing by second intention

Healing by second intention (Fig. 3.11) involves the following:

- Wound margins are unapposed due to extensive tissue damage.
- Tissue defect fills with granulation tissue.
- Epithelial regeneration to cover surface.

Wounds are healed by either first or second intention healing processes. The type of healing process depends on the extent of tissue damage:
- Minimal tissue loss—involves healing by first intention.
- Extensive tissue loss—involves healing by second intention.

- Granulation tissue eventually contracts resulting in scar formation.

Scar formation

Myofibroblasts within granulation tissue are attached to one another and to adjacent extracellular matrix. Their contraction draws together surrounding the matrix thus reducing the size of the defect.

Patterns of chronic inflammation

Fibrinous inflammation

This is the deposition of increased amounts of fibrin on the tissue's surface, e.g. in acute pleurisy secondary to acute lobar pneumonia. Presence of fibrin tends to inhibit resolution.

Suppurative inflammation

Characterized by the production of pus, usually caused by infection with pyogenic bacteria such as *Staphylococcus aureus* and *Streptococcus pyogenes*. Pus becomes surrounded by a 'pyogenic membrane' of

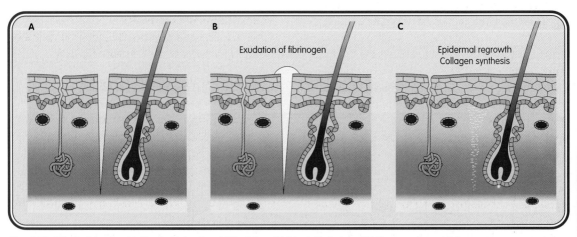

Fig. 3.10 Skin incision healed by first intention. (A) Incision. (B) Weak fibrin join. (C) Strong collagen join.

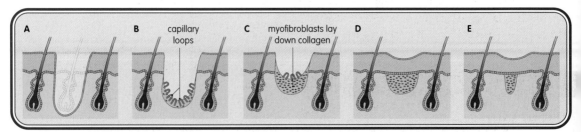

Fig. 3.11 Skin wound repaired by second intention. (A) Loss of tissue. (B) Granulation tissue. (C) Organization. (D) Early fibrous scar. (E) Scar contraction.

sprouting capillaries, neutrophil polymorphs and fibroblasts.

There are two types of suppurative inflammation: superficial, e.g. a boil, and deep-seated, e.g. an abscess within a hollow viscus such as the gall bladder. In the deep-seated type, mucosal layers of outflow tract may become fused with fibrin resulting in empyema. Fistulae—abnormal passages between mucosal surfaces—may form.

Haemorrhagic inflammation
If damage is severe, blood vessels within the area may rupture, e.g. haemorrhagic pneumonia.

Granulomatous inflammation
This is a form of chronic inflammation in which modified macrophages (epithelioid cells) aggregate to form small clusters or granulomas surrounded by lymphoid cells. It usually occurs in response to the presence of indigestible particulate matter within macrophages, for example:
- Micro-organisms resistant to intracellular cell killing, e.g. *Mycobacterium tuberculosis* and *M. leprae*.
- Foreign bodies—endogenous (e.g. bone, adipose tissue, uric acid crystals); exogenous (e.g. silica, suture materials, implanted prostheses).

There are some idiopathic causes, e.g. in Crohn's disease and sarcoidosis.

Granulomas commonly contain multinucleate giant cells—Langhans' giant cell, foreign body giant cell and Touton giant cell—formed either from the fusion of many macrophages or by nuclear division without cytoplasmic separation.

Ulceration
Ulcers are formed when the surface of an organ or tissue is lost due to necrosis and replaced by inflammatory tissue. The most common sites are the alimentary canal and the skin.

Chronic ulceration is a balance between tissue damage, e.g. by gastric acid, and tissue repair by the body's healing response, i.e. the chronic inflammatory response.

TISSUE NECROSIS

Cell death
Cells may be damaged either reversibly (sublethal damage) or irreversibly (lethal damage) (Fig. 3.12). The type of damage depends on:
- Nature and duration of injury.
- Type of cells affected.
- Regenerative ability of tissues.

Note that there are no absolute ultrastructural criteria by which reversible and irreversible cellular injury may be distinguished, and that there is a continuum from reversibly injured cell through to irreversible necrotically damaged cell.

Necrosis
Necrosis is the death of cells or tissues which are still part of the living organism.

Regardless of the cause of cell death, necrosis is the result of:
- Depletion of intracellular energy systems.
- Disruption of cytoplasmic organelles.
- Liberation of intracellular enzymes.
- Production of oxygen free radicals.
- Disintegration of nucleus.
- Alterations in the plasma membrane.

Mechanisms of cell death
The initiating mechanisms of cell death depend on the type of injury and are summarized in Fig. 3.13.

Histological types of necrosis
Coagulative necrosis
This is the most common form of necrosis, characteristically occurring in the heart, kidney and spleen, but it may occur in most tissues.

Dead tissue is initially swollen and firm, but later becomes soft as a result of digestion by macrophages. Dead cells retain 'ghost' outlines, and the necrotic area is highly eosinophilic.

It usually evokes an inflammatory response; damaged tissue is removed by phagocytosis and repaired or regenerated.

Colliquative necrosis
This characteristically occurs in the brain due to minimal supporting stroma. Necrotic neural tissue undergoes total liquefaction, and a glial reaction occurs around the periphery with eventual cyst formation.

Caseous necrosis (caseation)
Commonly seen in TB. Histologically, the complete loss

of normal tissue architecture is replaced by amorphous, granular and eosinophilic tissue. There are variable amounts of fat and an appearance reminiscent of cottage cheese, hence the term caseation.

Gangrene

Necrotic tissue is invaded by putrefactive organisms, notably clostridia. The tissue appears green or black due to the breakdown of haemoglobin.

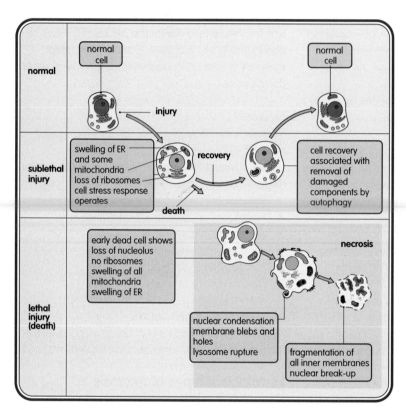

Fig. 3.12 Relationships between sublethal and lethal cell damage.

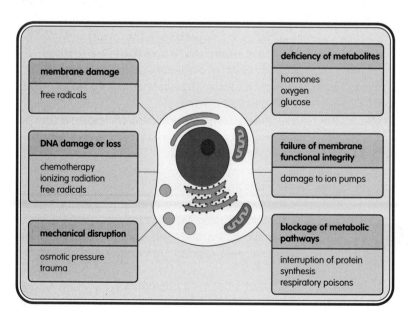

Fig. 3.13 Mechanisms of cell death.

Dry gangrene

An example is ischaemic necrosis of the toes which is common in elderly people with gradual arterial occlusion. The putrefactive process is very slow, and only small numbers of putrefactive organisms are present.

Wet gangrene

Examples are ischaemic necrosis of the bowel (clostridia are common in the bowel), strangulation of the viscera, or occlusion of the leg arteries in obese diabetic patients. Tissues are moist at the start of the process due to either oedema or venous congestion.

Gas gangrene

This is a primary infection of healthy tissue resulting in putrefactive necrosis.

Fibrinoid necrosis

This occurs in malignant hypertension, where increased arterial pressure results in necrosis of the smooth muscle wall. Plasma leaks into the media with consequent deposition of fibrin, hence fibrinoid necrosis. The histological appearance of the vessel wall is strongly eosinophilic. Actual necrosis is usually inconspicuous.

Fat necrosis

Adipose tissue damage may be due to:
- Direct trauma—release of triglycerides following trauma elicits a rapid inflammatory response. Fat is phagocytosed by neutrophils and macrophages, which ultimately results in fibrosis.
- Enzymatic lipolysis—in acute pancreatitis, lipases liberated from damaged acini act on fat cells in the peritoneal cavity thus:

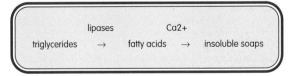

Fig. 3.14A Enzymatic lipolysis.

Insoluble calcium salts appear as whitish chalky areas scattered within otherwise normal adipose tissue.

Apoptosis

Apoptosis is an energy dependent mechanism of cell death for the deletion of unwanted individual cells; it is also known as 'programmed cell death'. Inhibition of apoptosis results in cell accumulation, e.g. neoplasia, whereas increased apoptosis results in cell loss, e.g. atrophy.

Apoptosis can be either physiological (i.e. associated with the maintenance of organ size in adults, and organ development and remodelling in the embryo) or pathological (i.e. in response to irreparable DNA damage thereby preventing the perpetuation of a genetically abnormal cell).

Stages of apoptosis

The process of apoptosis occurs in the following four stages.

Priming

This is the synthesis of enzymes needed to cause cell dissolution, e.g. proteases and nucleases. There are no structural cellular changes.

Enzyme activation

Endonucleases cleave chromatin, resulting in DNA fragmentation. Proteases degrade the cytoskeleton, resulting in cell shrinkage. The plasma membrane and organelles remain intact.

Fragmentation of the cell

The cell is fragmented into apoptotic bodies. Each fragment contains viable mitochondria and intact organelles. The presence of intact plasma membranes around apoptotic bodies explains the absence of any inflammation.

Phagocytosis

Apoptotic fragments are phagocytosed and destroyed by adjacent cells. Surrounding cells then move together to fill vacant space.

A comparison of cell death by apoptosis and necrosis is given in Fig. 3.14.

Comparison of cell death by necrosis and apoptosis		
Feature	**Necrosis**	**Apoptosis**
occurrence	pathological conditions	physiological or pathological conditions
number of cells involved	more than one cell in a group	single cells
cellular status	cell membrane broken	cell membrane remains whole
appearances	swelling and lysis of cells	shrinkage and fragmentation of cells
surrounding response	inflammatory cells (e.g. neutrophils and/or macrophages) present	none
destiny of dead cells	phagocytosed by inflammatory cells	phagocytosed by adjacent cells in the same tissue
biochemical mechanism	loss of feedback control within the cell (not energy dependent)	fragmentation of DNA by endonucleases (energy-using process)

Fig. 3.14 Comparison of cell death by necrosis and apoptosis.

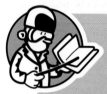

- ○ **Describe the mechanisms of acute inflammation: vascular response and cellular events.**
- ○ **What are the chemical mediators of inflammation?**
- ○ **Describe the mechanisms of chronic inflammation.**
- ○ **Briefly describe wound healing by primary and secondary intention, and scar formation.**
- ○ **What are the key differences between acute and chronic inflammation?**
- ○ **Tissue necrosis—describe the mechanisms of cell death, the differences between sublethal and lethal cell injury, and the difference between necrosis and apoptosis.**
- ○ **What are the histological types of necrosis?**

4. Infectious Disease

GENERAL PRINCIPLES OF INFECTION

Infection and colonization

Infection is the invasion of the body's internal tissues by micro-organisms, whereas colonization is the inhabitation of external body surfaces—skin, GI tract, external genitalia and vagina—by normally harmless micro-organisms.

Koch's postulates

To establish that a given disease has an infective cause, the postulates stated by the German bacteriologist Robert Koch (1843–1910) must be fulfilled. These are:

- The infectious agent should be found in all cases of the disease, and in parts of the body affected by the disease.
- The infectious agent associated with the disease can be isolated from the lesions of an infected person and grown in artificial culture media.
- The cultivated infectious agent can reproduce the disease upon inoculation of a member of the same species.

Be aware that there are certain diseases to which one or more of these criteria cannot be applied but which can still be confidently attributed to a particular organism. For example, *Treponema pallidum* is the cause of syphilis but it cannot be grown in culture.

Pathogens and commensals

Pathogens are micro-organisms that are normally absent from the body but which have mechanisms to invade and cause infection. Commensals are those micro-organisms that constitute the normal flora of a healthy body. They do not normally cause disease and are often advantageous to the host by the production of nutrients such as B_{12} and by the exclusion of harmful bacteria.

The distinction between commensals and pathogens is not absolute. Many commensals are potential pathogens, i.e. they are harmless only so long as they are kept at bay by the host's defence mechanisms.

Other micro-organism characteristics

Pathogenicity

Pathogenicity is the capacity of a particular micro-organism to cause disease.

Virulence

Virulence is the degree of pathogenicity of a micro-organism measured by the severity of the ensuing infection. Micro-organisms are said to be highly virulent if a small number of microbes can cause severe disease.

Opportunistic infection

Opportunistic infection is an infection by organisms of low pathogenicity, usually due to impaired immune responses.

CATEGORIES OF INFECTIOUS AGENTS

Fig. 4.1 shows the classification of the major pathogens.

Viruses

Viruses carry nucleic acids but lack synthetic machinery, therefore they can only replicate within the host cell, i.e. they are obligate intracellular parasites (Fig. 4.2).

Viruses have the following characteristics:

- Consist of a nucleic acid core and protein coat (capsid), which together constitute the nucleocapsid.
- Some, but not all, viruses are enveloped by the membrane of host cell origin.

Classification of major pathogens					
	Viruses	Bacteria	Fungi	Protozoa	Helminths and ectoparasites
size	20–300 nm	0.1–~5 µm	2–10 µm	2–100 µm	0.5–35 cm
pro- or eucaryote	neither	procaryote	eucaryote	eucaryote	eucaryote
nucleic acid	DNA or RNA	DNA + RNA	DNA + RNA	DNA + RNA	DNA + RNA
replication	intracellular	intra- and/or extracellular	intra- and/or extracellular	intra- and/or extracellular	extracellular
external cell wall	no	yes (usually): peptidoglycan	yes: rigid chitin	no	no
reproduction	assembly	binary fission	binary fission and sexually	binary fission and sexually	sexually

Fig. 4.1 Classification of major pathogens.

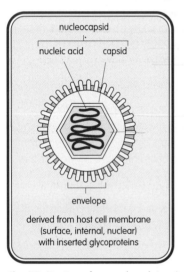

Fig. 4.2 Structure of an enveloped virus.

Classification of viruses based on nucleic acid type		
Virus type	Mode of replication	Examples
DNA viruses	utilize host cell polymerases for mRNA synthesis can remain in infected cell and establish persistent infections (latent, immortalizing viruses)	herpes simplex virus varicella-zoster virus adenovirus papillomavirus
RNA viruses	encode their own replicative enzymes for formation of more mRNA (Host enzymes cannot replicate RNA)	measles virus mumps virus influenza virus rabies virus poliovirus
retroviruses (RNA)	contain 'reverse transcriptase' enzyme for production of viral DNA viral DNA is inserted into host genome	HIV I and II HTLV I and II

Fig. 4.3 Classification of viruses based on nucleic acid type.

- Morphology is icosahedral, helical or complex.
- Classification is usually based on type of nucleic acid (Fig. 4.3).

Bacteria

Bacteria are divided into two broad groups—Gram-positive and Gram-negative—based on their reaction to the Gram stain (a staining procedure used with light microscopy).

Differential staining is obtained due to inherent differences in the structures of bacteria's cell walls.

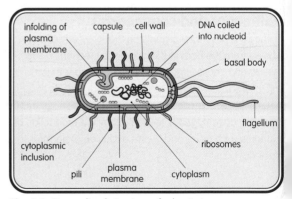

Fig. 4.4 Generalized structure of a bacterium.

Further classification is based on practical characteristics, i.e. size, shape, respiration and reproduction, and the analysis of biochemical and immunological criteria. A generalized structure of a bacterium is shown in Fig. 4.4, and an example of the characteristics used to classify bacteria is shown in Fig. 4.5.

Fungi

Fungi are unicellular, multicellular or multinucleate organisms (Fig. 4.6). They are eucaryotic but contain ergosterol instead of cholesterol in their plasma membranes.

Fungi have a well-defined cell wall composed of polysaccharides and chitin; they can be moulds, yeasts or dimorphic.

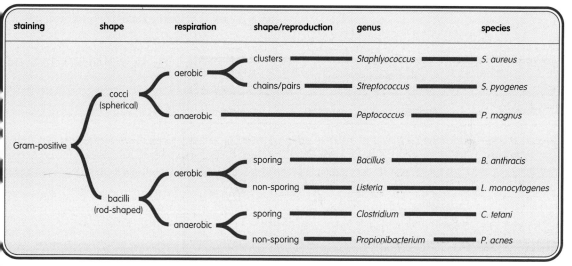

Fig. 4.5 The characteristics used to classify bacteria, using Gram-positive bacteria as an example.

Fig. 4.6 Classification of fungi.

Classification of fungi		
Yeast-like form	**Hyphal form**	**Dimorphic form**
single, rounded cells multiply by budding, e.g. *Candida albicans*, *Cryptococcus neoformans*	branching filaments interlaced to make mycelium or mould produce spores hyphae may be several hundred mm in length, e.g. *Aspergillus fumigatus*, dermatophytes	can assume either yeast or hyphal form depending on environment, e.g. *Histoplasma capsulatum*, *Blastomyces dermatidis*

Fungal infections are either superficial (e.g. involving the skin, hair, nails and mucous membranes) or systemic (e.g. involving the lungs, brain or heart) but the latter is usually only in the immunocompromised.

Protozoa

Protozoa are unicellular eucaryotes which may develop into cysts in harsh conditions. The main divisions of protozoa are shown Fig. 4.7.

Helminths and ectoparasites

Helminths are a group of parasitic worms, as shown in Fig. 4.8. Ectoparasites, e.g. bed bugs, crab louse, fleas, etc., are parasites that live on the outer surfaces of host.

Prions

Prions are not micro-organisms but are infectious proteins. Humans express normal prion proteins but their function is unknown. However, if an abnormal prion protein is inoculated into a normal host,

Fig. 4.7 Main divisions of protozoa.

Main divisions of protozoa			
Sporozoa	**Flagellates**	**Amoebae**	**Ciliates**
all are intracellular parasites, e.g. Plasmodium in red blood cells	move by beating one or more flagella, e.g. Trypanosoma	move by extending pseudopodia; they have no fixed shape, e.g. Entamoeba	move by beating many cilia, e.g. Balantidium

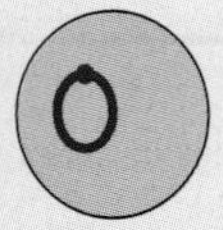

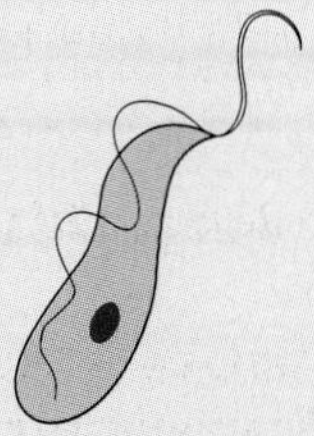

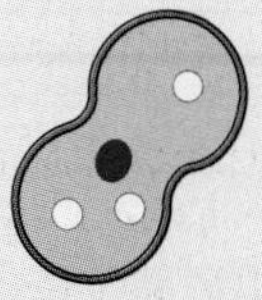

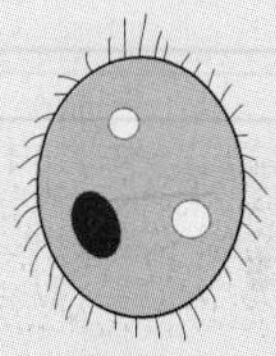

Fig. 4.8 Main groups of helminths (parasitic worms).

Main groups of helminths (parasitic worms)		
Nematodes (roundworms)	**Cestodes (tapeworms)**	**Trematodes (flukes)**
resistant cuticle; longitudinal muscles; complete digestive system; separate sexed reproductive system, e.g. *Ascaris lumbricoides, Strongyloides stercorali*	cellular epithelium; no digestive system; all hermaphrodites, e.g. *Taenia solium, Echinococcus granulosus*	cellular epithelium; circular and longitudinal muscles; incomplete digestive system; mostly hermaphrodites, e.g. *Schistosoma*

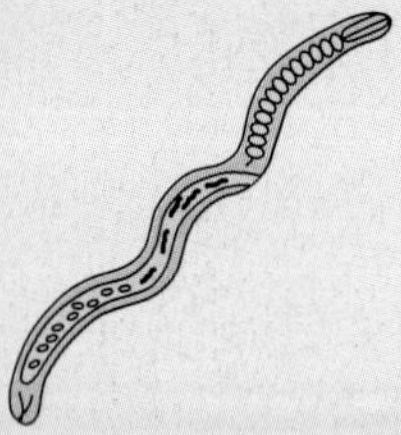

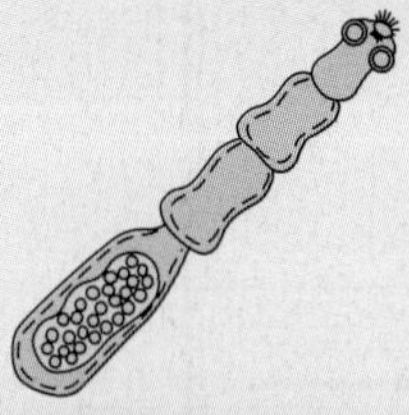

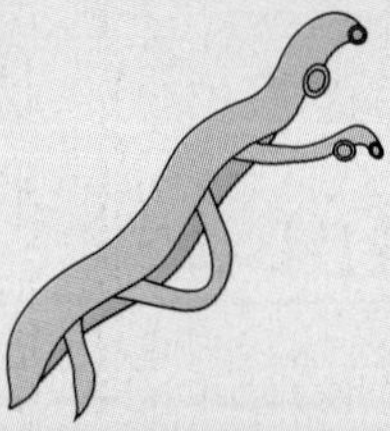

conformational changes are induced in the normal host prions resulting in their conversion to abnormal host prions.

These abnormal host proteins then induce further conformational changes in remaining normal host prions. Thus the original inoculated prion protein is able to catalyse a chain reaction in which host proteins become conformationally abnormal.

The net result is the formation of amyloid plaques of prion protein in the CNS. These plaques result in vacuolar spongiform degeneration of neuronal processes with neuronal loss and glial proliferation.

In humans, two forms prion protein disease exist: kuru ('laughing death') and Creutzfeldt–Jakob disease, which are always fatal, usually within six months.

MECHANISMS OF PATHOGENICITY

Host defences and routes of entry

The majority of infectious agents encountered by an individual are prevented from entering the body by a variety of biochemical and physical barriers (Fig. 4.9).

However, despite these defences, pathogenic micro-organisms possess efficient mechanisms for attaching to, and often penetrating, the body surfaces. If they are to be transmitted to a fresh host, the micro-organisms must also exit from the body.

The different routes of entry and exit of micro-organisms are outlined in Fig. 4.10.

Virus infections
Viral replication cycles

Fig. 4.11 outlines two types of viral replication cycles.

DNA viruses have their own DNA and use the host's cellular machinery to make more DNA, protein and glycoprotein. These are then reassembled into new virus particles prior to release from the cell.

RNA retroviruses first make viral DNA using viral 'reverse transcriptase'. Viral DNA is then inserted into the host genome prior to its transcription to form mRNA. Viral RNA is in turn translated into viral protein, which is packaged together with the RNA into new virus particles and released.

Release of new virus particles
Cell lysis (cytolysis)

Non-enveloped viruses, e.g. adenoviruses, are released directly into the extracellular environment by lysis of the host cell; their mode of release results in the death of the cell.

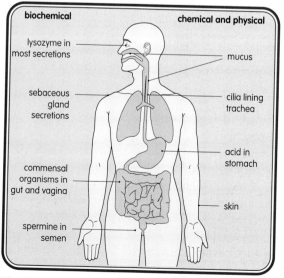

Fig. 4.9 Exterior host defences.

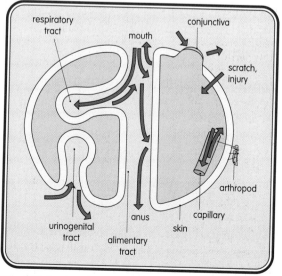

Fig. 4.10 Routes of entry and exit of micro-organisms.

29

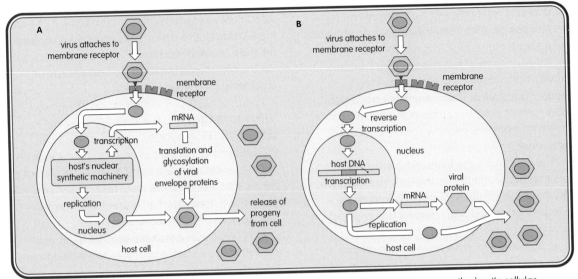

Fig. 4.11 Viral replication cycles. (A) DNA virus— DNA viruses have their own DNA. The viruses use the host's cellular machinery to make more DNA, protein and glycoprotein. These are then reassembled into new virus particles prior to release from the cell. (B) RNA retrovirus—RNA retroviruses first make viral DNA using viral 'reverse transcriptase'. Viral DNA is then inserted into the host genome prior to its transcription to form mRNA. Viral RNA is in turn translated into viral protein, which is packaged together with the RNA into new virus particles and released.

Budding

Enveloped viruses, e.g. HIV and herpesvirus, are released by 'budding' from the host cell membrane, thus:

- Nucleocapsid proteins are inserted into the host cell membrane.
- Modified area of host cell membrane extends out from cell surface, and is pinched off, i.e. budded, from the host cell enclosing the new viral particle.
- Mechanism does not cause the death of the cell, and so viral replication can continue.

Immune reaction to virally infected cells

Cytotoxic T cells kill virally infected cells as follows:
- Virally infected cells express viral peptides bound to MHC class I on their cell surfaces.
- Cytotoxic T cells (T_C) recognize viral antigen via T cell receptor.
- T_C cells secrete cytolysins, which results in the lysis of the virally infected cells.

Natural killer (NK) cells can do the same, but less effectively. The activity of these cells is enhanced by interferons produced by T_C and T_H cells. Interferons also prevent adjacent cells from becoming infected by intercellular viral transport.

Bacterial infections
Adherence

Certain bacteria are able to adhere specifically to epithelial cells by means of pili (also called fimbriae), which are are slender processes on the surfaces of some bacteria. Pili are coated with recognition molecules called adhesins. Specific interactions between adhesins of pili and molecules on the surface epithelial cells enable the bacterium to adhere to the host cell membranes.

Pili are more common in Gram-negative bacteria, although a few Gram-positive bacteria also possess them.

Exo- and endotoxins
Exotoxins

Exotoxins are proteins secreted by bacteria which are highly toxic to the host. The modes of action of some exotoxins are considered below:

- Enzymatic lysis, e.g. α-toxin (phospholipase C) of *Clostridium perfringens* breaks down host cell membranes.
- Pore forming, e.g. α-toxin of *Staphylococcus aureus* disrupts host cell membrane by pore formation.
- Inhibiting protein synthesis, e.g. diphtheria toxin.

- G protein hyperactivating, e.g. cholera toxin.
- Affecting synaptic transmission at neuromuscular junctions, e.g. tetanus and botulinum toxin.

Treating exotoxin with formaldehyde or high temperatures can denature the toxin forming toxoids, which can be useful for vaccination.

Endotoxins

Endotoxins are integral parts of bacterial cell walls, normally released only when the bacterium dies. They are typically lipopolysaccharides contained within the cell walls of Gram-negative bacteria. (But note that an exception is the protein endotoxin TSST1 produced by the Gram-positive *S. aureus*, causing toxic shock syndrome.)

These endotoxins are not in themselves toxic but induce toxic effects due to their potent activation of:
- The complement cascade, causing inflammatory damage.
- The coagulation cascade, causing disseminated intravascular coagulation.
- Tumour necrosis factor and interleukin-1 released from leukocytes, causing fever.

In overwhelming infections, the patient is said to suffer from endotoxic shock with fever, hypotension, and cardiac and renal failure.

Avoiding death by phagocytosis

Successful parasites have evolved numerous ingenious antiphagocytic devices:
- Phagocyte killing, e.g. via exotoxin release.
- Prevention of opsonization. The microbe produces protein which prevents interaction between opsonizing antibody and phagocyte.
- Preventing phagocyte contact. Some bacteria have an external capsule of polysaccharide which gives a slimy surface and provides protection against phagocytosis, e.g. *Streptococcus pneumoniae*.
- Protection against intracellular death. This allows the micro-organism to survive within the phagocyte as follows: inhibition of phagosome and lysosome fusion, e.g. mycobacteria; escape of microbe from phagolysosome into cytoplasm, resistance to killing by antioxidant production, e.g. mycobacteria, brucella and *Salmonella typhi*.

Antibiotic resistance and plasmids

Many bacteria are resistant to antibiotics. Resistance is conferred by genes which encode bacterial enzymes that block the effect of an antibiotic. These genes are not usually contained within the bacterial genome, but rather are contained within extrachromosomal DNA termed 'plasmids'. These plasmids are capable of self-replication and can be transferred from bacterium to bacterium.

Antibiotic-susceptible bacteria (those lacking plasmid conferring antibiotic resistance) can acquire plasmids from resistant bacteria and so gain antibiotic resistance. These newly resistant forms are then differentially selected under antibiotic treatment, the non-resistant bacteria being deleted from the population.

INFLAMMATORY RESPONSES TO INFECTION

Suppurative polymorphonuclear inflammation

This is characterized by the production of pus, such as in a boil, which is usually caused by infection with pyogenic bacteria (e.g. *Staphylococcus aureus, Streptococcus pyogenes*).

Chronic inflammation and scarring

This is caused by persisting reactions of tissue to injury, and occurs over weeks, months or even years. The cell-mediated immune response is characterized by lymphocytes, plasma cells and macrophages.

Infectious causes are micro-organisms resistant to phagocytosis or intracellular cell killing, e.g. *Mycobacterium tuberculosis* or *M. leprae*.

Granulomatous mononuclear inflammation

This is a form of chronic inflammation in which modified macrophages—epithelioid cells—aggregate to form small clusters or granulomas surrounded by lymphoid cells. It occurs in response to the presence of micro-organisms within macrophages which are resistant intracellular cell killing, e.g. *M. tuberculosis* or *M. leprae*.

Necrotizing inflammation
Gangrene
Here, necrotic tissue is invaded by putrefactive
organisms, notably clostridia. Tissue appears green or
black due to the breakdown of haemoglobin.

- Define 'infection', 'colonization', 'pathogen', 'commensals' and 'Koch's postulates'.
- What are the categories of infectious agents, their key features and main differences?
- Describe the host's defences against invasion and microbial routes of entry.
- Describe the mechanisms of viral infection and pathogenicity, and the immune responses of the host.
- Describe the mechanisms of bacterial infection and pathogenicity, intracellular evasion of phagocytosis and antibiotic resistance.
- Outline the inflammatory responses to infection.

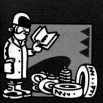

5. Inherited Disease

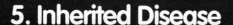

MOLECULAR BASIS OF INHERITED DISEASE

Genes code for polypeptides

Genes

A gene is a sequence of DNA that acts as the unit controlling the formation of a single polypeptide chain. Genes are composed of exons, introns and regulatory sequences.

Exons and introns

Exons (<u>ex</u>pressed sequences) are sequences of DNA that code for proteins ; introns (<u>in</u>tervening sequences) are sequences of DNA of unknown function that do not code for proteins.

Both exons and introns are transcribed into mRNA. A mechanism known as splicing is used to excise the non-protein-coding introns out of the mRNA prior to translation (protein synthesis). This mechanism, and the structure of a gene, is shown in Fig. 5.1.

Regulatory sequences

These are DNA sequences, known as promotor regions, that bind proteins (transcription factors) which control the expression of the gene, either by enhancing or inhibiting its expression.

Genes and their arrangement on genomic DNA

The human genome is the total DNA contained within a haploid set of human chromosomes. Each somatic cell therefore contains two copies of the human genome.

The human genome includes the genes themselves (an estimated 100 000 genes per haploid set of chromosomes) and repetitive sequences of DNA which are not transcribed but may have a role in chromosomal pairing, alignment and recombination.

Genomic DNA is packaged into chromosomes

The DNA double helix of a cell is coiled together with associated proteins, called histones, to form a chromosome (Fig. 5.2).

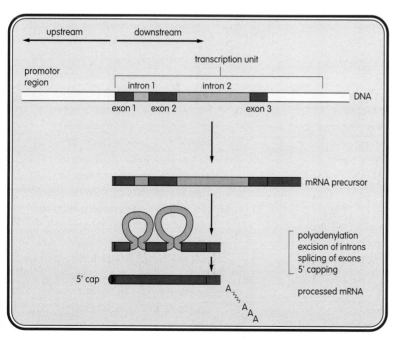

Fig. 5.1 Structure of a gene and the splicing of precursor mRNA.

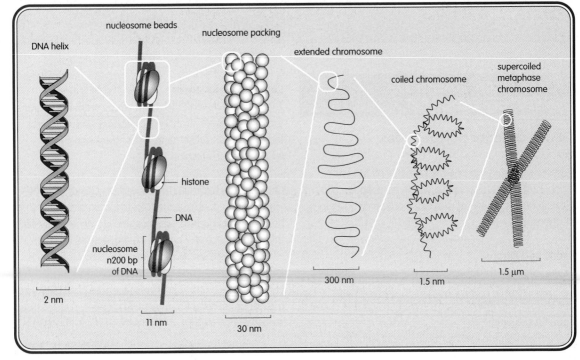

Fig. 5.2 The packaging of DNA and histones into chromosomes.

The chromosome set of an individual, described in terms of both the number and structure of the chromosomes, is called the karyotype.

Each somatic human cell nucleus contains 23 pairs of chromosomes, of which 22 are autosomal chromosomes (numbered 1 to 22 according to size). The remaining pair comprises the sex chromosomes: XX in females, XY in males.

Pairs of chromosomes of similar shape and size, and which have identical gene loci (regions of a chromosome occupied by a particular gene), are known as homologous pairs. One of each homologous pair is maternal in origin, the other paternal.

Single gene inheritance

This is the inheritance of a disorder in which there is a mutation in one or both members of a pair of genes. Single gene disorders are governed by Mendelian inheritance.

Multifactorial inheritance

This is the inheritance of a disorder in which there is both a genetic and an environmental contribution.

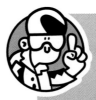

The '–ploid' suffix is used to denote the number of sets of chromosomes within the nucleus in the following ways:

- Haploid—Cells that have a single set of unpaired chromosomes. Gametes have haploid nuclei.
- Diploid—Cells that have a single set of paired chromosomes. Somatic cells have diploid nuclei.
- Polyploid—Cells in which there are more than twice the haploid number of chromosomes, e.g. triploid (69 chromosomes) and tetraploid (92 chromosomes).
- Euploid—Chromosome numbers are multiples of the haploid set.
- Aneuploid—Chromosome number is not an exact multiple of the haploid number, e.g. trisomy 21.

Mitosis and meiosis

Mitosis

Mitosis is the process whereby a somatic cell, which is diploid, undergoes a doubling of the DNA content and then divides to form two daughter cells (also diploid) which are identical to each other and to the parent cell.

Meiosis

Meiosis is the process whereby a germline cell (diploid) undergoes two successive nuclear divisions without an intervening period of DNA replication. The daughter cells have haploid nuclei and are genetically different to each other and to the parent cell.

Diversity is generated by either homologous recombination, i.e. the exchange of genetic material between homologous chromosomes, or by the independent assortment of chromosomes.

An overview of mitosis and meiosis is shown in Fig. 5.3; Fig. 5.4 provides a comparison of these processes.

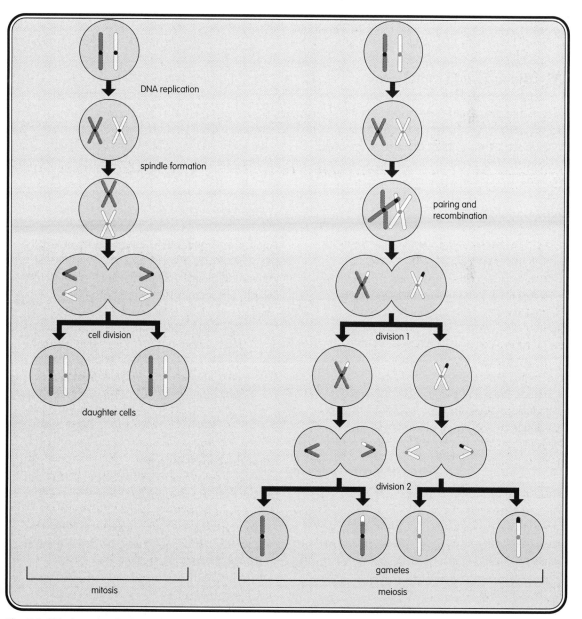

DNA replication

spindle formation

pairing and recombination

cell division

division 1

daughter cells

division 2

gametes

mitosis

meiosis

Fig. 5.3 Mitosis and meiosis.

Comparison of the processes of mitosis and meiosis		
	Mitosis	**Meiosis**
cell type	somatic cell (diploid)	germline cell (diploid)
function	to produce genetically identical cells for growth, differentiation and repair	to halve the chromosome number to generate genomic diversity
cell division/cycle	involves one division	involves two successive divisions (meiosis I and meiosis II)
frequency	line of somatic cells may divide many times	germline cell undergoes meiosis only once
result	diploid somatic cell identical to parent genome	haploid reproductive gamete different genome to parent

Fig. 5.4 Comparison of the processes of mitosis and meiosis.

DNA damage and mutations

A mutation is a permanent alteration in DNA due to some change in a nucleotide sequence or a rearrangement of DNA within the chromosome.

There are two basic types: single gene mutations, and chromosome mutations due to chromosome breakage (see below).

Gene mutations

Point mutations

These are single nucleotide substitutions. They can result in one of the following:

- The substitution of a single amino acid, e.g. point mutation in β-globin gene results in sickle cell anaemia:

    GAG   →   GTG
    glutamate   valine

- The introduction of a stop codon, e.g. in β-thalassaemia; this results in the formation of a truncated β-globin protein which is rapidly degraded:

    CAG   →   UAG
    glutamine   STOP!

- The creation or removal of intron splice sites, e.g. in Tay–Sachs disease; a point mutation in the intron of a hexosaminidase gene results in the loss of a splice site causing a deficiency of the enzyme:

    GT   →   CT
    splice site   loss of splice site

- An alteration in gene expression; point mutations in promoter sites can interfere with the binding of transcription factors resulting in decreased mRNA and protein synthesis, e.g. mutation in factor IX promoter prevents binding of transcription factor, resulting in a 70% decrease in the production of factor IX.

Small insertions/deletions (10 base pairs or less)

The addition or removal of nucleotides can result in frameshifts (change in reading frame), which result in proteins of abnormal structure, for example

    Tay–Sachs disease   →   no hexaminidase
    (4bp insertion)   produced

    cystic fibrosis   →   no frameshift but
    (3bp deletion)   deletion of single
                           phenylalanine
                           amino acid (ΔF_{508})

Large insertions/deletions

Insertion or deletion of larger sequences of DNA can result in the following disorders:

- Duchenne muscular dystrophy: the majority of cases are caused by deletions of dystrophin gene.
- α-Thalassaemia: many cases are due to the entire deletion of one of the α-globin genes.
- Haemophilia A: approximately 1% of cases are due to the insertion of the L1 element (long repetitive sequence of 6000bp) into the factor VIII gene.

How gene mutations occur

They occur through:

- Errors introduced during DNA replication.
- Exposure to chemical mutagens, e.g. base analogues (mimic bases but pair improperly); alkylating agents (addition of alkyl groups to bases prevents pairing); intercalating agents (intercalate with DNA distorting structure); other agents that act directly on DNA.
- Exposure to UV or ionizing radiation.
- Deamination of methylated cytosines.

Repair and proof-reading mechanisms

DNA proof-reading enzymes

DNA proof-reading enzymes correct more than 99.9% of errors introduced during DNA replication. However, despite such an efficient system, a single base pair error is introduced for approximately every 10^9 to 10^{10} base pairs replicated.

DNA repair enzymes

DNA repair enzymes are responsible for the correction of environmentally induced gene mutations. There are two types of repair mechanisms:

- Damaged DNA is directly repaired.
- Damaged region is removed (excised), then DNA synthesis fills in the gap.

However, if the DNA damage is too extensive for repair, then the cell is deleted by apoptosis.

Genetic nomenclature

Chromosomal nomenclature

Individual chromosomes can be identified by light microscopy from the differential staining of proteins contained within the chromosome. The labelling system runs as follows:

- The short arm of the chromosome is called 'p'.
- The long arm of the chromosome is called 'q'.
- The arms are divided into regions, bands and sub-bands according to their staining pattern.

Thus, band Xp25.2 is to be found in the short arm 'p' of the X chromosome, in region 2, band 5, sub-band 2.

Karyotype nomenclature

Karyotypes are described using a shorthand system of symbols, thus:

- Total number of chromosomes and sex chromosome constitution:
  46, XY—Normal male.
  47, XXY—Male with Klinefelter's syndrome.
- Additional or lost chromosomes are indicated by + or −, as follows:
  47, XX, +21—Female with trisomy 21; this is Down syndrome.
  46, XX, 8p+ —Additional unidentified material on short arm of chromosome 8.
- Description of structural rearrangement and its location on the chromosome: the commonest abbreviations are del (deletion), ins (insertion), inv (inversion) and t (translocation):
  46, XY, t(9;22)(q34;q11)—Translocation between chromosomes 9 and 22 involving the long arms; this is the Philadelphia chromosome seen in chronic myeloid leukaemia.
  46, XX, del(5)(p25)—Deletion on the short arm of chromosome 5 (at position p25); this is cri du chat syndrome.

CHROMOSOMAL DISORDERS

These disorders generally cause (multiple) congenital malformations and mental retardation. They are present in 6 per 1000 live births and in >20% spontaneous abortions.

Some of the more common disorders are shown in Fig. 5.5. There are two basic types:

- Numerical (i.e. there are too many or too few chromosomes: trisomy, monosomy, polyploidy)
- Structural (i.e. the result of chromatin breakage with loss, gain or rearrangement of chromosomal material).

See Fig. 5.6 for an overview of the aetiology of chromosomal disorders.

Mendelian inheritance

Mendelian inheritance describes the inheritance patterns of single gene defects. More than 4000 single-gene traits have been listed. The risks of inheriting a particular trait can be calculated by knowing the mode of Mendelian inheritance and the details of the family pedigree.

There are three basic types of Mendelian inheritance patterns: autosomal dominant, autosomal recessive, and X-linked disorders.

The main types of structural chromosomal disorders are:

○ **Translocation**—Part of a chromosome is transferred to another part of the same chromosome or to a different one. This changes the order of the genes on the chromosomes and so can lead to serious genetic disorders, e.g. chronic myeloid leukaemia.

○ **Inversion**—A section of the chromosome is inverted resulting in a block of genes in reverse order within that chromosome.

○ **Deletion**—Loss of part of a chromosome resulting in the loss of many genes.

○ **Duplication**—Duplication of part of a chromosome.

Autosomal dominant disorders

Autosomal dominant disorders have the following characteristics:

- They are caused by a mutation in one or both members of a pair of autosomal genes.
- Both heterozygotes and homozygotes manifest the disease, but the majority are heterozygotes.
- Males and females are equally affected.
- Defective genes usually code for structural proteins.

The pattern of inheritance of an autosomal dominant disorder is shown in Fig. 5.7.

An affected parent (heterozygote) with a normal partner has a 50% chance that their offspring will be affected.

All offspring of a homozygous parent will be affected.

Penetrance

Usually, all individuals known to possess the dominant mutant gene manifest the disease; this is known as complete penetrance. Occasionally, individuals with the dominant mutant gene do not manifest its phenotype—this is known as incomplete, or reduced, penetrance.

Autosomal recessive disorders

Autosomal recessive disorders are

- Caused by a mutation in both members of a pair of

Types of chromosomal disorders			
Types of disorder	**Example**		**Outcome**
Numerical			
polyploid	triploidy	69 chromosomes	lethal
aneuploid	trisomy of X chromosome 21	ΛΛΛ	Down syndrome
	monosomy of chromosome	X	Turner's syndrome
	47 chromosomes (XXY)	X Xλ	Klinefelter's syndrome
Structural			
deletion	terminal deletion 5p	X←	cri du chat syndrome
	interstitial deletion 11p	X←	found in Wilms' tumour
inversion	pericentric inversion 9	X	normal phenotype
duplication	isochromosome X (fusion of long arms with loss of short arms)	X q/q	infertility in females
ring chromosome	ring chromosome 18	O	mental retardation syndrome
fragile site	fragile X	X	mental retardation syndrome
translocation	reciprocal	XX	balanced translocations cause no abnormality; unbalanced translocations cause spontaneous abortions or syndromes of multiple physical and mental handicaps
	robertsonian	V 14 X 13	

Fig. 5.5 Types of chromosomal disorders. (Adapted with permission from *ABC of Clinical Genetics*, 2nd edn, by H.M. Kingston, BMJ, 1994.)

autosomal genes.
- Manifested only by homozygotes.
- Carried by heterozygotes.
- Equally prevalent in males and females.
- Defective genes usually code for enzymes or ion channels.

Patterns of inheritance for an autosomal recessive disorder

Fig. 5.8 shows the pattern of autosomal recessive inheritance.

Aetiology of chromosomal disorders	
Congenital	**Acquired**
majority	rare
occurs during gametogenesis	occurs during life
affects all cells of body usually presents with abnormal mental and/or physical development	restricted to abnormal (neoplastic) tissue
examples: • Down syndrome • Klinefelter's syndrome	examples: • chronic myeloid leukaemia • Burkitt's lymphoma

Fig. 5.6 Aetiology of chromosomal disorders.

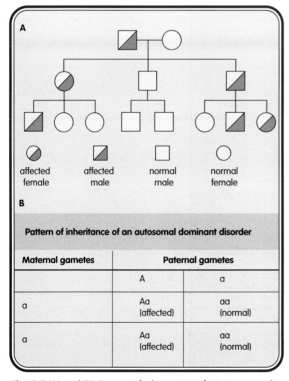

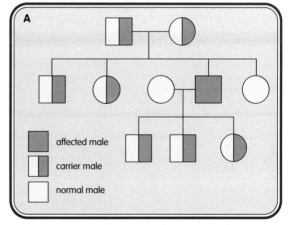

Pattern of inheritance of an autosomal dominant disorder

Maternal gametes	Paternal gametes	
	A	a
a	Aa (affected)	aa (normal)
a	Aa (affected)	aa (normal)

Fig. 5.7 (A) and (B) Pattern of inheritance of an autosomal dominant disorder.

	Pattern of autosomal recessive inheritance	
Gametes	**Gametes**	
	A	a
A	AA (affected)	Aa (carrier)
a	Aa (carrier)	aa (normal)

Fig. 5.8 (A) and (B) Pattern of autosomal recessive inheritance.

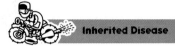

For two unaffected heterozygous (carrier) parents there is a:

- 25% chance of producing an affected homozygous child (AA).

- 50% chance of producing an unaffected heterozygous (carrier) child (Aa).
- 25% chance of producing an unaffected child with normal genes (aa).

Examples of autosomal disorders	
Recessive	**Dominant**
cystic fibrosis	achondroplasia
Friedreich's ataxia	adult polycystic kidney disease
galactosaemia	Huntington's disease
glycogen storage diseases	Marfan's syndrome
homocystinuria	myotonic dystrophy
sickle cell disease	neurofibromatosis
Tay–Sachs disease	osteogenesis imperfecta
Wilson's disease	von Willebrand's disease

Fig. 5.9 Examples of autosomal disorders.

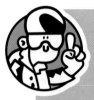 **For X-linked disorders, it is important to note that:**
- **The X chromosome of the male *always* comes from mother.**
- **A defective gene cannot therefore be transmitted from father to son; this is the hallmark of X-linked disorders.**
- **Males cannot be carriers without having the disease.**

Comparison of autosomal dominant and recessive disorders	
Dominant	**Recessive**
heterozygotes affected	heterozygotes not affected (symptomless carriers)
homozygotes affected (but often not compatible with life)	homozygotes affected
males and females equally affected	males and females equally affected
at least one parent shows overt disease	both parents may be symptomless carriers
50% chance of affected offspring if one parent affected	25% chance of disease in children of symptomless carriers
not usually transmitted by individual without disease	commonly transmitted by individuals without disease (carriers)
no association with consanguinous marriages	associated with consanguinous marriages

Fig. 5.10 Comparison of autosomal dominant and recessive disorders.

Comparison of X-linked dominant and recessive diseases		
	X-linked dominant	**X-linked recessive**
sex ratio of affected individuals	f > m by 2:1	m >> f
male to male transmission	never	never
male to female transmission	all daughters affected	all daughters carriers
female to female transmission	50% chance of all daughters affected	50% chance of all daughters carriers

Fig. 5.11 Comparison of X-linked dominant and recessive diseases.

Fig. 5.9 gives some examples of autosomal disorders, and Fig. 5.10 gives a comparison of autosomal dominant and recessive disorders.

X-linked disorders
These disorders are due to the inheritance of a mutated gene on an X chromosome. X-linked disorders can be recessive or dominant (Fig. 5.11 and Fig. 5.12)

Patterns of inheritance of X-linked recessive disease
Fig. 5.13 shows an example of X-linked recessive inheritance pattern of a carrier mother, and Fig. 5.14 shows an example of X-linked recessive inheritance pattern of an affected father.
The exceptions are:
- Heterozygous females occasionally show features of the condition. This is due to non-random X chromosome inactivation, i.e. the chromosome that carries the mutant allele remains active in most cells.
- Rarely, a homozygous affected state may occur in female offspring of affected fathers and carrier mothers; there is a 50% chance of this.

X-linked dominant disease
This is shown by examples in the following figures:
- X-linked dominant inheritance pattern of an affected father is shown in Fig. 5.15.
- X-linked dominant inheritance pattern of an affected mother is shown in Fig. 5.16.

Examples of X-linked disorders	
Recessive	**Dominant**
glucose-6-phosphatase deficiency red–green colour blindness Duchenne muscular dystrophy haemophilia A and B Becker muscular dystrophy	vitamin D resistant rickets orofaciodigital syndrome incontinentia pigmenti

Fig. 5.12 Examples of X-linked disorders.

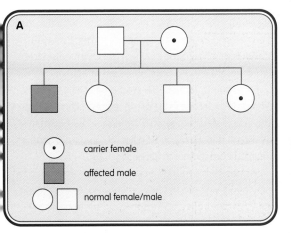

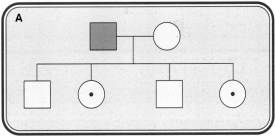

B	X-linked recessive inheritance of carrier mother		
Paternal Gametes	**Maternal Gametes**		
	X*	X	
X	XX* (carrier female)	XX (normal female)	
Y	X*Y (affected male)	XY (normal male)	

Fig. 5.13 (A) and (B) X-linked recessive inheritance pattern of carrier mother. Offspring of female carrier: 50% chance of sons being affected; 50% chance of daughters being carriers.

B	X-linked recessive inheritance of affected father		
Gametes	**Gametes**		
	X	X	
X*	XX* (carrier female)	XX* (carrier female)	
Y	XY (normal male)	XY (normal male)	

Fig. 5.14 (A) and (B) X-linked recessive inheritance pattern of affected father. Offspring of affected male: all sons normal; all daughters carriers.

41

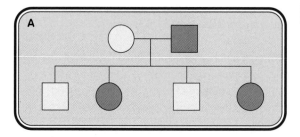

Fig. 5.15(A) and (B) X-linked dominant inheritance pattern of affected father. Offspring of affected male: all sons normal; all daughters affected.

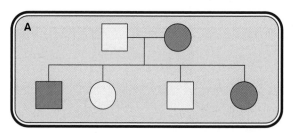

Fig. 5.16 (A) and (B) X-linked dominant inheritance pattern of affected mother. Offspring of affected female: 50% chance of producing affected sons; 50% chance of producing affected daughters.

NON-MENDELIAN INHERITANCE

Trinucleotide repeat disorders

This is a group of disorders caused by the disruption of specific genes with trinucleotide repeat expansions (e.g. CAG CAG CAG CAG etc.). Fig. 5.17 gives some examples of this.

Normal copies of the genes responsible for these disorders contain 6 to 50 trinucleotide repeat sequences which are stable and have low mutation rates. However, in affected individuals, the number of repeats are:

- Outside the normal range.
- Have high mutation rates.
- Unstable, i.e. the disorder becomes more severe in successive generations of a family due to an increase in the number of repeats in offspring; this phenomenon is known as anticipation.

Genomic imprinting

Genomic imprinting is a phenomenon by which certain genes function differently depending on whether they are maternal or paternal in origin. It contrasts with Mendelian inheritance in which genes inherited from either parent should have an equal effect.

For example, Prader–Willi syndrome versus Angelman's syndrome: deletions in the q11-13 region of chromosome 15 may cause either Prader–Willi syndrome or Angelman's syndrome depending on whether the abnormal gene is inherited from mother or father (Fig. 5.18).

Prader–Willi syndrome has also been diagnosed in individuals who do not have a chromosome deletion but in whom both chromosomes 15 are maternally derived (uniparental disomy). This suggests that Prader–Willi syndrome is caused by a deficiency of 15q11-13 of paternal origin.

Normal human development therefore requires the gene in the region of 15q11-13 to be inherited from each parent.

Mitochondrial inheritance

Mitochondria contain their own DNA genome (16 kbase pairs) and there are up to ten copies of mitochondrial genome per mitochondrion. As there are hundreds of mitochondria per cell, then there are more than 1000 copies of mitochondrial genome per cell.

The main function of mitochondrial genes is to synthesize oxidative phosphorylation proteins. Mutations of mitochondrial DNA are therefore more likely to affect the brain, skeletal muscle, cardiac muscle and the eye as these contain abundant mitochondria and rely on aerobic oxidation for ATP production.

Examples of diseases caused by mitochondrial inheritance are shown in Fig. 5.19.

Aetiology of mitochondrial mutations

Mitochondrial mutations are usually sporadic but sometimes inherited. All inherited mitochondrial disorders are maternal in origin as the oocyte contributes cytoplasm and mitochondria to the zygote. Furthermore all offspring of a carrier mother will carry the mutation, whereas all offspring of a carrier father will be normal.

Heteroplasmy and mitochondrial inheritance

All cells of an affected individual are heteroplasmic, i.e. they contain a mixture of mutant and normal mitochondrial DNA. With successive cell divisions some cells will remain heteroplasmic but others may drift towards homoplasmy for the mutant or normal DNA. Therefore, the severity of mitochondrial diseases is extremely variable and depends on the relative proportions of normal to mutant DNA.

Note that not all disorders of mitochondrial function are due to defects of the mitochondrial genome; some are due to defects of the nuclear genome.

Examples of trinucleotide repeat disorders		
Trinucleotide repeat disorder	**Trinucleotide repeat**	**Number of repeats in genes of affected individuals**
myotonic dystrophy	CTG	50–1000+
fragile X syndrome	CGG	200–1000+
Huntington's disease	CAG	40–80

Fig. 5.17 Examples of trinucleotide repeat disorders.

Comparison of Prader–Willi and Angelman's syndromes		
	Prader–Willi syndrome	**Angelman's syndrome**
origin of mutated chromosome	paternal chromosome	maternal chromosome
symptoms	severe neonatal hypotonia failure to thrive later onset of obesity mental retardation characteristic facial appearance small hands and feet hypogonadism	severe mental retardation microcephaly ataxia epilepsy absent speech

Fig. 5.18 Comparison of Prader–Willi syndrome and Angelman's syndrome.

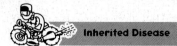

Examples of diseases caused by mitochondrial inheritance	
Disorders	**Symptoms**
Leber's hereditary optic neuropathy (Leber's optic atrophy)	acute visual loss and other neurological symptoms
MERRF	**M**yoclonic **E**pilepsy with **R**agged **R**ed **F**ibres in skeletal muscle
MELAS	**M**yo**E**ncephalopathy, **L**actic **A**cidosis, **S**troke-like episodes

Fig. 5.19 Examples of diseases caused by mitochondrial inheritance.

You must be able to:

- Describe how genes code for polypeptides and how they are packaged into chromosomes.
- Outline the key differences between mitosis and meiosis.
- Describe the different types of gene mutations.
- Describe genetic nomenclature.
- Give examples of chromosomal disorders and describe their aetiology.
- Give examples of autosomal dominant, autosomal recessive, X-linked dominant and X-linked recessive disorders.
- Describe the inheritance of trinucleotide repeat disorders, genomic imprinting disorders and disorders of mitochondrial inheritance.

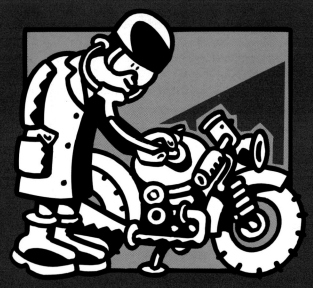

SYSTEMIC PATHOLOGY

6. Pathology of the Nervous System

DISORDERS OF THE CENTRAL NERVOUS SYSTEM

Common pathological features

Intracranial herniation

Intracranial herniation is the movement of part of the brain from one space to another with resultant damage. It usually occurs following a critical increase in intracranial pressure caused by an expanding lesion, e.g. tumour or haematoma. However, it may be inadvertently precipitated by withdrawing cerebrospinal fluid (CSF) at lumbar puncture.

Fig. 6.1 shows a diagrammatical representation of the sites of intracranial herniation.

Cerebral oedema

This is an abnormal accumulation of fluid in the cerebral parenchyma. It is usually the result of breakdown of the blood–brain barrier, and may occur following damage initiated by several different causes:

- Ischaemia, e.g. from infarction.
- Trauma, e.g. from head injury.
- Inflammation encephalitis or meningitis.
- Cerebral tumours (primary or secondary).
- Metabolic disturbances, e.g. hyponatraemia or hypoglycaemia.

The condition results in cerebral swelling and is associated with raised intracranial pressure.

Treatment is by minimizing the formation of oedema by use of osmotic agents or steroids.

Hydrocephalus

Hydrocephalus is an increase in the volume of CSF within the brain resulting in the expansion of the cerebral ventricles. It can be due to one of three mechanisms:

- Obstruction to flow of CSF (commonest form).
- Impaired absorption of CSF at arachnoid villi (rare).
- Overproduction of CSF by choroid plexus neoplasms (very rare).

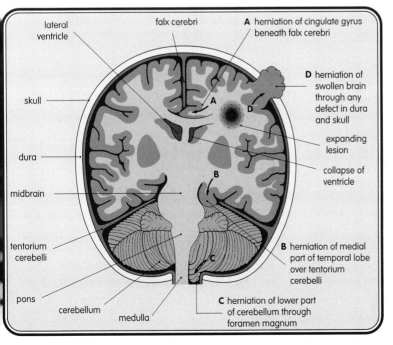

lateral ventricle
falx cerebri
A herniation of cingulate gyrus beneath falx cerebri
skull
D herniation of swollen brain through any defect in dura and skull
expanding lesion
collapse of ventricle
dura
midbrain
tentorium cerebelli
pons
cerebellum
medulla
B herniation of medial part of temporal lobe over tentorium cerebelli
C herniation of lower part of cerebellum through foramen magnum

Fig. 6.1 Sites of intracranial herniation. (A) Herniation of the cingulate gyrus beneath the falx cerebri. (B) Herniation of the medial part of the temporal lobe over the tentorium cerebelli. (C) Herniation of the lower part of the cerebellum through the foramen magnum. (D) Herniation of swollen brain through any defect in the dura and skull.

Obstructive hydrocephalus is by far the commonest form of hydrocephalus. It is commonly subdivided into:

○ **Non-communicating hydrocephalus—Obstruction** within the ventricular system leading to blockage of CSF flow from the ventricles to the subarachnoid space.

○ **Communicating hydrocephalus— Extraventricular obstruction** within subarachnoid space.

Obstructive hydrocephalus is either congenital or acquired.

Congenital hydrocephalus
This occurs in 1 per 1000 births. The principal causes are congenital malformations, for example:
- Arnold–Chiari malformation (see pp. 49).
- Congenital stenosis of the cerebral aqueduct.
- Atresia of the foramina of Magendie and Luschka (Dandy–Walker syndrome).
- Some genetic causes associated with X-linked inheritance.

Acquired hydrocephalus
This may result from any lesion which obstructs the CSF pathway such as:
- Tumours: especially if located in the posterior fossa as the fourth ventricle aqueducts are easily obstructed.
- Scarring: postinflammatory fibrosis of the meninges, at exit foramina, following meningitis or subarachnoid haemorrhage.
- Haemorrhage: intraventricular or in the posterior fossa.

Diagnosis
Severe forms of congenital hydrocephalus may be diagnosed antenatally via ultrasound. Less severe forms may present with considerably enlarged heads at birth.

In acquired hydrocephalus, enlargement of the head is prevented by the inability of the skull to expand but this leads to massive dilatation of the ventricles resulting in increased intracranial pressure.

Associated features are dementia with gait disturbances and incontinence.

Treatment and management
A ventricular shunt with one-way valve system can be inserted to drain CSF into the peritoneum.

Prognosis
Untreated patients may suffer irreversible brain damage, and the condition is often fatal.

Special types of hydrocephalus
Secondary or compensatory hydrocephalus
Here, an increase in CSF occurs as a compensatory measure following loss of brain tissue, e.g. due to infarction or atrophy. There is no associated increase in CSF pressure.

Normal pressure hydrocephalus (intermittent pressure hydrocephalus)
This is a rare condition of progressive dementia associated with ventricular dilatation. Random sampling shows normal CSF pressure but continuous monitoring reveals intermittent increases.

Malformations, developmental disease and perinatal injury
Neural tube defects
These are the commonest congenital abnormalities of the CNS and are caused by defective closure of the midline structures over the neural tube.

Anencephaly
This is a common neural tube defect which manifests as an absence of the cranial vault and failure of development of the cerebral hemispheres. The condition is invariably fatal and often results in spontaneous abortion.

Encephalocele
Ossification defects in the bones of the skull result in herniation of the brain and meninges. This condition occurs in 1 per 8000 live births. The types are occipital, frontal, orbital and nasal. The commonest form is occipital with herniation of the posterior cerebral hemispheres and their coverings through a defect in the skull.

Spina bifida

Spina bifida is a neural tube defect of the spinal cord resulting from defective development and defective closure of the neural tube and vertebral arches. Most common in the lumbar region.

There are two types: spina bifida occulta and spina bifida cystica.

Spina bifida occulta

This is present in 1–2.5% of the population, and is usually asymptomatic. The meninges and cord are normal but there is abnormal development of the vertebral arches. There may be an associated sinus track to the skin surface, or subcutaneous lipoma.

Spina bifida cystica

This is present in 1 per 800 live births (females > males and appears in two forms, one is much more common than the other:

- Meningocele (10%): abnormal development of the vertebral arches with cystic outpouching of the meninges covered by skin. Spinal cord may be normally or abnormally formed.
- Meningomyelocele (90%): abnormal development of the vertebral arches with cystic outpouching of the meninges, nerve roots and abnormally developed spinal cord.

Diagnosis can be made *in utero* by ultrasonography and by increased amounts of α-fetoprotein in amniotic fluid.

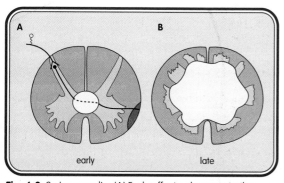

Fig. 6.2 Syringomyelia. (A) Early effects: damage to the decussating sensory fibres, with loss of temperature and touch in local segments. (B) Late effects: destruction of grey matter and gradual affection of long tracts with loss of local reflexes, severe sensory loss and spastic paralysis.

Complications

The complications are:

- Neurological deficit: paraplegia, absence of sphincter control and neurogenic atrophy of lower limb muscles.
- Meningitis.
- Renal problems: recurrent urinary tract infections, chronic pyelonephritis and renal failure.

Associated malformations

These are hydrocephalus (25%) and Arnold–Chiari malformation (see below).

Posterior fossa abnormalities
Arnold–Chiari malformation

This is the second most common developmental abnormality of the CNS and it is the commonest congenital malformation of the posterior fossa (at 1 per 1000 births). It involves prolongation of the cerebellum downwards through the foramen magnum. It commonly results in obstructive hydrocephalus and is nearly always associated with lumbar myelomeningocele.

Dandy–Walker malformation

This is a form of hydrocephalus resulting from obstruction of the foramina of Luschka and Magendie (the exit foramina of the fourth ventricle). The fourth ventricle is distended and forms a cyst-like structure between the cerebellar hemispheres; the cerebellar vermis may be absent or hypoplastic.

Syringomyelia and hydromyelia

Syringomyelia is a rare condition in which a cyst (syrinx) develops within the spinal cord, usually posterior to the central canal (Fig. 6.2). The cavity is lined by gliosis (astrocytes). It is most common in the cervical spinal cord but may extend into the medulla (syringobulbia).

Hydromyelia is the term used to denote cases in which the dilatated central canal contains CSF, and is lined by ependyma.

The causes of these conditions are either:

- Acquired (majority of cases): secondary to trauma or ischaemia, or occurring in association with tumours of the spinal cord.
- Congenital: may be associated with maldevelopment of the cord or other developmental abnormalities of the craniocervical junction, especially in Arnold–Chiari syndrome.

The clinical manifestations are muscle weakness and atrophy in the upper limbs due to compression of the anterior horn cells. There is loss of the sensations of pain and temperature, but with preservation of those of position and vibration, due to damage to nerve fibres crossing the cord in the lateral spinothalamic tracts.

Surgery may arrest or alleviate symptoms by decompression or by draining the fluid in the cystic cavity.

Perinatal injury
Cerebral palsy

Cerebral palsy describes brain malformation or damage affecting motor areas of the brain. It is the leading cause of crippling handicap in children, affecting 2 per 1000 live births. Damage may occur during fetal life, may be birth related, or may occur postnatally (Fig. 6.4).

The different types of cerebral palsy are outlined in Fig. 6.3.

Ischaemia and hypoxia

Ischaemia and hypoxia are major causes of severe perinatal brain damage. Perinatal hypoxia is usually due to asphyxiation associated with the trauma of birth, whereas perinatal ischaemia is commonly caused by intracranial haemorrhages.

Premature infants are highly susceptible to developing intracranial haemorrhages due to disturbances in the cerebral circulation possibly caused by in-utero hypoxia/ischaemia.

In full-term infants, intracranial haemorrhages with the formation of small haematomas may occur during difficult deliveries, although this is less common now due to improved obstetric care.

Mortality is high; one-third of survivors may develop cerebral palsy, epilepsy or mental retardation.

Traumatic injuries to the CNS
Skull fractures

Skull fractures occur in approximately 80% of fatal cases of head injuries. The importance of skull fractures cannot be overemphasized due to the increased incidence of intracranial haematoma (1 in 4 versus 1 in 6000!). The most common are linear fractures of the vault of the skull (62%); such fractures may extend into the base of the skull causing cranial nerve laceration.

The other types of skull fracture are:

- Penetrating: increased risk of infection due to tearing the dura.
- Compound: increased risk of infection due to laceration of the scalp and tearing of the dura.
- Depressed: increased incidence of epilepsy.
- Comminuted (fragmented): increased incidence of massive brain damage.

Parenchymal damage
Concussion

This is an abrupt transient loss of consciousness due to temporal neuronal dysfunction following a relatively slight impact. It is caused by an enormous but short-lived increase in pressure within the cranium at time of impact. Full recovery usually ensues although repeated concussion may result in permanent brain damage.

Types of cerebral palsy and their associated characteristics	
Type	**Characteristics**
spastic cerebral palsy (70%)	hypertonia, ankle clonus and extensor plantar response
dystonic (athetoid) cerebral palsy (10%)	irregular, involuntary muscle movements
ataxic cerebral palsy (10%)	hypotonia, weakness, uncoordinated movements and intention tremor
mixed cerebral palsy (10%)	–

Fig. 6.3 Types of cerebral palsy and their associated characteristics.

Causes of cerebral palsy
cerebral malformation
cerebrovascular accident
hypoglycaemia
hypoxia
infection
kernicterus (bilirubin-induced brain damage)
poisoning
toxins
trauma (peri- and postnatal)

Fig. 6.4 Causes of cerebral palsy.

Contusions and lacerations

A contusion is a bruise with extravasation of blood but with the pia-arachnoid intact. A laceration is where the pia-arachnoid is torn.

Both are focal types of brain damage occurring at the moment of injury, caused by striking the brain against adjacent bone. They are most common at the frontal and occipital poles and mainly affect the crests of gyri. Both lesions are characteristically haemorrhagic.

Types of contusion:

- Fracture contusion: occurs at site of fracture.
- Coup contusion: occurs at point of impact in absence of fracture.
- Contrecoup contusion: occurs diametrically opposite site of impact.
- Herniation contusion: occurs when the hippocampi or cerebellar tonsils (or both) are impacted and bruised by the free edge of the tentorium and foramen magnum respectively.
- Gliding contusion: occurs at superior margins of the cerebral hemispheres; usually caused by interference of the dura with a rotational movement of the brain.

Diffuse axonal injury

The condition is produced as a result of rotational movements of the brain within the skull during angular acceleration or deceleration. It often occurs in the absence of any skull fracture and cerebral contusions.

There are two main features:

- Small haemorrhagic lesions in the corpus callosum and dorsolateral quadrant of brainstem (macroscopic).
- Widespread tearing of axons (microscopic).

This type of injury occurs in almost 50% of patients with severe head injury and in almost all fatal head injuries. It is associated with head injuries involving vehicular accidents.

Traumatic vascular injury

Bleeding from craniocerebral trauma is often associated with high mortality and may take place in one or more of the potential spaces surrounding the brain, e.g. extradural and subdural.

Extradural (epidural) haemorrhage

This type occurs in 2% of all head injuries and in 15% of fatal cases. Haemorrhage occurs between the skull and dura and gradually strips dura from bone forming a large, saucer-shaped haematoma (Fig. 6.5).

This injury is almost always the result of skull fracture, usually a linear fracture of the thin squamous part of the temporal bone, which contains the middle meningeal artery.

It is associated with a post-traumatic lucid interval of several hours followed by a rapid increase in intracranial pressure.

Subdural haemorrhage

Haemorrhage occurs between the dura and the outer surface of the arachnoid membrane. It is usually due to a rupture of the small bridging veins or the venous sinuses. The resulting haematoma is often extensive because of the loose attachment of the dura and arachnoid membranes.

Subdural haemorrhage may be acute or chronic. Acute subdural haemorrhage:

- Is associated with severe head injury, subarachnoid haemorrhage and cerebral contusions.
- Presents with rapid increase in intracranial pressure.

Chronic subdural haemorrhage has the following characteristics:

- More common in the very young and elderly.
- Usually occurs as a result of minimal trauma, or as a

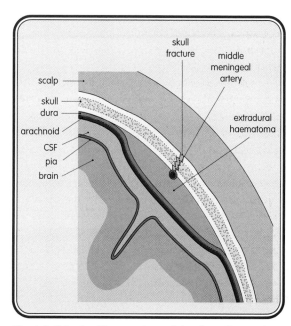

Fig. 6.5 Extradural haemorrhage. Taken from Stevens & Lowe, *Pathology*, Mosby.

result of cerebral atrophy (in the elderly), which causes a gradual widening of the subdural space leading to rupture of the bridging veins.
- Blood typically accumulates slowly over a period of days or weeks.
- Presents with personality change, memory loss and confusion.

Subarachnoid haemorrhage

Arterial rupture is usually secondary to superficial contusions or lacerations of the brain. Small amounts of blood can be disposed of by arachnoid granulations. Larger haemorrhages cause arachnoid fibrosis leading to meningeal irritation and raised intracranial pressure. It can also occur as a result of hypertension, aneurysms, embolisms or infarction.

Intracerebral haemorrhage

This is caused by direct rupture of the intrinsic cerebral vessels at the time of injury.

Resulting haematomas are classified into three types:
- Solitary: occur in association with cortical contusions; common in temporal and frontal poles.
- Multiple: associated with severe contrecoup lesions; often fatal.
- Burst lobe: intracerebral or intracerebellar haematoma in continuity with subdural haematoma; most common in temporal and frontal lobes; rapidly fatal.

Spinal cord injuries

Most spinal injuries occur in males aged under 40 years. Road traffic accidents account for more than 80% of such injuries.

There are two types of spinal cord injuries—open and closed.

Open injuries

These are rare and are a direct trauma to the spinal cord and nerve roots. They can be either perforating (i.e. with extensive disruption and haemorrhage) or penetrating (i.e. with incomplete cord transection—Brown–Séquard's syndrome).

Closed injuries

These are in the majority and are associated with fracture or dislocation of the spinal column causing compression of the cord by distortion of the spinal canal.

Primary damage:
- Contusions.
- Nerve fibre transection.
- Haemorrhagic necrosis.

Secondary damage:
- Extradural haematoma.
- Infarction.
- Infection.
- Oedema.

The consequences depend mainly on the site and severity of the lesion. Cervical lesions result in tetraplegia; lower thoracic lesions result in paraplegia.

Cerebrovascular disease

Cerebrovascular disease is the third leading cause of death in the UK.

Stroke is a common outcome of cerebrovascular disease, and is defined as a sudden event in which a neurological deficit occurs over minutes or hours and lasts for longer than 24 hours.

If CNS disturbance lasts for less than 24 hours, then the condition is termed a transient ischaemic attack.

The incidence is 1 or 2 per 1000 per year but is much higher in the elderly, affecting males > females.

Causes of stroke are:
- Cerebral infarction (80%).
- Intracerebral haemorrhage (10%).
- Subarachnoid haemorrhage (10%).

Pathological effects occur due to extensive hypoxic neuronal damage. The area of brain affected can be readily localized since the blood supply of the brain has a fairly constant anatomic distribution. Fig. 6.6 shows the territories of the major arteries.

Clinical features of stroke depend on localization and the nature of the lesion. Risk factors are atheroma, heart disease, hypertension and diabetes mellitus.

Hypoxia, ischaemia and infarction

Cerebral infarction is the process whereby a focal area of necrosis is produced in the brain in response to a decreased supply of oxygen (and glucose) in the territory of a cerebral arterial branch.

There are two main causes of infarction:
- Hypoxia: the reduction of oxygen supply to tissues

despite an adequate blood supply, e.g. following respiratory arrest.

- Ischaemia: blood supply to tissues is absent, or severely reduced, usually as a result of constriction or obstruction of a blood vessel.

Ischaemia accounts for the majority of cases of cerebral infarction.

Mechanisms of ischaemia
Ischaemia may be caused by:

- Vascular disease – e.g. thrombosis, embolic occlusion or vasculitis.
- Cardiac disease – e.g. prolonged hypotension or cardiac embolism.
- Trauma – head injury leading to vascular occlusion, dissection or rupture.

Fig. 6.7 shows the pathological features of cerebral infarction.

Strokes caused by cerebral infarction clinically present with slowly evolving signs and symptoms.

Atraumatic haemorrhage
Intracerebral haemorrhage
The majority of intracerebral haemorrhages are thought to arise from Charcot–Bouchard microaneurysms associated with hypertension and diabetic vascular disease. These haemorrhages occur most frequently in the basal ganglia (80%), brainstem, cerebellum and cerebral cortex.

The resulting haematoma acts as a space-occupying lesion leading to increased intracranial pressure and herniation. The clinical picture is often indistinguishable from a cerebral infarction, but the

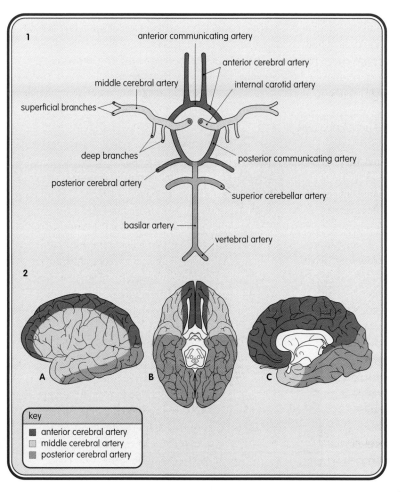

Fig. 6.6 Territories of the major arteries. (1) Main cerebral arteries forming circle of Willis. (2) Their territories: (A) Lateral view. (B) Inferior view. (C) Medial view. (Reproduced from Anderson's *Pathology*, Mosby.)

Pathological features of cerebral infarction		
Time	Macroscopic	Microscopic
before 24 h	no naked eye abnormalities	some neuronal damage
after 24 h	softening and swelling (oedema) of affected tissue	line of demarcation between normal and abnormal myelin in white matter
after a few days	necrotic tissue	infiltrating macrophages proliferating astrocytes and capillaries
after weeks/months	fluid-filled cystic cavity with gliotic wall	necrotic tissue removed thickened capillary walls only astrocytes remain

Fig. 6.7 Pathological features of cerebral infarction.

raised intracranial pressure commonly gives rise to sudden headache, vomiting and impairment of consciousness. Mortality is about 80%.

Subarachnoid haemorrhage

This can occur at any age but is an important cause of death and disability in the 20–40 year age group. The majority of subarachnoid haemorrhages are caused by saccular berry aneurysms, which develop at proximal branch points in the major cerebral vessels on the circle of Willis (Fig. 6.8).

These aneurysms occur in 1–2% of the population but are more common in the elderly; and hypertensive patients are more likely to have aneurysms than normotensive ones.

The clinical picture is one of sudden onset of severe headache accompanied by neck pain/stiffness and vomiting.

Only 30–40% survive for a few hours; among those who survive longer, there is a 30% mortality rate within the first month.

Hypertensive cerebrovascular disease

Systemic hypertension can affect the CNS resulting in neurological dysfunction, thus:

- Atheroma of the larger cerebral vessels leads to a loss of autoregulation of cerebral blood flow.
- Aneurysms, both saccular and microaneurysms, may cause spontaneous intracerebral haemorrhage.
- Encephalopathy: pathogenesis is uncertain but damage to the blood–brain barrier leads to forced cerebral hyperperfusion.

Infections of the CNS
Acute pyogenic (bacterial) meningitis

This is infection of the leptomeninges—pia and arachnoid mater—and the CSF, which diffusely affects the whole meninges and subarachnoid space. Organisms which typically cause this condition vary between age groups (Fig. 6.9).

The clinical features are headache, drowsiness, vomiting, fever and neck stiffness.

There are four possible mechanisms of meningeal infection:
- Direct spread—From penetrating trauma (e.g. compound skull fractures) or adjacent focus of infection (e.g. sinusitis, middle ear or mastoid infection).
- Blood-borne spread—From septicaemia or septic emboli from other infections such as bacterial endocarditis.
- Iatrogenic infection—Following the introduction of organisms into CSF at lumbar puncture.
- Congenital abnormalities, e.g. meningomyeloceles.

The complications are:
- Ventriculitis.
- Intracerebral abscess (see below).
- Cerebral infarction.
- Subdural empyema.
- Epilepsy.

Diagnosis and management—The CSF is cloudy due to increased numbers of neutrophils (>1000 cells/mm^3) with increased protein and decreased glucose concentrations. Treatment is with vigorous antibiotic therapy.

Prognosis—Mortality ranges from 3% for *Haemophilus influenzae* to 60% for *Streptococcus pneumoniae*, and is highest in the very young and the elderly.

Aseptic (viral) meningitis

This is the commonest cause of meningitis. It is a benign and self-limiting illness, usually less severe than bacterial meningitis. It may occur as a complication of viral infection, e.g. mumps or measles.

Common causative organisms

The common causative organisms are enteroviruses (e.g. echoviruses, coxsackieviruses and polioviruses) and mumps virus.

The illness clinically presents with acute onset of headache, irritability and rapid development of meningeal irritation.

Diagnosis and management—The CSF contains excess lymphocytes but normal glucose and protein. Treatment is symptomatic

Prognosis—Complete recovery usually occurs without specific therapy.

Brain abscess

A brain abscess is a severe focal infection of the brain and is typically 1–2 cm across. It starts as an area of cerebritis—inflammation of the brain parenchyma—and develops into a pus-filled cavity walled off by gliosis and surrounded by cerebral oedema. It often results in raised intracranial pressure.

The aetiology of brain abscesses is as follows:
- Middle ear infection (60%): temporal lobe and cerebellar abscesses.
- Frontal sinusitis (20%): frontal lobe abscess.
- Bacteraemia/septicaemia (10%): usually frontal lobe abscess.
- Penetrating skull trauma.
- Secondary to meningitis.
- Unknown causes.

Common causative organisms are *Streptococcus vividans, Staphylococcus aureus*

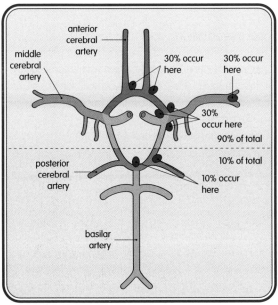

Fig. 6.8 Berry aneurysms—approximate frequency and distribution. The dotted line separates anterior from posterior circulation. (After Anderson's *Pathology*, Mosby.)

Fig. 6.9 Meningitis-causing bacteria.

Meningitis-causing bacteria			
Neonates	Infants	Young adults	Elderly
Escherichia coli group B Streptococcus Listeria monocytogenes	Neisseria meningitidis Haemophilus influenzae Streptococcus pneumoniae	N. meningitidis S. pneumoniae	S. pneumoniae N. meningitidis L. monocytogenes

and *Klebsiella*, but it may also be caused by fungal infection.

The clinical presentation is similar to that of acute bacterial meningitis but focal neurological signs, epilepsy and fever are common manifestations

Complications include:

- Meningitis.
- Intracranial herniation.
- Focal neurological deficit.
- Epilepsy.

Treatment is with antibiotic therapy at an early stage, with surgical aspiration or excision of the capsule.

Prognosis—Overall mortality is about 10%.

Subdural empyema

This is a collection of pus in the subdural space and is relatively uncommon. In adults it usually results from frontal sinusitis, whereas in infants it is usually secondary to meningitis.

Clinically, patients with subdural empyema are usually very ill. The pus spreads rapidly on the surface of a hemisphere, producing hemiparesis, raised intracranial pressure, fits and meningism.

Chronic meningoencephalitis

Tuberculous meningitis

This is meningitis due to infection by *Mycobacterium tuberculosis*. It is rare in the UK but a major problem in developing countries.

The disorder is almost always secondary to tuberculosis elsewhere in the body; infection usually reaches the CNS via the bloodstream.

Pathogenesis—Granulomatous inflammation affects the basal meninges, large arteries and cranial nerves.

It clinically presents with slow-onset, subacute meningitis. It may be accompanied by isolated cranial nerve palsies.

Hydrocephalus may result from impaired reabsorption of CSF or obstruction of CSF outflow from the fourth ventricle.

CSF shows an initial increase in polymorphs, then an increase in lymphocytes.

Prognosis—Untreated, the disease is usually fatal. Intensive treatment with antituberculous drugs lowers mortality to 15–20%.

Chronic meningitis

This is a rare condition, which usually occurs in the middle-aged and elderly. *Neisseria meningitidis* is the commonest cause. The patient can be unwell for weeks or even months with recurrent fever, sweating, joint pains and transient rash.

Neurosyphilis

This is caused by invasion of the CNS by *Treponema pallidum* weeks, months or years after initial infection. Meningitic illness occurs in only approximately 25% of cases of syphilis. It is usually mild or even asymptomatic but may be severe with transient cranial nerve palsies and convulsions.

Lyme disease

This disorder is caused by the tick-borne spirochaete *Borrelia burgdorferi*. It is a systemic illness characterized by skin lesions and neurological features.

Viral encephalitis

This is a virally induced diffuse inflammation of the brain, which is usually concomitant with inflammation of the meninges. It is a common complication of many viral illnesses. Common causative viruses are:

- Arboviruses.
- Herpes simplex virus I and II.
- Measles.
- Cytomegalovirus.
- Polio and enterovirus.
- Rabies.
- HIV.

Most cases are mild and self-limiting. However, some cases (e.g. those involving herpes simplex virus type I and rabies) result in extensive tissue destruction and may be fatal.

Mortality for the more severe type is 50%, and the majority of survivors have severe, permanent brain damage.

Fungal infections

These are relatively rare and occur mainly in the immunosuppressed (e.g. associated with chemotherapy, steroid treatment, AIDS), but some organisms, e.g. *Cryptococcus neoformans*, can produce disease in the absence of immunosuppression.

The spread can be haematogenous (e.g. from the lungs, which is the most common) or direct (e.g. from the nose and paranasal sinuses, which is rare).

Causative organisms are:
- *Cryptococcus neoformans*: fungal meningitis.
- *Aspergillus fumigatus*: fungal abscesses usually accompanied by pulmonary infection.
- *Candida albicans*: fungal abscesses.
- Phycomycosis: thrombosis and associated infarction; commonly affects uncontrolled diabetics.

Protozoal infection
Toxoplasmosis
This is caused by infection with *Toxoplasma gondii* and is acquired by eating poorly cooked infected meat or food contaminated with feline faeces. It has two forms: congenital and acquired.

The incidence of congenital toxoplasmosis shows geographical variation, e.g. 1 per 4000 births in the US; 1 per 100 births in France. The organism is transmitted to the fetus through the placenta during maternal infection.

The infection can cause:
- Abortion or stillbirth.
- Severe brain damage leading to early death.
- Moderate brain damage and chorioretinitis; compatible with life but with permanent disability.

Acquired toxoplasmosis is the commonest opportunistic infection of the CNS in adults with AIDS. It results in:
- Necrotizing cerebritis.
- Chronic abscesses.
- Meningoencephalitis.

However, in healthy subjects, it rarely causes cerebral symptoms.

Other protozoan organisms that may cause infection of the CNS are:
- Amoeba.
- *Plasmodium falciparum*.
- Trypanosomes.

Progressive multifocal leukoencephalopathy
Multifocal destruction of oligodendrocytes results in demyelination with minimal inflammation and minimal damage to axons. It is caused by DNA papovavirus, usually JC and SV40 virus, and occurs in association with underlying diseases such as AIDS, chronic lymphocytic leukaemia, carcinoma, and systemic lupus erythematosus.

Patients present with progressive dementia. The disease is progressive and death usually occurs within a few months.

Subacute sclerosing panencephalopathy
This subacute encephalitis occurring in children is due to persistent measles infection. It presents with progressive neurological dementia, and death usually occurs within two years of onset.

Spongiform encephalitis (Creutzfeldt–Jakob disease)
This is rapidly progressive dementia, ataxia, and myoclonus, and is rare in the UK (at 1 per 1 000 000 per year). The infectious agent is not precisely known but is most likely to be non-nucleic acid transmission by prion (for proteinaceous infectious agent) protein. The condition has an incubation period of up to 30 years but it is always fatal, usually within six months.

A recently described variant appears to be the human manifestation of bovine spongiform encephalopathy.

Demyelination and degeneration
Demyelinating diseases
This group of diseases has a common factor of primary damage to myelin of nerves while the axons and nerve cells remain relatively intact.

Multiple sclerosis (MS)
This is the commonest demyelinating disorder of the CNS affecting 50 per 100 000 in the UK. Peak incidence is between 20–40 years with a slight female predominance.

MS is characterized by relapsing and remitting episodes of immunologically mediated demyelination within the CNS. Recovery from each episode of demyelination is usually incomplete leading to progressive deterioration. The aetiology is unknown but current theories are:
- Myelin abnormality.
- Autoimmune disorder.
- Toxin damage.
- Viral infection of the CNS, e.g. measles.

Pathogenesis—Acute demyelination occurs in the

central white matter in discrete areas known as plaques. Abnormalities are confined to the CNS; the peripheral nervous system (PNS) is usually spared.

Common sites are the optic nerve, brainstem, cerebellum, periventricular regions and cervical spinal cord.

Fig. 6.10 gives a list of the clinical manifestations of MS and their causes.

Diagnosis and management—Clinical evaluation and CT/MRI scanning to show areas of demyelination within the brain. CSF examination shows increased lymphoid cells and oligoclonal bands of IgG. There is no specific treatment but corticosteroids may accelerate remission in relapse.

The disease's progress is variable. In about 5% of patients the disease is rapidly progressive and fatal within five years. However, others may survive for more than 20 years with only minor disability.

Degenerative disorders
Cortical
Alzheimer's disease
This is the commonest cause of dementia in Western countries. In the UK it affects 5% of people over 65 years, and 15% of people over 80 years; females > males. Also significant is the subgroup of early onset (40–60 years).

The aetiology and pathogenesis are unknown; some cases (5%) are familial but most (95%) are sporadic. Current theories are:
- Infectious agents.
- Toxins, e.g. aluminium.
- Traumatic injury.

Macroscopically, there is marked atrophy, especially of the frontal lobes; the brain is reduced in weight to 1000 g or less. There is a loss of cortical grey and white matter.

Histological hallmarks are as follows:
- Senile plaques, composed of an extracellular core of amyloid protein (10–150 nm diameter) surrounded by dystrophic neurites; occur most frequently in the hippocampus, cerebral cortex and deep grey matter.
- Neurofibrillary tangles: abnormal tangles of insoluble cytoskeletal-like proteins (paired helical filaments) that form within the neurons of the brain.
- Neuropil threads: distorted, twisted and dilated dendritic processes and axons of cerebral cortex found around amyloid plaques.

Clinically, there is failure of memory and disturbance of emotions.

Prognosis—Progressive physical decline with poor food intake and inability to walk. Death is commonly due to the development of pneumonia.

Pick's disease
Progressive dementia with the development of severe memory and speech impairment. This is a rare condition whose peak incidence is at 60 years old.

The aetiology is unknown, and the majority of cases are sporadic, with some familial cases (autosomal dominant).

The morphological changes include:
- Extreme atrophy of the cortex in areas of the frontal and temporal lobes.
- Compensatory hydrocephalus occurs as a consequence of atrophy.
- Affected areas show neuronal loss and reactive gliosis.

Fig. 6.10 Clinical manifestations of MS and their causes.

Clinical manifestations of MS and their causes	
Manifestations	**Causes**
Early clinical symptoms • blurring of vision • incoordination • abnormal sensation	optic nerve disease cerebellar peduncle disease disease of long ascending sensory tracts
Late stages • blindness, paraplegia and incontinence • ataxia • intellectual dysfunction	spinal tract involvement spinal and cerebellar involvement loss of hemispheric white matter

- Surviving neurons contain characteristic intracytoplasmic inclusions (Pick's bodies), containing filamentous material.

Prognosis—Most patients die within 2–5 years of diagnosis.

Basal ganglia
Parkinsonism
This term is used to refer to patients whose clinical presentation is one of akinetic rigidity and rest tremor. The causes of are:
- Parkinson's disease.
- Postencephalitic parkinsonism.
- Neuroleptic drugs.
- Cerebral anoxia.

Parkinson's disease
This is characterized by rest tremor, slowness of voluntary movement and rigidity. It occurs in 1 per 1000 adults but 1 per 200 over the age of 65. The aetiology is unknown.

Pathogenesis:
- The disorder shows degeneration of pigmented dopaminergic neurons of the substantia nigra, the locus caeruleus and several other brainstem nuclei.
- Degeneration of these cells causes disease by reducing the amount of dopamine in the corpus striatum.
- Surviving cells in the substantia nigra contain eosinophilic spherical inclusions (Lewy bodies), which contain cytoskeletal filaments.

The disease can be symptomatically treated with drugs, such as L-dopa, that correct neurotransmitter imbalance. Eventually there is failure of response to treatment, and patients die from wasting and poor nutritional intake.

Huntington's disease
This inherited autosomal dominant disorder is characterized by chorea and progressive dementia. It has a delayed onset of usually between 30–50 years with a prevalence in the UK of 1 per 20 000.

Disease is caused by a trinucleotide repeat sequence in a gene located on chromosome 4. The greater the number of repeats, the earlier the onset and the more severe the disease. Function of the protein encoded by the gene is unknown.

Morphological features are:
- Cerebral atrophy: most marked in the caudate nucleus and adjacent putamen.
- Neuronal loss accompanied by reactive fibrillary gliosis.
- Atrophy accompanied by compensatory hydrocephalus with enlargement of lateral ventricles.

Affected individuals develop choreiform movements, jerking and progressively severe dementia, and die as a result of severe mental and physical incapacity.

The average duration of the disease, from the onset of symptoms to death, is about 15 years.

Spinocerebellar degenerative diseases
This is a group of familial diseases in which there is loss of cerebellar cortical neurons together with degeneration of spinal cord tracts.

Friedreich's ataxia
This is the most common form of spinocerebellar degeneration. It is an autosomal recessive condition resulting in degeneration of posterior columns, corticospinal and spinocerebellar tracts in the spinal cord. It usually presents in childhood with progressive ataxia of gait and limbs.

Cardiomyopathy is present in 65% of patients and death (from cardiac failure) usually occurs during the fourth decade.

Motor neuron disease
A progressive neurodegenerative disease characterized by the selective loss of motor neurons from the spinal cord, brain stem and motor cortex. Its prevalence is 5 per 100 000 of the population, with male incidence greater than female.

The majority of cases are sporadic but 5% of cases are familial—mutation of superoxide dismutase gene.

It eventually progresses to severe paralysis with loss of swallowing and respiration leading to death in 2–3 years.

(In the US, motor neuron disease is known as Lou Gehrig's disease.)

Metabolic disorders and toxins
Vitamin deficiencies
Vitamin B$_1$ (thiamine) deficiency
This is common in chronic alcoholics, resulting in:
- Wernicke's encephalopathy: memory impairment,

ataxia, visual disturbances and peripheral neuropathy.
- Korsakoff's psychosis: confused state, memory loss and confabulation.

If both occur, it is known as Wernicke–Korsakoff syndrome.

Vitamin B$_{12}$ (cyanocobalamin) deficiency
This produces weakness and paraesthesia in the lower limbs due to subacute combined degeneration of the spinal cord (Fig. 6.11). Replacement therapy at an early stage reverses the degenerative process but long-

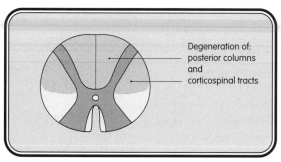

Degeneration of:
posterior columns and
corticospinal tracts

Fig. 6.11 Subacute combined degeneration of the spinal cord. Degeneration of posterior columns leads to sensory loss (vibration and proprioception) causing ataxia. Degeneration of corticospinal tracts leads to upper motor neuron damage causing spastic paralysis.

standing cases show irreversible axonal damage with reactive gliosis.

Iodine deficiency
Severe iodine deficiency causes hypothyroidism; it is the most important endocrine disorder to affect the CNS in children. In the fetus, severe iodine deficiency causes cretinism characterized by dwarfism, mental defect and spastic diplegia. This can be prevented by iodine supplements during pregnancy.

Toxins
Carbon monoxide
Carbon monoxide (CO) binds irreversibly to haemoglobin, rendering erythrocytes incapable of oxygen transport. CO poisoning therefore results in brain damage due to hypoxia. This poisoning may be accidental or associated with attempted suicide.

The amount of HbCO with corresponding clinical symptoms are as follows:
- >20%—Dyspnoea and slight headache.
- 30%—Severe headache, fatigue, and impaired judgement.
- 60–70%—Loss of consciousness.
- >70%—Rapidly fatal.

Pathogenesis—Hypoxia results in neuronal necrosis with a predilection for globus pallidus. Other selectively vulnerable regions are the hippocampus, and cerebral and cerebellar cortices.

Consequences of excess ethanol intake on the central nervous system		
Disease	**Features**	**Mechanism**
fetal alcohol syndrome	cerebral malformations facial and somatic malformations growth retardation	direct toxicity
acute intoxication	cerebral oedema petechial haemorrhages	direct toxicity
cerebral and cerebellar atrophy	neuronal loss	direct toxicity
nutritional disorders	Wernicke's encephalophathy	deficiency of vitamin B$_1$
hepatocerebral syndromes	hepatic encephalopathy chronic hepatocerebral degeneration	hepatic toxicity with secondary effects on CNS
demyelinating disorders	central pontine myelinolysis	electrolyte disturbances

Fig. 6.12 Consequences of excess ethanol intake on the CNS. (Adapted with permission from *General and Systematic Pathology*, 2nd edn, by J.C.E. Underwood, Churchill Livingstone, 1996.)

Methanol

Methanol is highly toxic to the CNS. It is lipid soluble, so therefore readily diffuses into the CSF and aqueous humour in concentrations higher than in plasma.

Methanol is metabolized into formic acid and formaldehyde. It is the formaldehyde that is thought to be the mediator of toxic effects. There are two types of methanol poisoning:
- Acute: sudden death with multiple haemorrhagic lesions in the cerebral hemispheres.
- Chronic: atrophy of retinal ganglion cells with secondary degeneration of the optic nerve.

Ethanol

The consequences of excessive ethanol intake on the CNS are manifold (Fig. 6.12).

Neoplasms of the CNS
Gliomas

Gliomas are tumours that arise from glial supportive tissue of brain. They are the most common primary brain tumours, accounting for 50% of all CNS tumours.

Astrocytoma

This is a glioma derived from astrocytes, and is more common in children, usually occurring in the cerebellum. It accounts for 10% of all primary tumours in adults, usually in the cerebral hemispheres.

Common types of astrocytomas (grade):
- Benign juvenile pilocytic astrocytoma (grade I).
- Astrocytoma (grade I/II).
- Anaplastic astrocytoma (grade III).
- Glioblastoma multiforme (grade IV).

Prognosis depends on the degree of tumour differentiation and the size of the neoplasm:
- Grade I: survival times of 20–30 years are possible.
- Grade IV: 20% survive for 1 year.

Oligodendrogliomas

These ill-defined, slow-growing tumours arise from oligodendrocytes in the white matter of the cerebral hemispheres, especially the temporal lobe. They account for 5% of all primary CNS neoplasms in adults but are rare in children.

The prognosis is relatively good.

Ependymoma

This arises from the ependymal cells lining the ventricle and central canal of the spinal cord. It is the most common tumour of the spinal cord, accounting for 5% of all primary CNS neoplasms. It is common in children and young adults.

The majority are benign ependymomas, of which there are three types:
- Myxopapillary ependymoma: common in the spinal cord.
- Papillary ependymoma: rare; located in the cerebellopontine angle.
- Subependymoma: located in the fourth ventricle, extending into the cisterna magna.

Neuronal tumours

Rare tumours of relatively low malignancy, these occur most commonly in children. There are three types:
- Central neurocytoma: neoplasms of small mature neurons occurring within the ventricles.
- Ganglioneuroma: a tumour of differentiating neuronal cells.
- Ganglioma: a mixture of neoplastic neuronal and glial cells (usually astrocytes).

Medulloblastoma

This tumour of primitive neuroepithelial cells arises in the cerebellum in children, in whom it is the commonest CNS tumour. It is malignant, with a rapid growth rate; obstruction of the fourth ventricle results in hydrocephalus.

Other tumours
Primary brain lymphomas

Associated with immunosuppression, especially AIDS, most are high grade, non-Hodgkin's lymphomas of B cell type with a poor prognosis.

Germ cell tumours

These rare tumours are seen mainly in children; males > females. Most arise near the pineal gland and behave as malignant teratomas.

Meningiomas

These account for approximately 15% of adult intracranial tumours; females > males. Tumours arise from the arachnoid mater and are usually benign but may invade adjacent bone resulting in erosion and hyperosteosis. Meningiomas produce symptoms by compression of brain tissue rather than by invasion.

Metastatic tumours

The CNS is a common site for metastasis and tumours are usually multiple. They may arise from haematogenous or direct spread. The cerebellum is the preferred site but they can affect any part of the brain as well as other intracranial structures, especially meninges (hence malignant meningitis).

The commonest neoplasms to metastasize to the CNS are:

- Breast carcinomas.
- Bronchus carcinomas.
- Kidney carcinomas.
- Colon carcinomas.
- Malignant melanoma.

DISORDERS OF THE PERIPHERAL NERVOUS SYSTEM

Disorders of peripheral nerves are termed neuropathies and can be predominantly sensory, predominantly motor or mixed depending on which nerves are affected.

- Describe the common pathological features of the CNS.
- What are the congenital malformations and developmental diseases of the CNS?
- Give examples of types of traumatic injury that affect the CNS.
- What is the pathogenesis of cerebrovascular disease?
- Name the infections of the CNS.
- Give examples of diseases of demyelination and diseases of degeneration.
- Name the vitamin deficiencies and toxins that damage the CNS.
- Name the neoplasms of the CNS.

Hereditary neuropathies
Hereditary motor and sensory neuropathies (HMSN)
Peroneal muscular atrophy, HMSN I + II (Charcot–Marie–Tooth disease)

This disorder is characterized by pronounced atrophy of calf muscles with associated sensory deficits as a result of slowly progressive symmetric neuropathy. It is the commonest of the hereditary neuropathies, and is usually autosomal dominant. It impedes ambulation and causes foot deformities (pes cavus) but does not shorten the lifespan.

Fig. 6.13 provides a table of the different types of peroneal muscular atrophy and their characteristics.

Dejerine–Sottas disease (HMSN III)

This severe, chronically progressive symmetric peripheral neuropathy is caused by hypertrophy of peripheral nerves followed by gradual axon degeneration. There is delayed onset of motor skills (e.g. in walking) and gradual progression to wheelchair confinement in young adult life.

Hereditary sensory and autonomic neuropathies (HSAN)

This group of autosomal inherited diseases produce mainly sensory and autonomic neuropathies. There are three major types as described in Fig. 6.14.

Note that:
- Disorders affecting many peripheral nerves are termed polyneuropathies, and usually cause symmetrical deficits.
- Disorders affecting only one (mononeuropathy) or a few (multiple mononeuropathies) peripheral nerves typically cause asymmetrical deficits.
- Radiculopathies are disorders of nerve roots.

Fig. 6.13 Different types of peroneal muscular atrophy and their characteristics.

Different types of peroneal muscular atrophy and their characteristics		
	HMSN I	HMSN II
type of neuropathy	demyelinating neuropathy	axonal neuropathy
relative occurrence	75%	25%
type of axonal loss	large calibre axons	large and small calibre axons
nerve conduction velocity	impaired (<30 m/s)	normal (>45 m/s)
time of onset	early (first decade)	later (second decade)
effects	severe distal wasting in legs	weakness and wasting less marked

Types of hereditary sensory and autonomic neuropathies (HSANs)			
	HSAN I	HSAN II	HSAN III
clinical syndrome	ulcerative acropathy due to numbness	congenital sensory neuropathy	familial dysautonomia
eponym	Morvan's	Giacci's	Riley–Day
inheritance	autosomal dominant	autosomal recessive	autosomal recessive
affected neurons	degeneration of large myelinated fibres of both peripheral nerves and posterior columns of spinal cord	degeneration of large and small myelinated fibres	degeneration of non-myelinated fibres with preservation of myelinated fibres loss of neurons of autonomic ganglia

Fig. 6.14 Types of hereditary sensory and autonomic neuropathies.

Traumatic neuropathies

Lacerations

Laceration refers to a jagged tear of the peripheral nerve in which there is partial or complete loss of continuity of the nerve. It occurs most commonly from a penetrating injury such as a knife wound, or a misplaced intramuscular injection, or from bone fractures.

Avulsion

This is the tearing of nerve fibres from the surface of the spinal cord or from a muscle. It may be partial or complete depending on whether all or only some of the rootlets contributing to the spinal nerve are involved.

Nerve roots may be avulsed from the spinal cord in two ways:

- Tensile stresses from cervical plexus transmitted centrally can stretch and finally avulse the nerve roots.
- A spinal cord injury such that displacement of the

cord acts directly on the nerve roots between their attachment to the cord and their entry into the intravertebral foramen.

Both laceration and avulsion injuries cause the severed ends of the damaged nerve to retract and then to undergo Wallerian degeneration forming a traumatic neuroma. Subsequently, the proximal portion of the nerve develops neuritic sprouts which, if sited in proximity to the severed distal nerve, may reinnervate by regrowth along the nerve sheath.

If continuity of the nerve is completely interrupted, basal laminae sheaths no longer form continuous tubes to guide regeneration sprouts and so the potential for recovery is limited.

Compression/entrapment neuropathy

Compressed nerves undergo segmental demyelination with decreased nerve conduction velocity. If compression

Common sites of nerve compression are:
- **Nerve roots in the intervertebral foramina by prolapsed intervertebral discs or osteophytes due to osteoarthritis of the spine.**
- **Median nerve in carpal tunnel at the wrist.**
- **Ulnar nerve in flexor carpal tunnel at medial epicondyle of humerus.**
- **Common peroneal nerve at the neck of the fibula.**

is prolonged or severe, axonal degeneration may occur. Symptoms of nerve compression are paraesthesia, anaesthesia and loss of muscle strength.

Carpal tunnel syndrome

This is a disorder in which the size of the carpal tunnel is significantly reduced causing compression of the median nerve. Causes include inflammation of the flexor retinaculum, arthritic changes, etc.

Saturday night palsy

Radial nerve compression (in the middle of the arm), which may result from improper positioning of the upper limb during sleeping, especially in intoxicated persons.

Inflammatory neuropathies

Guillain–Barré syndrome (acute inflammatory demyelinating polyradiculopathy)

This is the commonest form of acute neuropathy caused by immune-mediated demyelination of peripheral nerves, usually occurring 2–4 weeks after viral illness.

Affected patients develop motor neuropathy with lesser sensory changes due to widespread demyelination of the peripheral nerves. Recovery (i.e. remyelination) occurs over 3–4 months and is usually complete.

Infectious neuropathies

Leprosy (Hansen's disease)

A chronic granulomatous disease caused by *Mycobacterium leprae*. It is the commonest cause of peripheral neuritis worldwide, affecting about 10 million patients in total.

The clinicopathological features of leprosy are dependent on the host's response to infection, with a spectrum of disease ranging from tuberculoid to lepromatous form (Fig. 6.15).

Comparison of peripheral nerve damage by lepromatous and tuberculoid forms of leprosy		
	Lepromatous	**Tuberculoid**
immune mechanism	minimal immune response (occurs in patients with low cellular immunity)	vigorous T cell mediated (delayed) hypersensitivity
spread of organisms	bacteraemia occurs in peripheral sites	bacteraemia rare
distribution in nerves	widely disseminated diffuse nerve involvement	one or a few sites (asymmetrical)
nerve enlargement and damage	intense infiltration of nerves by vacuolated macrophages	hallmark of nerve involvement is discrete, well-formed granulomas
neurological deficit	sensory and motor involvement patchy loss of sensation	sensory, motor and autonomic involvement peripheral nerve palsies anaesthetic areas prone to injury and secondary infection
prognosis	progressive and lethal	progression slow, but immune response produces extensive destruction of tissue resulting in severe disfigurement eventually heals spontaneously

Fig. 6.15 Comparison of peripheral nerve damage by lepromatous and tuberculoid forms of leprosy.

Varicella-zoster virus (VZV)

An invasion of cutaneous sensory nerves during primary infection with VZV (chicken pox) leads to infection of the dorsal root ganglia where the virus enters a latent state. Reactivation of VZV may occur years later causing shingles. The reason for reactivation is unknown but there is increased incidence in the immunocompromised.

In shingles, VZV migrates down the nerves into the skin and causes vesicular lesions identical to those of chickenpox but confined to one or two adjacent dermatomes usually on the trunk.

Metabolic and toxic neuropathies
Peripheral neuropathy of diabetes mellitus

This occurs in both type I and II diabetes mellitus with a prevalence of 10–60% clinically, but up to 100% when evaluated by nerve conduction studies. There is increased prevalence with increased duration of the disease.

Pathogenesis

Vascular occlusion of the blood vessels supplying the nerves results in neuronal atrophy.

There are four types:
- Symmetrical and predominantly sensory polyneuropathy.
- Autonomic neuropathy.
- Proximal painful motor neuropathy.
- Cranial mononeuritis (mainly CN III, IV and VI).

Metabolic and nutritional causes

Uraemic neuropathy in renal failure

Approximately 60% of patients with chronic renal failure have symptoms of uraemic neuropathy at onset of dialysis. It is expressed as pain and paraesthaesia with the lower extremities preferentially involved. Dialysis usually improves symptoms.

Thyroid dysfunction

Mild chronic sensorimotor neuropathy is sometimes seen in both hypothyroidism (more commonly) and hyperthyroidism.

Vitamin deficiencies

Vitamin deficiencies are important causes of peripheral neuropathies. Especially important are deficiencies of vitamins B_1 (thiamine), B_{12}, B_6 (pyridoxine), and E.

Toxic neuropathies

Many toxins cause damage to peripheral nerves. The most common toxins are:
- Drugs: isoniazides, sulphonamides, vinca alkaloids, dapsone and chloroquine.
- Alcohol: in cases of chronic abuse.
- Industrial toxins: acrylamide, hexane, organophosphates, lead, arsenic, mercury.

Most toxins produce a 'dying back' pattern of axonal damage resulting in a distal symmetric pattern of sensorimotor involvement. There is a 'stocking glove' distribution at onset but continued exposure to the toxin extends the deficit to the lower calves and forearms.

Neuropathies associated with malignancy (metastatic neuropathy)

Cancer patients frequently have neurological symptoms caused by direct infiltration of individual nerves or plexuses.

Neoplasms of peripheral nerves
Schwannoma

This benign neoplasm is derived from Schwann cells of the nerve sheaths. It is the most common tumour of the peripheral nerves; it is more common in adults, and females > males.

It arises from the intracranial roots, spinal nerves and peripheral nerves with a predilection for the sensory nerves. The commonest site within the cranium (80–90% of all schwannomas) is the vestibular branch of CN VIII in the region of cerebellopontine angle—acoustic neuroma.

Nerve compression may occur particularly intracranially or in spinal nerve foramina.

Macroscopically, tumours are firm and encapsulated. Microscopically, there are two types: Antoni type A and Antoni type B.

Antoni type A is a densely packed spindle cell tumour, has long oval nuclei, and has palisading of cells.

Antoni type B has loosely packed spongy tumours, small round nuclei, and is sparsely cellular.

Schwannoma tumours are usually a mixture of these two types and contain prominent, thick-walled blood vessels. Most can be removed as benign tumours without damaging the underlying axon.

Neurofibroma

A neoplasm derived from neural crest cells of the epi- and endoneurium, this arises from small nerves, deep major nerves and nerves of retroperitoneal tissues and GI tracts. Cranial and spinal nerves are rarely affected.

The macroscopic appearance is as follows:

- Nodular lesions: discrete tumours forming a defined mass either within the skin (dermal neurofibroma) or along the nerve trunk.
- Plexiform lesions: diffuse, spindle-shaped expansions of the nerve, which affect the nerve over a wide area.

Microscopically, tumour cells have attenuated cytoplasmic processes and spindle-shaped nuclei set in a wavy arrangement of collagen bundles.

Neurofibroma can arise spontaneously but the occurrence is enhanced by neurofibromatosis type 1. The nerve fibres are intimately intermingled with the tumour mass, therefore the tumour cannot be removed without sacrificing the nerve. Malignant changes may occur.

Malignant peripheral nerve sheath tumour (MPNST)

This is rare and about 50% of cases are associated with neurofibromatosis type 1 where they originate in a pre-existing neurofibroma. It arises from the peripheral mixed motor and sensory nerves; cranial nerve involvement is rare.

Malignant transformation is usually heralded by rapid enlargement and pain. Neoplasms behave as sarcomas and are frequently fatal.

Neurocutaneous syndromes

Neurofibromatosis type I (von Recklinghausen's disease)

An autosomal dominant disorder affecting 1 in 3000. Expression of the disease is variable but commonly causes formation of multiple benign but disfiguring tumours of the skin and nerves—neurofibromas.

It is associated with hamartomas of the iris, pigmented skin lesions (*café-au-lait* spots) and with many other neoplasms. There is an increased risk of development of MPNST.

Neurofibromatosis type II (bilateral acoustic neurofibromatosis)

An autosomal dominant disorder affecting 1 in 100 000. Clinical features are development of bilateral

Schwannomas on CN VIII as well as a propensity to develop other neoplasms, especially meningiomas and gliomas.

Patients present with tinnitus, deafness or signs of an intracranial mass compressing the lower cranial nerves and brainstem.

Tuberous sclerosis

An autosomal dominant disease causing epilepsy and mental retardation, affecting 1 in 100 000. The brain shows characteristic tubers—firm, white nodules approximately 1–3 cm in size at the crest of gyri. Caused by hamartomatous overgrowth of neurons and astrocytes, it is also associated with retinal hamartomas and skin lesions (angiofibromas).

Von Hippel–Lindau disease

This is an autosomal dominant disease, characterized by:

- Multiple haemangiomas of the retina and brain.
- Benign neoplasms (haemangioblastoma) of the cerebellum.
- Cysts in the kidney and pancreas.
- Increased incidence of renal adenocarcinoma and phaeochromocytoma.
- Polycythaemia: haemangioblastoma is associated with erythropoietin production.

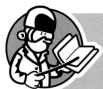

- **Name the different types of hereditary neuropathies.**
- **What are the causes and outcomes of traumatic neuropathies?**
- **Outline the pathololgy of Guillain–Barré syndrome (inflammatory neuropathy).**
- **Name infections that can cause neuropathies.**
- **Give types of metabolic and toxic neuropathies.**
- **Name the neoplasms of the peripheral nerves.**

DISORDERS OF THE AUTONOMIC NERVOUS SYSTEM

Disorders of the sympathetic nervous system

Horner's syndrome

An uncommon condition caused by loss of sympathetic innervation to the eye. It is characterized by:

- Pupillary constriction (miosis) due to unopposed action of the pupillary constrictor.
- Partial ptosis (drooping) of the upper eyelid due to paralysis of smooth muscle fibres contained in the levator muscle of the upper eyelid.
- Enophthalmos (eye sunken into socket).
- Loss of sweating on affected side of the face.

Lesions affecting any part of the sympathetic pathway (Fig. 6.16) may produce Horner's syndrome:

- Brainstem—Tumours, vascular lesions or syringobulbia.
- Cervical cord—Tumours or syringomyelia.
- Cervical sympathetic chain—Pancoast tumours (apical tumours of the lung) frequently invade adjacent sites; invasion of the superior cervical sympathetic ganglion often results in Horner's syndrome.

Trauma/surgical section of the sympathetic trunk

Surgical sympathectomies are sometimes performed for the relief of such conditions as:

- Raynaud's phenomenon: pallor, pain and numbness of the fingers caused by vasospastic constriction of the digital arteries; sympathectomy is performed to improve limb perfusion.
- Causalgia: severe burning pain that occurs following injury to the major peripheral nerves of the limbs (e.g. median, ulnar, sciatic) due to disturbances of sympathetic reflexes.

The consequences of both traumatic or surgical section of the sympathetic chain depend on the level of the section, but may cause:

- Loss of blood pressure control → syncope (fainting).
- Impairment of sweating → hyperpyrexia.
- Impairment of bladder and bowel functions.
- Interruption of pathway to erectile tissue → impotence.

Phaeochromocytoma

This is a rare tumour arising from chromaffin cells of the adrenal medulla, occurring in 1 in 1000 cases of hypertension. The majority are sporadic but about 10% are familial. Most are benign but about 5% are malignant.

Effects are those of hypersecretion of catecholamines, i.e. hypertension, hypermetabolism, and hyperglycaemia. There is also pallor, headaches, sweating, and nervousness.

It may be associated with other endocrine neoplasias, namely:

- Multiple endocrine neoplasia syndrome (especially medullary carcinoma of the thyroid).
- Von Recklinghausen's disease.
- Von Hippel–Lindau syndrome.

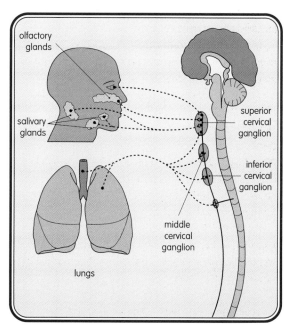

Fig. 6.16 Sympathetic innervation to the eye and face showing the relationship of the sympathetic trunk to the apex of the lungs.

It is diagnosed by increased amounts of urinary excretion of catecholamine metabolite vanillylmandelic acid (VMA).

Surgical removal of the tumour relieves hypertension and other effects.

Diseases of the parasympathetic nervous system
Effects of ablation of parasympathetic innervation

The commonest site of parasympathetic ablation is the vagus nerve (vagotomy) for treatment of duodenal ulcers. This is less common now due to the awareness of bacterial aetiology (*Helicobacter pylori*) of intestinal ulcers.

Beneficial effects
Of benefit is the reduction of acid and pepsin secretion by abolishing direct vagal drive (and to a minor degree by reducing antral gastrin secretion).

Harmful effects
Impairment of antral motility is caused by abolishing receptive relaxation in the gastric corpus, and reducing the power of antral contractions.

The harmful effects of truncal vagotomy can now be largely overcome by performing a selective vagotomy instead, but this is less effective and has a higher incidence of ulcer recurrence.

- **Truncal vagotomy means a section of the trunk of the vagus nerve.**
- **Selective vagotomy means a vagotomy where only those vagal fibres that pass to the body of the stomach are divided, while those supplying the antrum, pylorus and other abdominal viscera are spared.**

- **What are the characteristics and causes of Horner's syndrome?**
- **Give indications for performing sympathectomies and describe their effects.**
- **Describe the pathology of phaeochromocytomas.**
- **What are the effects of vagotomies?**

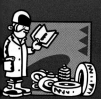

7. Pathology of the Cardiovascular System

CONGENITAL ABNORMALITIES OF THE HEART

Overview

Congenital heart abnormalities are relatively common, affecting about 8 per 1000 live births.

Causes

Sporadic

These are the majority of cases and no teratogenic factors can be identified.

Maternal factors

There is an increased incidence associated with certain maternal factors including:

- Maternal rubella infections.
- Chronic alcohol abuse.
- Intrauterine radiation.
- Drugs.

Genetic or chromosomal abnormalities

These are associated with an increased incidence of congenital heart malformations. An example of this is Down syndrome.

Clinical features

Most cardiac abnormalities become apparent at or shortly after birth usually by some manifestation of heart failure such as cyanosis, breathlessness, feeding difficulties, or a failure to thrive.

Types

Congenital heart defects may be divided into two main groups depending on whether the lesions cause:

- Abnormal shunting of blood between the two sides of the heart, either left-to-right shunts which are more common because of higher pressure in the left side of the heart; or right-to-left shunts caused by an increased resistance to blood moving on from the right side of the heart.
- Obstruction to blood flow.

Left-to-right shunts

These are malformations that result in the shunting of blood from the left side of the heart to the right; they are the most common group of congenital heart abnormalities. Shunting is from left to right because of the higher pressures in the left side of the heart. These defects are not associated with clinical cyanosis as the blood does not bypass the lungs.

Fig. 7.1 lists the prevalence of left-to-right shunts.

Ventricular septal defect

This defect of the interventricular septum is the commonest cardiac abnormality, accounting for approximately 25–30% of all cases of congenital heart disease (Fig. 7.2). The interventricular septum can be divided into a membranous (fibrous) portion and a muscular portion.

Most congenital defects are perimembranous, i.e. occurring at the junction of the membranous and muscular portions.

There are small and large defects:

- Small defects: often confined to the tiny membranous area.
- Larger defects: also involve the muscular wall of the septum.

The size and site of the defect determine the extent of shunting of blood from left to right. Defects may present as cardiac failure in infants, or as a murmur in older children or adults.

Physical signs include:

Prevalence of left-to-right shunts	
Type	**% of all CHD abnormalities**
ventricular septal defect	25–30
atrial septal defect	10–15
patent ductus arteriosus	10
atrioventricular septal defect	5

Fig. 7.1 Prevalence of left-to-right shunts. CHD = Congenital heart disease.

- Pansystolic murmur: caused by flow from the high-pressure left ventricle to the low-pressure right ventricle during systole.
- Tachypnoea.
- Indrawing of the lower ribs on inspiration.

Management—Small defects need no treatment and often close spontaneously. Larger defects are associated with persistent cardiac failure, and so need surgical repair.

Atrial septal defect

This is a common congenital heart defect, affecting females more than males by 2:1. There is a defect of the interatrial septum causing chronic shunting to the right with gradual enlargement of the right side of the heart and of the pulmonary arteries (Fig. 7.3). The lesion is usually located at the level of the fossa ovalis which is incompletely closed (ostium secundum defect).

Clinical features—Most children are free of symptoms for many years and the condition is often detected at routine clinical examination or following a chest radiograph. Some children present with dyspnoea, chest infections, cardiac failure or arrhythmia (e.g. atrial fibrillation).

The characteristic physical signs are the result of the

volume overload of the right ventricle, as follows:
- Systolic flow murmur over the pulmonary valve.
- Wide splitting of the second heart sound: caused by the delayed closure of the pulmonary valve, which is a result of the increased stroke volume and right bundle branch block.
- Diastolic rumbling murmur due to the increased flow across the tricuspid valve.

Atrial septal defects should be closed surgically. Untreated, right ventricular hypertrophy and pulmonary hypertension inevitably develop, and shunt reversal may eventually occur.

Long-term prognosis following surgical intervention is excellent unless pulmonary hypertension has developed. Pulmonary hypertension and shunt reversal are contraindications to surgery.

Patent ductus arteriosus

This is persistence of an embryological connection between the aorta and the pulmonary trunk (or left main pulmonary artery), as shown in Fig. 7.4. Patent (open) ductus arteriosus occurs in about 10% of all cases of congenital heart disease, affecting females more than males. There is a recognized association with maternal rubella.

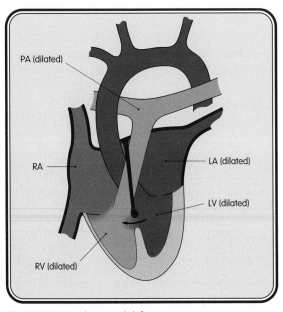

Fig. 7.2 Ventricular septal defect.

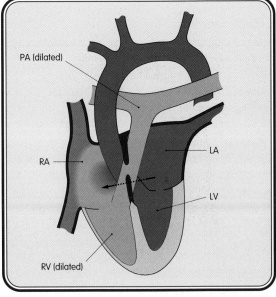

Fig. 7.3 Atrial septal defect.

> Understanding the embryonic development of the heart will enable you to get to grips with the congenital abnormalities that occur.

Embryology

In intrauterine life, the duct allows oxygenated placental blood to flow from the pulmonary artery to the aorta, thereby bypassing the lungs.

At birth, the pulmonary vascular resistance declines, blood is diverted to the lungs for oxygenation and the ductus arteriosus closes within the first few days of life.

However, if the ductus remains patent, blood is continually shunted from the aorta to the pulmonary artery, and as much as 50% of the left ventricular output may be recirculated through the lungs, with a consequent increase in the work of the heart.

Clinical features—The symptoms are proportional to the size of the left-to-right shunt. Small shunts are asymptomatic, whereas larger shunts produce retarded growth and development, with eventual cardiac failure. A continuous 'machinery' murmur can be heard, which is loudest at the time of the second heart sound.

A patent ductus usually requires surgical treatment in childhood.

Atrioventricular septal defect

This is a septal defect with both an atrial and a ventricular component caused by failure of the endocardial cushions to fuse together. An atrioventricular canal persists resulting in a single heart chamber partially separated by abnormal valve leaflets.

Right-to-left shunts

Defects leading to permanent right-to-left shunts are less common (than those the other way round), and result in the blood bypassing the lungs to enter the systemic circulation with the development of cyanosis.

Tetralogy of Fallot

This is the commonest cause of cyanosis in infancy (<1 year), occurring in about 1 in 2000 live births. The abnormality consists of four (hence 'tetra-') defects (Fig. 7.5):

- Ventricular septal defect.
- Overriding aorta, which sits astride the ventricular septal defect so that it receives blood from both right and left ventricles.

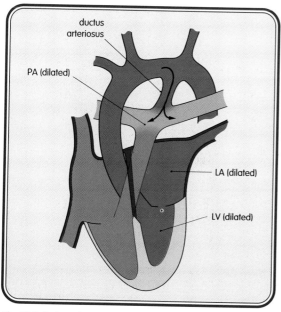

Fig. 7.4 Patent ductus arteriosus.

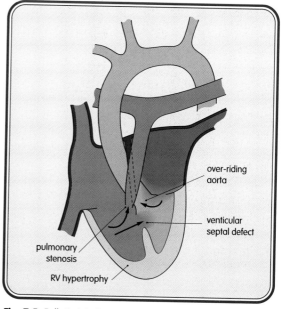

Fig. 7.5 Fallot's tetralogy.

- Pulmonary stenosis, usually due to thickening of the subvalvar muscle in the pulmonary outflow tract but sometimes associated with fused stenotic valve cusps.
- Right ventricular hypertrophy.

Aetiopathogenesis—Defects are caused by the abnormal embryological development of the bulbar septum which normally separates the ascending aorta from the pulmonary artery and which aligns and fuses with the interventricular septum.

Pulmonary stenosis leads to inadequate perfusion of the lungs, and the overriding aorta receives blood from both the right and left ventricles. The net result is that the systemic circulation contains deoxygenated blood, causing cyanosis in affected individuals.

Clinical features are:

- Cyanosis, especially after feeding or a crying attack. In older children cyanosis causes stunting of growth, digital clubbing, and polycythaemia. Some children characteristically obtain relief by squatting after exertion.
- Loud ejection systolic murmur: either from ventricular septal defect or pulmonary stenosis.

Before the advent of surgical treatment most patients died well before adult life. Most cases are now surgically corrected by closing the ventricular septal defect, rechannelling the flow into the aorta from the left ventricle only, and relieving the pulmonary stenosis. Complications include bacterial endocarditis, and consequent cerebral infarction or brain abscess.

Transposition of the great arteries

This is a complex malformation in which connections between the right and left ventricle, aorta and pulmonary artery are disordered, the aorta emanating from the right ventricle, and the pulmonary artery from the left (Fig. 7.6).

Postnatal survival is possible only if there is one or more of the following:

- Atrial septal defect.
- Ventricular septal defect.
- Patent ductus arteriosus.

Surgical correction is possible.

Persistent truncus arteriosus

Both the aorta and pulmonary artery develop from a single tube, the truncus arteriosus. Persistence of the truncus is caused by failure of the conotruncal ridges to fuse and to descend towards the ventricles. The result is that the pulmonary artery arises some distance above the origin of the undivided truncus.

Persistent truncus is always accompanied by a defective interventricular septum since the ridges also participate in the formation of the interventricular septum. The undivided truncus therefore overrides both ventricles and receives blood from both sides.

Tricuspid atresia

This rare disorder is caused by an absent tricuspid orifice. The defect is always associated with:

- Patent foramen ovale.
- Ventricular septal defect.
- Underdevelopment of the right ventricle.
- Hypertrophy of the left ventricle.

Blood is shunted first from the right atrium to the left, and then a small proportion is shunted from the left ventricle to the right through ventricular septal defect. Some of the

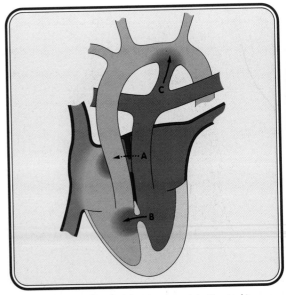

Fig. 7.6 Transposition of the great vessels. Survival is possible only if other shunts are present at either the atrial (A), ventricular (B) or ductus (C) level.

deoxygenated blood enters the systemic circulation resulting in cyanosis.

Surgical correction may be possible.

Total anomalous pulmonary venous connection

Here, pulmonary veins do not open into the left atrium but into either the right atrium, systemic veins or both. There is always an atrial septal defect resulting in right-to-left shunting with mixing of saturated and desaturated blood in the atria.

The increased pulmonary flow leads to pulmonary vascular disease.

Obstructive congenital defects

Coarctation of the aorta

This is a stenotic narrowing of the aorta, usually located at, or just beyond, the site of the ductus arteriosus (Fig. 7.7). About 50% of affected individuals have an associated bicuspid aortic valve.

This defect accounts for up to 5% of all forms of congenital heart disease, and affects 1 in 4000 live births, male incidence being greater than female by 2:1.

Clinical features—Stricture produces:

- Hypertension proximal to the stenosis, leading to symptoms such as headache and dizziness.

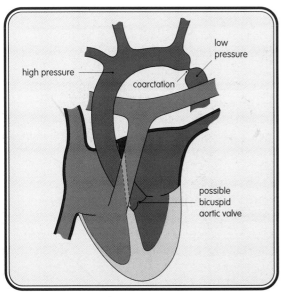

Fig. 7.7 Coarctation of the aorta.

- Hypotension distal to the stenosis, leading to generalized weakness and poor peripheral circulation.

Characteristically, the blood pressure is raised in the upper body but is normal or low in the legs:

- Upper body: abnormally large arterial pulsations may be seen in the neck, and severe hypertension leads to the development of collateral circulations involving pericapsular and intercostal arteries, which become dilated and tortuous, and may be visible or even palpable in older children and adults.
- Lower body: femoral pulses are weak and delayed.

A systolic murmur may sometimes be heard posteriorly over the coarctation. An ejection systolic murmur may be present in the aortic area due to the bicuspid valve.

Pathological complications—In untreated severe cases death may occur in several ways:

- Left ventricular failure, following prolonged hypertension.
- Dissection of the aorta, particularly in patients with associated bicuspid aortic valves.
- Bacterial endocarditis, usually at the site of aortic constriction.
- Cerebral haemorrhage.

A rare variant is the so-called 'infantile preductal coarctation', in which there is stenosis of a long segment of the aorta between the left subclavian artery origin and the ductus arteriosus, which remains patent. Systemic circulation to the lower part of the body often depends on a right-to-left shunt through the patent ductus causing peripheral cyanosis.

Pulmonary artery stenosis or atresia with intact ventricular septum

This presents as a narrowing (stenosis) or fusion (atresia) of the trunk of the pulmonary artery. In atretic cases, the patent foramen ovale forms the only outlet for blood from the right side of the heart. The ductus arteriosus is always patent and represents the only access route to the pulmonary circulation.

Aortic stenosis and atresia
Semilunar aortic valves are stenosed or even atretic. If fusion is complete, the aorta, left ventricle and left atrium are markedly underdeveloped. This is usually accompanied by an open ductus arteriosus which delivers blood into the aorta. The condition is associated with severe cyanosis.

Fig. 7.8 gives a summary of congenital cardiac malformations.

- **Name the congenital abnormalities that cause left-to-right shunts.**
- **Describe the effects of atrial septal defects.**
- **Name the congenital abnormalities that cause right-to-left shunts.**
- **Describe the anomalies of tetralogy of Fallot.**
- **Name the congenital abnormalities that cause obstruction to blood flow.**
- **Explain the clinical effects of coarctation of the aorta.**

Summary of congenital cardiac malformations

left-to-right shunts
- ventricular septal defect
- atrial septal defect
- patent ductus arteriosus
- atrioventricular septal defect

right-to-left shunts
- tetralogy of Fallot
- transposition of the great arteries
- persistent truncus arteriosus
- total anomalous venous connection

obstructive congenital defects
- coarctation of the aorta
- pulmonary artery stenosis/atresia
- aortic stenosis/atresia

Fig. 7.8 Summary of congenital cardiac malformations.

ATHEROSCLEROSIS, HYPERTENSION AND ISCHAEMIC HEART DISEASE

Definitions and concepts
Arteriosclerosis
This is an imprecise term meaning thickening and loss of elasticity of the arteries caused by any condition.

Atherosclerosis
This is the commonest form of arteriosclerosis and is defined below. Atherosclerotic lesions are called atheromas.

The terms 'arteriosclerosis' and 'atherosclerosis' are often confused. They are not synonymous and should not be used interchangeably.

Commonest types of arteriosclerosis
There are many types of arteriosclerosis; three of the most common are outlined below.

Atherosclerosis
A degenerative disease, this involves the intima of large- and medium-sized arteries.

Mönckeberg's medial calcific sclerosis
This degenerative disease affects the media of medium-sized muscular arteries, particularly in the limbs. Calcification of the vessels occurs, but the lumen is not decreased.

Arteriolosclerosis (arteriolar sclerosis)
With thickening of the walls of small arteries and arterioles in response to systemic hypertension, this particularly affects the kidneys, pancreas, gall bladder, small intestine, adrenals and retina.

Consequences of arteriosclerosis
The consequences are:
- Vessel thickening → narrowing of lumen → poor tissue perfusion.

- Inelasticity of vessels → predisposition to vessel rupture and haemorrhage.
- Alterations in vascular endothelium → increased predisposition to thrombosis.

Factors that accelerate arteriosclerosis

Arteriosclerotic changes, in mild form, represent the response of the arterial wall to wear and tear, progressing gradually with age. However, certain diseases are known to accelerate and aggravate arteriosclerosis, e.g. hypertension and diabetes.

Atherosclerosis

A degenerative disease of large- and medium-sized arteries (but not veins), this is characterized by the focal accumulation of lipid-rich material in the intima of arteries and associated cellular reactions. Although essentially a disease of the tunica intima, atherosclerosis also has an impact on the structure and function of the underlying tunica media.

Atherosclerotic lesions are found to some extent in virtually every adult over the age of 40 as well as in many younger individuals. Its consequences account for half of all deaths in the Western world.

Commonly affected arteries are:
- Aorta (especially the abdominal aorta).
- Coronary arteries.
- Cerebral arteries.
- Common iliac/femoral arteries.

Atherosclerosis is rare in the arteries of the upper limb and in the pulmonary arteries (unless pulmonary hypertension is also present).

Epidemiological studies have identified risk factors associated with atheroma development. These can be broadly classified into:
- Constitutional risk factors, i.e. risk factors inherent to an individual.
- Hard risk factors: direct association with atherosclerosis.
- Soft risk factors: direct association with ischaemic heart disease → indirect association with atherosclerosis.

Constitutional risk factors are:
- Age: atherosclerotic lesions increase in number with increasing age.
- Gender: up to the age of 55; males >

females by 2:1, due to the protective effect of oestrogens; over 55 years the male to female ratio is equal.
- Familial traits: familial increase in predisposition is often associated with familial hyperlipidaemia.
- Race: wide interracial variations exist in the incidence of atheroma, but this may be due to dietary differences. The condition is relatively uncommon in Chinese, Japanese and Africans.

Hard risk factors lead to an increased severity of atherosclerosis:
- Hyperlipidaemia (increased serum levels of cholesterol or LDL): usually diet dependent but may also occur as a result of some forms of familial hyperlipidaemia (types II and III).
- Hypertension: increased blood pressure, especially diastolic blood pressure.
- Diabetes mellitus: probably an effect of hypercholesterolaemia.
- Cigarette smoking: there is a strong link between smoking and deaths from coronary artery disease; the mechanism is unclear.

Soft risk factors lead to an increased incidence of ischaemic heart disease:
- Lack of exercise: exercise decreases the incidence of sudden death from ischaemic heart disease but it is not clear whether it reduces atherosclerosis formation.
- Obesity: this may be a reflection of diet and resultant hyperlipidaemia.
- Stress and personality traits: linked to deaths from ischaemic heart disease.

Pathogenesis

Pathogenesis of the characteristic lipid plaques, which appear in atherosclerosis, is uncertain; several theories have been proposed:
- Response to injury hypothesis.
- Thrombogenic hypothesis.
- Clonal proliferation hypothesis.
- Lipid infiltration/insudation hypothesis.

Response to injury hypothesis

This is the most widely accepted theory, and it proposes that the first step in formation of the atheromatous plaque, is chronic, low-grade endothelial injury.

Endothelial injury may itself be induced by:
- Cigarette smoking.
- Hypertension.
- Hyperlipidaemia: direct endothelial damage; promotion of platelet attachment.

Stages of development in atherosclerosis

Atherosclerotic plaques (atheromas) develop as follows:
1. Endothelial injury results in platelet adhesion to damaged endothelium; diffusion of plasma proteins (including LDL) into the intima of arteries; migration of monocytes into the intima of arteries.
2. Platelets release platelet-derived growth factor (PDGF), leading to a proliferation of intimal smooth muscle cells (myointimal cells).
3. Myointimal cells deposit excess collagen and elastin in the intima.
4. Macrophages phagocytose LDLs and then release free lipid.

The stages of plaque development are shown in Fig. 7.09. Fig. 7.10 provides a summary of the events involved in pathgenesis.

Other theories of pathogenesis

Thrombogenic hypothesis

This has the following characteristics:
- Repeated episodes of mural thrombosis.
- Organization of thrombi produces elevated plaques.
- Lipid is thought to be derived from platelet membranes and/or leukocytes stimulated to proliferate by PDGFs.
- Not proven by studies.

Clonal proliferation hypothesis

This hypothesis runs as follows:
- Primary event is smooth muscle proliferation.
- Endothelial injury is a secondary phenomenon.
- Clonal proliferation of smooth muscle in plaques.

Lipid infiltration/insudation hypothesis

This hypothesis runs as follows:
- Increased uptake of LDLs from plasma.
- LDLs in intima are then chemically oxidized to act as toxic, proinflammatory and chemotactic factors.

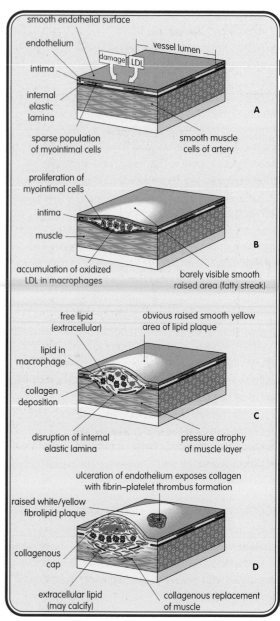

Fig. 7.9 Atheroma formation. (A) Endothelial injury—Allows entry of cholesterol-rich, low-density lipoproteins (LDLs) into the intima. (B) 'Fatty streaks'—Barely visible pale bulges form as a result of phagocytosis and accumulation of lipid by intimal macrophages. (C) Lipid plaques—Raised, yellow lesions within the intima consisting of free lipid released by macrophages, and collagen deposited by myointimal cells. (D) Fibrolipid plaques—Increased collagen deposition → dense fibrous plaque → pressure atrophy of the underlying media and elastic lamina → weakening of the arterial wall. The endothelium often ulcerates, allowing platelet aggregation and thrombosis.

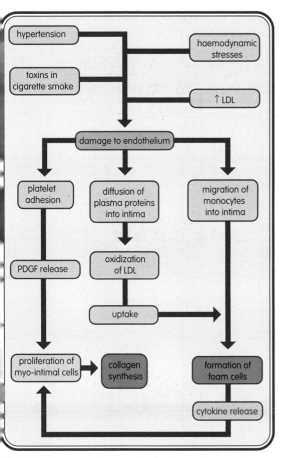

Fig. 7.10 Summary of events involved in pathogenesis.

Management of atherosclerosis
- Reduction or avoidance of risk factors.
- Antihyperlipidaemic drugs to lower serum lipid and cholesterol.
- Anticoagulants, e.g. aspirin to prevent thrombotic complications.

Mönckeberg's medial calcific sclerosis
This is a degenerative disease affecting the media of medium-sized muscular arteries, particularly in the limbs. Vessel walls become calcified, appearing tortuous and hard but with no associated decrease in lumen diameter (pipe-stem arteries). The disorder does not by itself produce ischaemia.

Hypertension
Elevated blood pressure is an important and treatable cause of cardiac failure and is a major risk factor for atherosclerosis and cerebral haemorrhage. Any increase in blood pressure is associated with an increased risk of disease. There are therefore no thresholds below which a person has no risk of developing disease in which blood pressure is a pathogenic factor, and definitions of hypertension are arbitrary.

Functional or operational definition
Hypertension is a sustained rise of the systemic blood pressure above 160 mmHg systolic and/or above 95 mmHg diastolic.

Borderline hypertension is 140–160 mmHg systolic and/or 90–95 mmHg diastolic.

Aetiological classification
Hypertension can be classified into two main types according to its aetiology (Fig. 7.11):
- Primary (essential or idiopathic) hypertension: elevation of blood pressure with age but with no apparent cause; this accounts for 90% of all cases.
- Secondary hypertension: elevated blood pressure due to an identifiable cause; this accounts for 10% of hypertension.

Pathological classification
Hypertension can also be classified according to the clinical course of disease:
- Benign hypertension: stable elevation of blood pressure over many years.
- Malignant (accelerated) hypertension: dramatic elevation of blood pressure over a short period of time.

Benign hypertension
Here, vessel changes develop gradually in response to a persistent stable elevated blood pressure; it affects males more than females. Histologically, it is characterized by:
- Hypertrophy and thickening of muscular media.
- Thickening of elastic lamina.
- Fibroelastic thickening of intima.
- Hyaline deposition in arteriole walls (hyaline arteriolosclerosis).

The effects are:
- Reduced size of vessel lumen leads to tissue ischaemia.

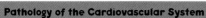

Causes of hypertension	
Primary hypertension: unknown aetiology but probably multifactorial involving…	
genetic predisposition	strong familial association
socio-economic factors	related to social deprivation
dietary factors	obesity, high salt intake, high alcohol, caffeine intake
hormonal factors	abnormalities in renin–angiotensin–aldosterone system
neurological factors	excessive sympathetic nervous system activity
Secondary hypertension: secondary to…	
renal disease	parenchymal disease, e.g. chronic pyelonephritis, glomerulonephritis, polycystic kidneys, amyloidosis vascular disease, e.g. stenosis of renal artery
adrenal disorders	phaeochromocytoma, Cushing's syndrome, Conn's syndrome (primary hyperaldosteronism), congenital adrenal hyperplasia
other endocrine disorders	thyrotoxicosis, hypothyroidism, acromegaly, hyperparathyroidism, diabetes with renal involvement
cardiovascular disorders	coarctation of the aorta, arteriovenous fistulae and shunts
drugs	e.g. oral contraceptives, anabolic steroids, corticosteroids, adrenaline and related sympatheticomimetic drugs
pregnancy	± pre-eclampsia

Fig. 7.11 Causes of hypertension.

- Increased rigidity leads to limited capacity for expansion and constriction.
- Increased fragility of vessels leads to an increased risk of haemorrhage (especially cerebral).

After many years of benign progression, 5% of such patients enter an accelerated malignant phase.

Malignant hypertension

Here, there are acute destructive changes occurring in the walls of small arteries when blood pressure rises suddenly and markedly. There are two main effects: necrosis of the vessel wall (i.e. fibrinoid necrosis of vessels) and infiltration of necrotic media by fibrin (i.e. fibrinoid necrosis of vessels).

Destructive changes lead to cessation of blood flow through the small vessels with multiple foci of tissue necrosis, e.g. in the glomeruli of the kidney.

See Fig. 7.12 for a table of the features of malignant and benign hypertension.

Complications and effects of hypertension
Vascular effects

Hypertension accelerates atherosclerosis and causes thickening of the media of muscular arteries, particularly the smaller arteries and arterioles.

The normal flow of protein into the vessel wall is increased resulting in intramural protein deposition termed hyaline in benign hypertension, and fibrinoid in malignant hypertension:

- Hyaline deposition: a common feature of ageing arteries; refers to the homogenous appearance of vessel walls due to infiltration by plasma proteins.
- Fibrinoid deposition: a combination of fibrin with necrosis of the vessel wall.

Heart

The left ventricle undergoes hypertrophy due to the increased work load, causing increased susceptibility to spontaneous arrhythmias. Ischaemic heart disease due to accelerated atherosclerosis is a common complication of hypertension.

Brain
Intracerebral haemorrhage is a frequent cause of death in hypertension. Small vessel damage within the cerebral hemispheres results in the development of microinfarcts which form hypertensive lacunae, i.e. small areas of brain destruction filled with fluid.

Kidneys
Arteriolosclerosis leads to progressive ischaemia of nephron and chronic renal failure. This is termed benign hypertensive nephrosclerosis, and is a common cause of chronic renal failure in the middle-aged and elderly population.

See Fig. 7.13 for a table of the complications and effects of hypertension.

Features of benign and malignant hypertension		
	Benign	**Malignant**
incidence	very common (at least 5% of UK population)	rare
age	begins at <45 years but prolonged into 6th and 7th decades	young adults (25–35 years)
gender	females > males	females = males
aetiology	majority of cases due to primary hypertension	majority of cases secondary to renal disease (few cases arise out of benign essential hypertension)
disease progression	very slow (many years)	rapid (months to 1–2 years)
blood pressure	very slow rise diastolic = 90–120 mmHg	rapid rise diastolic ≥ 120 mmHg
arterial changes	potentiates atheroma → accelerated arteriosclerosis	intimal fibrous thickening → accelerated arteriosclerosis
arteriole changes	hyaline thickening with narrowed lumen	fibrinoid necrosis of vessel wall lumen occluded by thrombus affects mainly kidney and abdominal viscera

Fig. 7.12 Features of benign and malignant hypertension.

Complications and effects of hypertension		
	Benign	**Malignant**
vessels	hyaline deposition due to infiltration by plasma proteins	fibrinoid deposition due to combination of fibrin deposition and necrosis of vessel wall
heart	hypertrophy of left ventricle → ↑ susceptibility to spontaneous arrhythmias heart failure in 60% of cases ischaemic heart disease	hypertrophy of left ventricle → ↑ susceptibility to spontaneous arrhythmias focal myocardial necrosis acute heart failure ischaemic heart disease
brain	cerebral haemorrhage	encephalopathy (fits and loss of consciousness) due to cerebral oedema cerebral haemorrhage
kidney	nephrosclerosis, but not usually serious	severe renal damage; death in uraemia
other organs	no significant damage	focal necrosis, e.g. perforation of gut

Fig. 7.13 Complications and effects of hypertension.

Pulmonary hypertension

Definition and causes

This is defined as pulmonary arterial pressure in excess of 30 mmHg. See Fig. 7.14 for a list of the causes.

Effects of pulmonary hypertension

With acute onset, there is a massive transudation of fluid from the pulmonary capillaries into the alveoli, leading to shortness of breath and expectoration of bloodstained, watery fluid.

Chronic onset has three effects:

- Hyperplastic arteriosclerosis: muscular hypertrophy, intimal fibrosis and dilatation of the pulmonary arteries.
- Necrotizing arteriolitis: increased pressure within the pulmonary arteries causes weakening of the vessel wall with repeated episodes of haemorrhage into the alveolar spaces which contain haemosiderin-laden macrophages.
- Cor pulmonale: right ventricular hypertrophy and dysfunction as a result of increased workload.

Effects of diabetes mellitus on the vessels

Diabetics suffer from an increased severity of atherosclerosis and microangiopathy, in which small vessel wall thickening is attributed to a marked expansion of the basement membrane termed hyaline arteriolosclerosis.

Vessel damage is probably due to the increased plasma levels of cholesterol and triglycerides. Clinical sequelae of diabetic vessel damage are described in Chapter 11.

Ischaemic heart disease (IHD)

A condition caused by a reduction or cessation of the blood supply to the myocardium (myocardial ischaemia). This is usually as a result of atherosclerosis, although in rare cases it may be caused by coronary embolism, arteritis or ostial obstruction. The left ventricle is more prone to ischaemia due to its greater bulk and work requirement, and its higher oxygen demand.

Causes of pulmonary hypertension	
Mechanism	**Example**
precapillary causes • increased pulmonary blood flow	left-to-right shunts, e.g. atrial septal defects, ventricular septal defects
capillary causes • destruction of lung capillary bed	emphysema interstitial fibrosis of lungs
• mechanical arterial occlusion	recurrent pulmonary emboli
• alveolar hypoxia causing pulmonary vasoconstriction	high altitude obesity chronic obstructive airways disease
postcapillary causes • pulmonary venous congestion	mitral valve disease, e.g. stenosis chronic left ventricular failure
idiopathic causes • primary pulmonary hypertension	rare disease of young women due to increased tone in pulmonary vessels → progressive vascular changes and death

Fig. 7.14 Causes of pulmonary hypertension.

IHD is the commonest type of cardiac disease and a leading cause of death in the Western world accounting for about 30% of all male deaths and 23% of all female deaths. Risk factors to the development of ischaemic heart disease are as for those predisposing to development of atherosclerosis.

Effects

IHD results in four main syndromes:
- Stable angina (chronic manifestation).
- Unstable angina (acute manifestation).
- Myocardial infarction (acute manifestation).
- Sudden cardiac death (acute manifestation).

Angina pectoris

Angina pectoris is episodic chest pain caused by ischaemia of the myocardium (i.e. ischaemic heart disease). Ischaemia is usually the result of stenosis of one or more of the coronary arteries resulting in reduced blood flow to the myocardium.

Stenosis of the coronary arteries is typically the result of atherosclerosis, and these atheromatous plaques may be one of two types:
- Eccentric: fibrolipid plaques affecting only one side of the wall of a coronary artery. Improvement of flow at the site of such plaques may be achieved by vasodilator drugs producing relaxation of the unaffected part of the vessel wall.
- Concentric: collagenous plaques affecting the whole of the arterial wall circumference. As the whole wall is abnormal, drug therapy cannot improve flow over a narrowed segment.

Cardiac referred pain

Pain of angina (and myocardial infarction) commonly radiates from the substernal and left pectoral regions to the left shoulder and medial aspect of the left arm; this is known as cardiac referred pain.

Afferent fibres of the heart, and sensory fibres of affected cutaneous zones, enter the same spinal cord segments (T1 to T4/T5 on the left side) and ascend in the CNS along a common pathway. The brain is unable to discern the origin of the pain, hence the phenomenon of cardiac referred pain.

Less commonly, pain radiates to the right shoulder and arm with or without concomitant pain on the left side.

Types of angina
Stable angina

A predictable angina that occurs at a fixed level of exercise, as a result of an increased demand in myocardial work, usually in the presence of impaired perfusion by blood. It is caused by a fixed arterial obstruction, which limits any increase in coronary blood flow. Pain can usually be relieved by one or two minutes of rest. A stenosis of at least 75% of the lumen of the arteries is required to produce angina on exercise.

Unstable angina

Unstable anginal pain is unpredictable and not related to exercise. It reflects reversible ischaemia due to variable luminal stenosis of some segments of the coronary arteries—dynamic stenosis.

The condition may be caused by either variations in vasomotor tone in segments markedly stenosed by eccentric plaques or by active fissuring or rupture of plaques with intimal surface thrombus deposition, microembolization and occlusion.

Prinzmetal's angina (vasospastic angina)

This is angina at rest caused by an increase in the coronary vasomotor tone. The mechanism for coronary spasm is unknown. The disorder may occur in non-atheromatous arteries (where an increase in tone must be extreme to produce angina) or in atheromatous arteries (where even physiological changes in tone may produce a critical reduction in blood flow).

Prinzmetal's angina is particularly common in the early morning. Attacks are usually self-limiting and, although pain may be severe, they rarely lead on to myocardial infarction.

Management of angina
- Avoidance of risk factors for atherosclerosis (see p. 75).
- Drug therapy is a combination therapy with nitrates, β-blockers, and Ca^{2+} channel blockers.
- Surgery—Coronary angioplasty or coronary artery bypass is indicated when there are signs of progressive coronary occlusion which may lead to myocardial infarction, e.g. unstable angina which increases rapidly in severity over a period of days or stable angina which begins to occur at rest when previously only associated with exercise.

Myocardial infarction (MI)

This is necrosis of the myocardium as a result of severe ischaemia. MI is extremely common, accounting for 10–15% of all deaths and about 60% of sudden unexpected deaths. It typically affects the middle-aged, between 50 and 60 years, but 10% occur in 35–50 year olds. MI affects males more than premenopausal women (by 5:1) but there is an increasing incidence in women postmenopausally.

Clinical features are chest pain accompanied by breathlessness, vomiting and collapse or syncope. Pain occurs in the same sites as angina but is usually more severe and lasts for longer.

Types

There are two main types of MI:
- Regional (90% of cases): infarction occurs in the territory supplied by one major common artery.
- Diffuse (10% of cases): relates to problems of overall myocardial perfusion rather than to thrombotic occlusion in any one artery.

Regional MI

This involves only one segment of the ventricular wall. The cause of infarction is nearly always thrombus formation on a complicated atheromatous plaque.
Patterns of regional MI (Fig. 7.15):
- Full thickness infarct or transmural infarct, due to complete occlusion of an artery (no collateral supply).
- Subendocardial infarct, due to lysis of thrombus or due to collateral supply.

Diffuse MI

General hypoperfusion of the main coronary arteries usually as a result of an episode of hypotension causes a critical reduction in flow in arteries already affected by high-grade, atherosclerotic stenoses.

The pattern of diffuse MI differs from that of regional MI in that there is circumferential necrosis of the subendocardial zone (the region at the end of the arterial perfusion zone) due to failure of perfusion.

Site of myocardial infarction and vessel involvement

The site of regional MI depends on which vessel is involved, as shown in Fig. 7.16. The majority of infarcts affect the left ventricle and septal region; infarction of the right ventricle is relatively rare.

Histological changes following MI

MI induces acute inflammation, and the necrotic tissue is gradually replaced by a collagenous scar. The entire process from fibre necrosis to scar formation takes 6–8 weeks, the macroscopic and microscopic appearances of the infarct changing with time (Fig. 7.17).

Sequelae of MI

The effects and sequelae of MI are variable, and can be classified into:
- Immediate effects: sudden cardiac death (described below).
- Short-term complications: occurring in the first two weeks post MI.
- Long-term complications.

Short-term complications

There are six short-term complications:
- Arrhythmias due to the involvement of conduction tissue, leading to ventricular fibrillation, atrial fibrillation, heart block, and sinus bradycardia.
- Left ventricular failure: this is common with large areas of infarction; the necrotic wall softens in organization leading to cardiac dilatation.
- Rupture: this could be:
  - External (majority): blood bursts through the external wall into the pericardial cavity (haemopericardium); the sudden rise in

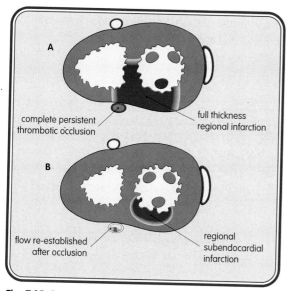

Fig. 7.15 Patterns of regional myocardial infarction (MI). (A) Transmural or full thickness infarct. (B) Regional subendocardial infarct.

intrapericardial cavity pressure prevents cardiac filling (cardiac tamponade), leading to rapid death.
- Internal (rarely): intracardiac rupture through septum leads to acquired septal defect causing a left-to-right shunt and development of left ventricular failure.
- Papillary muscle dysfunction: when one or more valve leaflets are unable to close during systole there is mitral valve incompetence.
- Mural thrombosis: on the inflamed endocardium over the area of infarction; there is a high risk of

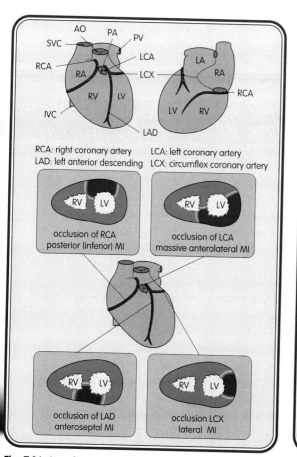

RCA: right coronary artery LCA: left coronary artery
LAD: left anterior descending LCX: circumflex coronary artery

occlusion of RCA posterior (inferior) MI

occlusion of LCA massive anterolateral MI

occlusion of LAD anteroseptal MI

occlusion LCX lateral MI

Fig. 7.16 Site of MI and vessel involvement.

Morphological changes occurring post MI		
time	macroscopic appearance	microscopic appearance
0–12 hours	not visible	infarcted muscle appears uncoloured on staining with nitroblue tetrazolium due to loss of oxidative enzymes; non-infarcted muscle stains blue
12–24 hours	pale with blotchy discoloration	infarcted muscle is brightly eosinophilic with intercellular oedema
24–72 hours	dead area appears soft and pale with a slight yellow colour	infarcted area excites an acute inflammatory response neutrophils infiltrate between dead cardiac muscle fibres
3–10 days	hyperaemic border develops around the yellow dead muscle	organization of infarcted area replacement with vascular granulation tissue
weeks to months	white scar	progressive collagen deposition infarct is replaced by a collagenous scar

Fig. 7.17 Morphological changes occurring post MI.

embolization producing infarction of various organs, e.g. cerebral, renal, splenic, mesenteric, and lower limbs.
- Acute pericarditis due to inflammation over the infarct surface.

Long-term complications
There are four long-term complications:
- Chronic intractable left-heart failure due to inadequate left ventricular pumping action; common when the infarct is extensive and full thickness.
- Ventricular aneurysm (in 10% of long-term survivors): gradual distension of the weakened fibrotic part of the left ventricular wall with thrombus formation, embolism or severe functional deficit.
- Recurrent MI: risk of developing a further episode due to underlying coronary artery insufficiency.
- Dressler's syndrome: a form of autoimmune-mediated pericarditis associated with a high ESR; develops in a very small number of cases after infarction.

Management is by investigations, i.e. ECG, chest X-ray (excluding aortic dissection), blood (increased ESR, cardiac enzymes), and treatment as follows:
- Oxygen to overcome lowered PO_2.
- Analgesia: morphine, diamorphine with antiemetics.
- Nitrates: sublingual glyceryl nitrates.
- Fibrinolytic therapy: should be considered within first 12 hours post infarction.
- Anticoagulation to prevent thromboembolic complications from prolonged immobilization.
- ACE inhibitors for patients with heart failure.
- Bed rest for the first 24–48 hours.

Sudden cardiac death
Sudden cardiac death is the most important immediate consequence of myocardial ischaemia and is usually due to ventricular fibrillation.

Arrhythmias causing ventricular fibrillation may be a result of:
- Previous ischaemic heart disease, e.g. angina or previous infarction; cardiac arrhythmias can arise from muscle adjacent to an area of old scarring.
- Acute myocardial ischaemia, which, due to a new thrombotic event, may precipitate arrhythmia.

Other causes of sudden death include ruptured or dissecting aneurysms of the aorta and pulmonary emboli.

- Define 'atherosclerosis' and list the risk factors implicated in its development.
- Describe the different types of hypertension.
- Describe the types of atheromatous plaques that occur in the coronary arteries.
- What is the difference between regional and diffuse myocardial infarction?
- Name the sites of myocardial infarction and name the vessel involved in each case.
- What are the complications of myocardial infarction?

DISORDERS OF THE HEART VALVES

Concepts of heart valve disease
Types of valve disorder:
- Stenosis: narrowing or abnormal rigidity of a valve.
- Regurgitation (or incompetence): failure of a valve to close fully.

Both types may coexist in one valve but one type is usually dominant.

Factors that may cause heart valve damage:
- Congenital abnormality.
- Postinflammatory scarring.
- Degeneration with ageing.
- Dilatation of the valve ring.
- Degeneration of collagenous support tissue of the valve.
- Acute destruction by necrotizing inflammation.

Commonly affected valves
The mitral and aortic valves are the most frequently

affected, the tricuspid and pulmonary valves only infrequently.

Fig. 7.18 gives an outline of the major causes and basic features of acquired valve disease.

Abnormalities of flow and their effects

Diseased valves often cause regurgitant jets of blood with concomitant development of endocardial lesions opposite the jet's site. These lesions (jet lesions) are typically seen on the septum opposite the aortic valve.

Degenerative valve disease

Calcific aortic stenosis

There are two types:

- Degenerative calcific aortic valve stenosis: calcification of the aortic valve associated with increasing age; typically affects the elderly.

- Bicuspid calcific aortic valve stenosis: calcification of the congenital bicuspid aortic valve; quite common, usually manifesting by 40–50 years of age.

In both types, the valves become thick and fibrotic with a fusion of the commissures. Large nodular masses of calcium may be found subendothelially within the sinuses of Valsalva behind the aortic cusps.

Effects

There are two effects:

- Aortic stenosis (i.e. thickening and fusion of valves) → decreased valve lumen → reduced systolic flow.
- Aortic regurgitation: increased rigidity of valves → failure to close properly → backflow into the left ventricle during diastole.

Major causes and basic features of acquired valve disease			
Valve lesion	**Causes**	**Effects**	**Physical findings**
mitral stenosis	rheumatic	left-sided cardiac failure with predisposition to atrial thrombosis left atrial hypertrophy and dilatation leads to: • pulmonary vascular congestion • pulmonary hypertension • right ventricular hypertrophy • 'nutmeg liver' and congested kidneys	loud S_1 opening snap diastolic rumble
mitral regurgitation	acute: • papillary muscle dysfunction • cusp damage by endocarditis chronic: • postinflammatory scarring, commonly rheumatic • left ventricular dilatation • floppy mitral valve syndrome	acute: • pulmonary oedema chronic: • left ventricle hypertrophy and dilatation • giant left atrium • progressive left-sided cardiac failure develops with time	pansystolic murmur widely split S_2
aortic stenosis	calcification of congenital bicuspid aortic valve rheumatic senile calcific degeneration	early: • asymptomatic but with slowly progressive left ventricular hypertrophy late: • left ventricular failure • low cardiac output → breathlessness • coronary artery insufficiency → angina • cerebrovascular insufficiency → syncope • sudden death	systolic ejection murmur reaching peak intensity in mid- or late systole
aortic regurgitation	rheumatic endocarditis senile calcification aortic root dilatation	left ventricular hypertrophy progressive left ventricular failure	diastolic murmur wide pulse pressure collapsing pulse

Fig. 7.18 Major causes and basic features of acquired valve disease.

Stenosis and regurgitation result in left ventricular hypertrophy, coronary insufficiency, and syncope or sudden death due to acute heart failure.

Mitral annular calcification
'Wear and tear' of the mitral valve with calcification of the valve leaflets. Massive calcification can immobilize the valve and predispose to the development of either thrombosis or bacterial endocarditis.

Myxomatous degeneration of the mitral valve ('floppy valve syndrome')
This is the idiopathic prolapse of the mitral valve leaflets. The leaflets are thickened and redundant, containing large amounts of mucopolysaccharides and abnormal collagen. It most commonly involves the posterior mitral leaflet which is soft and bulges upwards into the atrium during systole. Net result is mild valvular incompetence and increased risk of rupture of one of the chordae, which may lead to severe valvular incompetence.

Rheumatic heart disease
Rheumatic fever is an immune disorder that follows 2–3 weeks after a streptococcal infection, usually tonsillitis or pharyngitis.

Epidemiology
This disease occurs mainly in children aged 5–15 years, and was once prevalent in Europe, including the UK, and in the USA. Its incidence has decreased in the developed world, and is now most frequently seen in parts of central Africa, the Middle East and India. It is associated with poor nutrition and overcrowding.

Pathogenesis
Susceptible individuals develop antibodies to antigens produced by specific strains of streptococci; these antibodies then cross-react with host antigens. The disease is a systemic disorder affecting:
- Heart: pericarditis, myocarditis, and endocarditis (collectively known as pancarditis).
- Joints: polyarthritis.
- Skin: subcutaneous nodules and erythema marginatum.
- Arteries: arteritis.

The most important target organ is the heart. Repeated attacks of rheumatic fever lead to progressive fibrosis of the endocardium and valves, which is the main cause of chronic scarring of the valves.

Aschoff's nodules
These are areas of degenerate collagen surrounded by activated histiocytic cells and lymphoid cells. Lesions stimulate fibroblast proliferation and lead to scarring.

Acute rheumatic heart disease
In the acute phase, rheumatic fever causes a pancarditis, the components of which are described below:

Rheumatic pericarditis
Acute inflammation of pericardium with:
- Aschoff's nodules in the pericardium.
- Acute inflammatory exudate (serous type fluid with comparatively little fibrin or neutrophil components) leads to pericardial effusion and thus to distension of the pericardial cavity.

Rheumatic myocarditis
Usually mild but may produce left ventricular failure:
- Aschoff's nodules in the myocardium.
- Interstitial oedema.
- Mild inflammation occasionally with muscle fibre necrosis.

Rheumatic endocarditis
This manifests as follows:
- Aschoff's nodules in the endocardium produce an irregularity of the valves often with erosion of overlying endocardium, especially at the line of closure.
- Small aggregations of fibrin and platelets accumulate in these sites forming small vegetations.
- Aortic and mitral valves are most prone to develop severe lesions, probably because of higher pressures to which they are exposed and the more vigorous and traumatic valve closure.

During this acute phase, the greatest dangers to the patient are pericarditis and myocarditis, which, if severe, may result in heart block or heart failure; however these usually resolve without long-term ill effect.

Chronic rheumatic heart disease

The main morbidity of rheumatic fever is the long-term effects of the immune damage causing chronic scarring of valves. Chronic valvular heart disease develops in about 50% of those affected by rheumatic fever with carditis. Lesions may develop after 10–20 years in Western countries but much earlier in developing countries.

Pathogenesis

Endocardial valvular damage from the acute phase heals by progressive fibrosis. Valve leaflets and chordae tendinae become thickened, fibrotic and shrunken, often with fusion to their partners, and there is frequent secondary deposition of calcium.

Consequences of rheumatic fever

The consequences are:
- Thrombus deposition on the valve due to exposure of underlying collagen. Thrombi develop as irregular warty growths on valve leaflets, and are termed 'vegetations'.
- Increased predisposition to infective endocarditis.
- Stenosis and/or regurgitation: inflammation and thrombus formation on the valve cause collagenous scarring rendering it mechanically and functionally abnormal. Valves on the left side of the heart are more commonly affected than those on the right.

Once damage has developed, the altered haemodynamic stresses extend the damage even in the absence of continued autoimmune processes.

Frequencies of valve involvement

The frequencies of valve involvement are:
- Mitral valve alone—50%.
- Mitral and aortic—40%.
- Aortic valve alone—10%.

Infective endocarditis

This is an acute or subacute disease resulting from infection of a focal area of the endocardium. It can affect almost any age but with an increasing number in the elderly, with males outnumbering females by 3:1.

Morphological features

The characteristic lesions of endocarditis are termed vegetations, and are formed from deposits of platelets, fibrin and bacteria. The mechanism of formation is outlined in Fig. 7.19.

Almost all vegetation occurs on valve leaflets or chordae tendinae. The size varies from a small nodule to a large mass that may occlude the valve orifice. The mitral and aortic valves are the most commonly affected.

Causative organisms

Bacteria

The two groups of bacteria are:
- Pathogenic: *Staphylococcus aureus*, β-haemolytic streptococci, pneumococci, meningococci, *Escherichia coli*, etc.
- Low-grade pathogens: *Streptococcus viridans* (e.g. *S. mutans*), *S. faecalis*, *Staph. epidermidis*, *Haemophilus*, *Brucella*, mycobacteria, and various Gram-negative organisms.

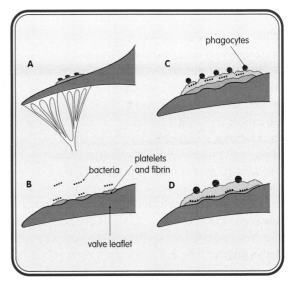

Fig. 7.19 Pathogenesis of vegetation formation in infective endocarditis. (A) Abnormality on endocardium of valve leaflet is coated with small deposits of platelets and fibrin (thrombus). (B) Circulating bacteria or fungi colonize the platelet thrombus. (C) Further layers of platelets and fibrin are deposited, and the micro-organisms proliferate in the superficial layer of the vegetation. They are separated from blood by a thin layer of fibrinous material, which protects against immune destruction but allows diffusion of nutrients. (Adapted with permission from *General and Systematic Pathology*, 2nd edn, by J.C.E. Underwood, Churchill Livingstone, 1996.)

Fungi

Fungi such as *Candida*, *Aspergillus*, etc., may cause endocarditis, particularly in drug addicts, the immunosuppressed or those with valve prostheses.

The type of causative organism responsible depends on whether the affected valve is structurally normal or abnormal.

Infection of structurally normal valves

Infective organisms are pathogenic and directly invade the valve causing rapid destruction. This is commonly seen in intravenous drug addicts, after open heart surgery, and following septicaemia from other causes.

Infection of structurally abnormal heart valves

Infective organisms are of low pathogenicity, and derived from normal commensal organisms of the skin, mouth, urinary tract and gut. Following trivial episodes of bacteraemia, organisms become enmeshed in platelet aggregates on the surface of the abnormal endocardium, growing to cause persistent infection.

The main underlying abnormalities in this group are:
- Congenital bicuspid aortic valves.
- Postinflammatory scarring.
- Mitral valve prolapse syndrome.
- Prosthetic valves.

Incidence has increased in Western countries in recent years, mainly as a result of patients surviving with structurally abnormal hearts and heart valves.

Types of infective endocarditis

Acute

The cause is usually a virulent organism, such as *Staphylococcus aureus*, but may affect either normal or abnormal heart valves.

The bacteria proliferate in the valve causing necrosis and the generation of thrombotic vegetations.

Consequently there is destruction of valve leaflets with perforation and acute disturbance of valve function leading to acute heart failure.

Prognosis—Disease is rapidly progressive and often fatal.

Subacute

The cause here is, typically, poorly virulent organisms, such as *Streptococcus viridans*, infecting structurally abnormal valves.

The bacteria proliferate slowly in the thrombotic vegetation on damaged valve surfaces. Gradual valve destruction occurs, stimulating further thrombus formation with the potential for systemic embolization.

Clinical features of endocarditis

- Systemic symptoms: fever, weight loss and malaise due to cytokine generation from low-grade infection.
- Skin petechiae and microhaemorrhages in the retina and skin, particularly around the finger nails (splinter haemorrhages); caused by the deposition of immune complexes (antibodies react with antigen of the infecting organism) in small vessels; they also cause a form of glomerulonephritis.
- Clubbing of fingers (cause unknown).
- Splenomegaly and anaemia due to persistent bacteraemia.

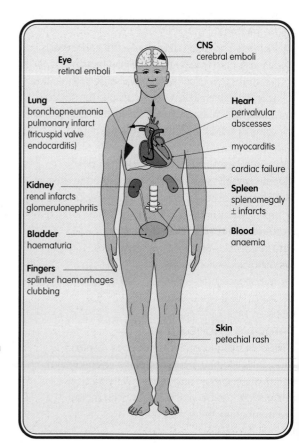

Fig. 7.20 Complications of infective endocarditis.

Sequelae (Fig. 7.20)

The sequelae are as follows:

- Valvular regurgitation due to gradual destruction of valves leading to cardiac failure.
- Perivalvular abscesses following extension of the infection into the valve ring and myocardium, producing sinuses, fistulae, septal defects and abnormalities of conduction.
- Mycotic aneurysms: infection of the muscular wall of a medium-sized artery caused by embolisms to the vasa vasorum.
- Multi-organ infarction: small emboli of infected thrombotic material enter systemic circulation producing infarction of many organs especially the brain, spleen, and kidneys. Infarcted organs may in turn become infected by organisms within the occluding thrombus.

Both rheumatic heart disease and infective endocarditis are common topics in examinations.

small intestine and with metastases in the liver), and can result in endocardial fibrosis of the tricuspid and pulmonary valves, in turn resulting in stenosis or incompetence.

Complications of artificial heart valves

The prosthetic valve diseases are:

- Thrombosis leading to valve obstruction or embolism.
- Valve failure due to mechanical breakage of the prosthesis, or tissue calcification and cusp rupture of bioprosthesis.
- Infective endocarditis from turbulence and prosthetic material; its incidence is 1–2% per year.
- Paravalvular leak: caused by poor surgical technique, or due to poor quality tissues, e.g. calcium, active infective endocarditis.
- Obstructive gradients: valve may be too small, or there may be tissue ingrowth of the pannus on to the valve ring.
- Haemolysis and rarely jaundice.

Precautions necessary to avoid them

The precautions are lifelong anticoagulation, and prophylactic antibiotic therapy to protect against infective endocarditis.

Non-bacterial thrombotic (marantic) endocarditis

This is inflammation of the valves with the formation of sterile thrombotic vegetations (marantic vegetations) on the closure lines of valve cusps. It occurs in severely debilitated patients with serious systemic disease.

Endocarditis of SLE (Libman–Sacks disease)

Thrombotic vegetations complicate systemic lupus erythematosus (SLE). This is seen in 50% or more of fatal cases of SLE. Valvular changes rarely give rise to any appreciable functional deficiency, but thrombotic material can fragment and cause embolic infarction.

Carcinoid heart disease

Carcinoid syndrome is caused by excess 5-hydroxytryptamine secretion by a tumour (usually of the

- o Define 'stenosis' and 'regurgitation'.
- o Describe the major causes and basic features of acquired valve disease.
- o Name three types of degenerative valve disease.
- o Define 'rheumatic fever'.
- o Describe the pathogenesis of chronic rheumatic heart disease.
- o Describe the aetiology and pathogenesis of infective endocarditis.
- o What is carcinoid heart disease?

DISEASES OF THE MYOCARDIUM

Concepts of myocardial disease
Cardiomyopathy
This is a group of disorders in which the structural or functional abnormality primarily affects the myocardium, but excluding myocardial impairment secondary to other cardiac conditions such as hypertension, valvular or coronary artery disease.

Effects of cardiomyopathy
Cardiomyopathies usually cause progressive development of cardiac failure. The time scale varies according to the cause of the disease, occurring over weeks or years. In some instances, sudden cardiac death is the first manifestation of disease.

> The terms 'cardiomyopathy' and 'myocarditis' are frequently confused. Myocarditis refers to inflammation of the myocardium and is a form of secondary cardiomyopathy, but is not synonymous with cardiomyopathy.

Classification
Cardiomyopathies can be grouped into two types according to aetiology:
- Primary idiopathic cardiomyopathies (aetiology unknown).
- Secondary cardiomyopathies (also known as specific heart muscle diseases): diseases of the heart muscle associated with or caused by a systemic disease.

Primary idiopathic cardiomyopathy
Primary cardiomyopathies follow three main patterns according to the dysfunction of the myocardium: dilated, hypertrophic or restrictive.

Dilated (congestive) cardiomyopathy
These are abnormalities of the myocardium causing poor systolic contraction and characterized by:
- Dilatation of the ventricles.
- Thin, stretched chamber walls.
- Hypocontractile muscle.

Aetiology is usually unidentifiable, but the condition occasionally represents end-stage myocardial damage for known causes including viral myocarditis and other forms of secondary cardiomyopathies.

Hypertrophic cardiomyopathy
A familial condition resulting in hyperkinetic systolic function with marked reduction in systolic volume and difficulty in diastolic filling. This is characterized by:
- Gross hypertrophy of the heart walls, particularly affecting the interventricular septum.
- Loss of the normal parallel orientation of hypertrophied muscle fibres—disorganized branching.

This condition may present in young adults and juveniles with sudden unexplained death on exertion. Less dramatic presentations include angina and breathlessness on exertion in a young person or repeated fainting attacks.

Restrictive cardiomyopathy
Abnormal stiffness of the myocardium results in impaired ventricular filling. The stiffness is caused by infiltration of the myocardium, for example:
- Amyloid in amyloidosis.
- Fibrosis in endomyocardial fibrosis (fibrosis of thrombotic material deposited on the endocardial surfaces).
- Haemochromatosis.

The condition causes high atrial pressures resulting in atrial hypertrophy → atrial dilatation → atrial fibrillation.

Secondary cardiomyopathies
Myocarditis
This rare disease is characterized by the presence of inflammatory cells in the myocardium.

Aetiology

The vast majority of cases of myocarditis are either infectious or immune-mediated.

The infectious causes are:

- Viruses: viral infection is the commonest cause of myocarditis in the UK. Coxsackie virus is the commonest culprit but it may also be caused by influenza, echovirus, HIV, CMV, poliomyelitis or mumps virus.
- Bacteria: direct infection (with chlamydia, rickettsia or pyogenic bacteria) or indirect toxin-mediated damage (e.g. diphtheria or typhoid).
- Fungi.
- Protozoa: toxoplasmosis; Chagas' disease due to *Trypanosoma cruzi*.
- Helminths.

The immune-mediated causes are:

- Poststreptococcal, e.g. acute rheumatic fever.
- Postviral.
- SLE.
- Drug hypersensitivity, e.g. sulphonamides, doxurubicin, cyclophosphamide.
- Transplant rejection.

Other less common causes include sarcoidosis (see Chapter 8) and giant cell myocarditis, an acute fulminating form of fatal acute myocarditis.

Other secondary cardiomyopathies

Other causes of secondary cardiomyopathies are listed in Fig. 7.21.

Neoplasms of the heart

Tumours or the heart are extremely rare.

Classification

Benign

There are two types of benign heart neoplasm: myxomas and connective tissue tumours.

Myxoma is the commonest primary heart tumour arising most often in the left atrium. It is composed of stellate cells in a myxoid matrix and is frequently pendunculated, having a soft and gelatinous appearance. It may cause interference to blood flow or act as a 'ball valve' obstruction, especially in the mitral valve. This is a rare cause of sudden death.

The connective tissue tumours are fibromas, lipomas and angiomas.

Malignant

Primary malignant tumours exist but are extremely rare. Examples include rhabdomyosarcomas, angiosarcomas and fibrosarcomas.

Secondary tumours can arise from direct or metastatic spread:

- Direct: local extension of tumours from adjacent structures, e.g. lung carcinoma (commonest tumour of heart), oesophageal carcinoma.
- Metastatic: carcinomas from any site, e.g. malignant melanoma, lymphomas.

Aetiology of secondary cardiomyopathies	
Causes	**Example**
infection and inflammation	myocarditis
multisystem disease	diabetes amyloidosis thyroid dysfunction haemochromatosis
toxic and metabolic disturbances	alcohol catecholamines drugs, e.g. adriamycin
primary muscle disorders	muscular dystrophy mitochondrial cytopathy

Fig. 7.21 Aetiology of secondary cardiomyopathies.

- Define 'cardiomyopathy'.
- What are the types and basic features of primary cardiomyopathies?
- List the causes of secondary cardiomyopathies.
- Define 'myocarditis' and explain its aetiology.
- What is the commonest primary heart tumour?

DISEASES OF THE PERICARDIUM

Accumulation of fluid in the pericardial sac
Pericardial effusion

This is the accumulation of fluid within the pericardial cavity. Effusions may be:

- Serous: transudate with low protein content (<2g/100 ml) and usually containing only very scanty mesothelial cells, caused by heart failure, hypoalbuminaemia or myxoedema.
- Serosanguinous: exudate with high protein content (>3 g/100 ml) occurring with infection, uraemia, neoplasia or connective tissue disorders.
- Chylous: accumulation of lymphatic fluid occurring in the presence of lymphatic obstruction of pericardial drainage, most commonly due to neoplasms and tuberculosis.

The aetiology is of two types: inflammatory (e.g. acute pericarditis) and non-inflammatory. Non-inflammatory has the following characteristics:

- ↑ Capillary permeability, e.g. severe hypothyroidism.
- ↑ Capillary hydrostatic pressure, e.g. congestive heart failure.
- ↓ Plasma oncotic pressure, e.g. cirrhosis and the nephrotic syndrome.

Pathophysiology—Large amounts of fluid eventually interfere with the heart's action.

Clinical effects depend on the increase in pressure within the pericardium which, in turn, depends on:

- Volume of effusion: the greater the volume the greater the increase in internal pressure.
- Rate at which the fluid accumulates. Sudden increase → marked elevation of pressure → severe cardiac chamber compression. Slow effusion (over weeks to months) → pericardium stretches → no elevation of pressure.
- Compliance characteristics of the pericardium: even small effusions may cause marked elevation of pressure if there is stiffness of the pericardium, e.g. in the presence of tumour or fibrosis.

The condition is often asymptomatic but may present with a dull constant ache in the left side of the chest. Unlike ischaemic cardiac pain, it is accentuated by inspiration, by movement and by lying flat.

Haemopericardium

This is the accumulation of blood in the pericardial sac. For its aetiology see Fig. 7.22 where the causes of haemopericardium are outlined. In most cases, death occurs rapidly due to the sudden rise in intrapericardial cavity pressure which prevents cardiac filling (cardiac tamponade), as little as 200–300 ml commonly being sufficient.

Cardiac tamponade

In this condition, fluid (of any kind) accumulates under high pressure compressing the cardiac chambers to such an extent that filling of the heart is severely limited.

Diagnosis

The physical signs are:
- Sinus tachycardia.
- Increased jugular venous pulse (often with a further rise on inspiration).
- Decreased systemic blood pressure (producing shock in severe cases).
- Cyclical decrease in systolic blood pressure during each inspiration: pulsus paradoxus.

Investigations include echocardiography (which shows the presence of pericardial effusion with right ventricular diastolic collapse) and cardiac catheterization combined with pericardiocentesis.

The management of cardiac tamponade depends on the extent of haemodynamic compromise. Severe cases may be rapidly fatal and require relief by emergency paracentesis; less critical cases require formal surgical drainage.

Aetiology of haemopericardium	
Causes	**Example**
rupture of heart	traumatic, e.g. stab wound spontaneous, e.g. myocardial infarct
rupture of intrapericardial portion of aorta	dissecting aneurysm syphilitic aneurysm traumatic
haemorrhagic tendencies	purpura scurvy hypoprothrombinaemia anticoagulant therapy

Fig. 7.22 Aetiology of haemopericardium.

Electromechanical dissociation (EMD)

This is a condition in which electrical activity is normal or near normal on ECG, but there is no effective cardiac output. It is associated with a poor prognosis as it is often due to cardiac rupture which is rarely amenable to treatment. However, treatable causes of EMD should not be overlooked and include:

- Cardiac tamponade.
- Hypovolaemia.
- Pneumothorax.
- Pulmonary embolism.

Pericarditis

Pericarditis, i.e. inflammation of the pericardium, is the main disorder of the pericardium. The condition is often complicated by the development of an effusion.

Acute pericarditis

Here, both pericardial surfaces (i.e. the heart and its sac) are coated with a fibrin-rich acute inflammatory exudate. The loss of smoothness leads to the clinical sign of a friction rub. The causes of acute pericarditis are listed in Fig. 7.23.

Variants can be:
- Serous.
- Serofibrinous or fibrinous.
- Suppurative (or purulent) pericarditis.
- Haemorrhagic.
- Caseous.

Remember the 'Five Is' of possible causes: infarctive, infective, injury, invasive, immunological.

Serous

Typically occurring with non-bacterial inflammations; exudate is a clear, straw-coloured, protein-rich fluid containing small numbers of immune cells and mesothelial cells. The volume produced is usually small and formed slowly, producing little effect on cardiac function. Fluid eventually reabsorbs with remission of disease and minimal adhesion formation.

Serofibrinous or fibrinous

The commonest morphological pattern, this occurs with rheumatic fever, myocardial infarction and in uraemia. Pericardial exudate contains plasma protein including fibrinogen, which may be converted into fibrin yielding a grossly rough and shaggy ('bread and butter') appearance. Portions of the visceral and parietal pericardium become fused and thickened.

The sequelae are:
- Resolution with digestion of fibrin.
- Further organization of fibrin → adhesion of

Fig. 7.23 Aetiology of acute pericarditis.

Aetiology of acute pericarditis	
infarction	myocardial infarction: local pericarditis over infarct is the commonest cause of pericarditis
infective	viral infections: second commonest cause, usually clinically mild, rarely requiring hospital treatment pyogenic: e.g. staphylococci, streptococci, haemophilus septicaemia or pneumonia tuberculosis: spread to pericardium from tuberculous lymph nodes in mediastinum; now rare
injury	postoperative: following open heart surgery pericarditis is diffuse, involving entire pericardial surface heals by fibrosis → obliteration of pericardial cavity
invasive	malignant pericarditis: usually due to infiltration of pericardium by local spread from a primary bronchial tumour; less commonly the cause is blood-borne metastases from a distant site, e.g. malignant melanoma
immunologic	immune pericarditis: associated with rheumatic fever or may present in patient with systemic autoimmune disease, e.g. SLE, rheumatoid disease

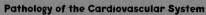

pericardial layers → dense scar that restricts movement and diastolic filling of cardiac chambers (constrictive pericarditis described below).

Suppurative (or purulent) pericarditis

This intense inflammatory response is almost always associated with a pyogenic bacterial infection. Serosal surfaces are erythematous and coated with thick creamy pus. The condition may be fatal. In survivors, typical sequelae are the organization and development of an adherent pericardium.

Haemorrhagic

Blood is mixed with inflammatory exudate. It is usually due to a neoplasm or fulminating bacterial infection.

Caseous

This is caused by tuberculosis infection either originating from pulmonary disease or mediastinal lymph nodes, or else blood borne. There is a fibrinous exudate with granulation tissue and areas of caseation covering the pericardial surfaces. It may occasionally be haemorrhagic and microscopically tuberculous caseating giant cells are seen.

The process heals by gross fibrosis often followed by calcification leading to constrictive pericarditis.

Clinical features

The clinical features of acute pericarditis are:
- Pleuritic chest pain.
- Fever.
- Pericardial friction rub.
- EKG abnormalities.

Chronic pericarditis

Adhesive pericarditis

Although fibrinous pericarditis may resolve completely, it occasionally results in fibrinous adhesions or even in complete obliteration of the pericardial sac.

Constrictive pericarditis

Gross fibrosis and calcification of the pericardium cause restriction of ventricular filling and interference with ventricular systole. The heart is effectively encased in a solid shell and filling is impaired. Calcification may extend into the myocardium producing impaired myocardial contraction.

This condition often follows tuberculous pericarditis but can also complicate haemopericardium, viral pericarditis, rheumatoid arthritis and purulent pericarditis.

Clinical features

In chronic pericarditis the fibrous tissue impairs venous return resulting in symptoms and signs of systemic venous congestion, namely raised jugular venous pressure, enlarged liver, and ascites.

Rheumatic disease of the pericardium

This is an acute form of pericarditis occurring with generalized pancarditis following streptococcal infection (see pp. 86–87).

- Describe the types of pericardial effusions, and list the aetiological factors involved.
- List the causes of haemopericardium.
- Define 'cardiac tamponade' and describe the physical signs.
- What is electromechanical dissociation? Name the causes.
- List the causes of acute pericarditis and describe the different types of inflammation.
- Describe the two types of chronic pericarditis.

ANEURYSMS

Definitions and concepts

Aneurysm

This is an abnormal localized, permanent, dilatation of an artery. Types of aneurysm are shown in Fig. 7.24:
- True aneurysms: wall is formed by one or more layers of the affected vessel. These can be saccular or fusiform.
- False aneurysms: wall is formed by connective tissue which is not a part of vessel; usually due to traumatic or infective rupture of vessel forming a blood-filled

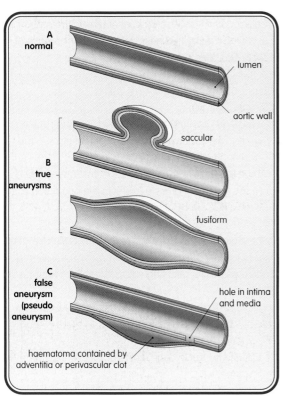

Fig. 7.24 Aortic aneurysms. (A) Normal. (B) True aneurysms. (C) False aneurysm (pseudo-aneurysm).

space limited by surrounding tissue (usually an organized haematoma).

True aneurysm morphology
Saccular aneurysms take the form of globular sacs, whereas fusiform aneurysms are spindle shaped due to long segments of the vessel wall being affected around the whole circumference.

Main causes of aneurysms
Any abnormality that weakens the media may produce an aneurysm:
- Atherosclerosis is the commonest cause, typically affecting the abdominal aorta causing thinning and fibrous replacement of media.
- Cystic medial degeneration: focal degeneration of media with formation of small cyst-like spaces filled with mucopolysaccharide. Aetiology may be idiopathic or associated with connective tissue diseases, e.g. Marfan's syndrome, and Ehlers–Danlos syndrome.

The condition is generally confined to the aorta and the origins of its major branches. Extensive disease leads to dissecting aneurysm.
- Infectious aortitis, e.g. syphilitic aortitis (rare, typically affecting the ascending and transverse portions of the aortic arch causing inflammatory destruction of media with fibrous replacement) and mycotic aneurysms (small saccular dilatations with destruction of the wall caused by bacteria in infected thrombus).
- Vasculitic syndromes (see pp. 97–99): inflammation of the vessels caused by immune complex deposition or cell-mediated immune reactions of the arterial wall leading to a weakening of vessel wall then aneurysmal dilatations.
- Congenital aneurysms.

Pathogenesis
The majority of aneurysms occur due to a weakening of the arterial wall with loss of elasticity and contractability. Stretching of the weakened wall is gradually progressive due to haemodynamic pressure forces producing an increased thinning of the wall until eventual rupture occurs.

The build-up of layers of thrombus within the lumen of the aneurysmal sac is protective, but not usually sufficient to repair the defect and reconstitute a normal lumen to the artery.

Main complications
The main complications of aneurysms are rupture and predisposition to thrombosis.

Abdominal aortic aneurysms (AAAs)
AAAs are more common in men, especially over 60 years of age.

Aetiology—Atherosclerosis is the commonest cause of abdominal aneurysms. However, they may also arise as a result of inflammation (vasculitis) or infection (mycotic aneurysms).

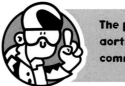
The pathology of abdominal aortic aneurysms is a common exam topic.

Site—The majority are situated below the origin of the renal arteries and are thus amenable to resection and replacement by graft.

Morphology—Atherosclerotic aneurysms produce a fusiform dilatation of the wall.

Symptoms and signs

The majority are asymptomatic, but occasionally patients are aware of a pulsatile mass. It is often first suspected because of aortic dilatation observed on radiographs, especially if walls of aneurysm are calcified. It may also come to attention by careful palpation during physical examination.

Symptoms may occur because of compression of neighbouring structures by expanding aneurysm, e.g. erosion of the vertebrae by a large abdominal aneurysm may cause back pain.

Confirmation of both types is achieved by ultrasonography, CT, MRI or arteriography.

Consequences

Rupture is the most devastating consequence and is often fatal. This may occur suddenly without warning or, alternatively, may slowly leak into the vessel wall resulting in pain and local tenderness.

Haemorrhage may occur into the retroperitoneal space, abdominal cavity or erode into the intestines resulting in massive GI bleeding.

Prognostic factors

Fifty per cent of all abdominal aortic aneurysms which are more than 6 cm in transverse diameter rupture within two years if not surgically resected. Aneurysms less than 6 cm across may also rupture, albeit less frequently.

Mortalities of emergency and elective surgery

Elective surgical repair has a much lower mortality than emergency surgery for rupture and is therefore recommended for most abdominal aortic aneurysms greater than 5 cm in diameter, or those expanding in diameter at a rate exceeding 1 cm per year. Mortality for surgical repair of abdominal aneurysms is also lower than that of thoracic aneurysms.

Aortic dissection

This is a tear in the intima of the aorta followed by the entry of blood into media with separation of a 'flap' of intima from the rest of the aortic wall. A false lumen is created, usually between the inner two-thirds and outer third of the medial thickness giving the appearance of a double-barrelled aorta.

Types of dissecting aneurysms

There are two types:

- Type A (66% of dissecting aneurysms) arise in the ascending aorta with or without extension into the descending aorta.
- Type B (33% of dissecting aneurysms) are confined to the descending aorta, distal to the origin of the left subclavian artery.

Epidemiology—There are approximately 600 cases per year in the UK, occurring most commonly between 50 and 70 years old, affecting males more than females by 2:1.

It is usually the result of cystic medial degeneration (see p. 95). Predisposing factors are:

- Hypertension.
- Connective tissue disorders (e.g. Marfan's syndrome).
- Pregnancy.
- Congenital abnormalities of the aortic valve.

Consequences

The false lumen inevitably ruptures, either:

- Externally—external rupture leads to massive fatal bleed into the thoracic cavity, or less commonly, the pericardial sac, pleural cavity, or abdomen.
- Internally—rarely, blood tracks back into the lumen by rupturing through the inner media and intima forming a double-channelled aorta.

The clinical features are characterized by:

- Severe pain: sudden onset in chest and back, often arising between the shoulder blades.
- Hypertension.
- Asymmetry of brachial, carotid or femoral pulses.
- Broadening of the upper mediastinum on chest radiograph.
- Distortion of aortic 'knuckle' (but not invariably) on chest radiograph.
- Commonly, left-sided pleural effusion.

Diagnosis is by CT or angiography.

Management depends on which type occurs:

- Type A requires emergency surgical repair under cardiopulmonary bypass.

- Type B requires control of hypertension with bedrest; surgical intervention may be needed if there is evidence of leakage, or of renal or bowel ischaemia.

Prognosis—This condition is fatal without treatment: 25% die within 24 hours, 50% within the week, and almost all by one year.

Syphilitic (luetic) aneurysms
Cardiovascular complications of untreated syphilis manifest one to three decades after initial infection and include:
- Inflammation of the arterial media (aortitis), primarily of the ascending aorta.
- Aneurysm formation due to deterioration of elastic fibres and weakening of media.
- Aortic regurgitation: dilatation of the aortic root weakens aortic valve support.
- Narrowing of coronary artery ostia by inflammation and aortic intimal proliferation leading to an increased rise of myocardial ischaemia.

These complications are now rare due to the early administration of antibiotic therapy.

- ⊙ **List the main causes of aneurysms.**
- ⊙ **Describe the features of abdominal aortic aneurysms.**
- ⊙ **What is meant by aortic dissection?**
- ⊙ **Describe the aetiology, predisposing factors and consequences of aortic dissection.**
- ⊙ **Name the two types of dissecting aneurysms and outline their management.**
- ⊙ **Describe the cardiovascular complications of untreated syphilis.**

INFLAMMATORY AND NEOPLASTIC VASCULAR DISEASE

Concepts and classification
Vasculitides
This is a group of disorders characterized by inflammation of the blood vessel walls (vasculitis). Vasculitis can affect capillaries, venules, arterioles, arteries and occasionally large veins.

Effect
The effects are:
- Mild cases: transient damage to the vessel wall produces leakage of red blood cells.
- Severe cases: irreversible vessel wall destruction resulting in ischaemia and organ damage with associated systemic disturbances.

Classification
Vasculitis can be classified either according to the size of the vessel affected (Fig. 7.25) or according to the pathogenesis of the inflammation (Fig. 7.26).

Mechanisms of pathogenesis
Idiopathic
The aetiology is unknown but the disorders (Fig. 7.26) are as follows:
- Giant cell arteritis (see below).
- Scleroderma (systemic sclerosis): vascular changes are similar to those of benign or malignant hypertension, but only about 25% are hypertensive. Condition is associated with progressive subcutaneous fibrosis leading to a marked tightening of the skin of the arms and hands; there is no effective treatment.
- Takayasu's (pulseless) disease: a rare inflammatory disorder of the aorta and its proximal branches typically affecting young or middle-aged females. Condition is characterized by severe necrotizing inflammation of all layers of affected vessel walls with fibrous replacement of muscle and reduction of lumen. It presents clinically with hypertension or ischaemic symptoms of the arms with loss of arm pulses.
- Kawasaki's disease: a disease of infants which affects the main aortic branch arteries particularly the coronary arteries; characterized by medial

Classification of vasculitis according to size of affected vessel	
Size of vessel	**Disorders**
large, medium and small	syphilitic aortitis Takayasu's disease giant cell arteritis Kawasaki's disease rheumatoid disease
medium and small	Wegener's granulomatosis polyarteritis nodosa Buerger's disease SLE
small	small vessel disease of arterioles, capillaries, and venules Henoch–Schönlein purpura

Fig. 7.25 Classification of vasculitis according to the size of the affected vessel.

Classification of vasculitis by pathogenesis	
Pathogenesis	**Disorders**
idiopathic	giant cell arteritis scleroderma (systemic sclerosis) Takayasu's (pulseless) disease Kawasaki's disease Buerger's disease
immune-mediated	polyarteritis nodosa Wegener's granulomatosis rheumatoid vasculitis SLE Henoch–Schönlein purpura
infectious	syphilitic aortitis bacterial aortitis

Fig. 7.26 Classification of vasculitis by pathogenesis.

fibroblastic thickening and sometimes aneurysm formation.

- Buerger's disease (thromboangitis obliterans): a rare disease with a strong association with smoking. Condition mainly affects the small arteries of the arms and lower leg which show intimal fibrosis, thrombus formation, and adventitial tissue changes affecting adjacent veins and nerves. Clinically, peripheral gangrene develops in the fingers and toes; disease is progressive and amputations are often required.

Immune-mediated vasculitis
Pathogenesis is due to immune complex formation between antigens and antibodies. Immune complexes become trapped in venule walls and activate complement producing a local, acute inflammatory response with neutrophil chemotaxis. Neutrophils release enzymes which destroy the vessel wall.

There are two main types:
- Hypersensitivity (neutrophilic) vasculitis: commonest pattern affecting capillaries and venules; usually manifests as a skin rash, often as a result of an allergy to a drug or occasionally arising as an allergic rash in viraemia or bacteraemia. It also occurs in Henoch–Schönlein purpura, serum sickness and cryoglobulinaemia.
- Multi-organ autoimmune diseases, e.g. SLE and rheumatoid disease (mainly affects the aorta).

Autoantibodies that react against neutrophils can be detected in 90% of patients with Wegener's granulomatosis and in other types of vasculitis. Identification of these antibodies in serum is used in diagnostic evaluation of patients with possible vasculitis.

Infectious vasculitis
These disorders (Fig. 7.26) include:
- Syphilitic aortitis: tertiary manifestation of syphilis typically affecting the ascending and transverse portions of the aortic arch causing inflammatory destruction of media with fibrous replacement.
- Other infections: bacteria in infected thrombi can cause destruction of vessel walls with the development of small saccular dilatations and mycotic aneurysms.

Giant cell (temporal) arteritis
This systemic disease mainly involves arteries in the head and neck region, particularly the temporal arteries (hence alternative name of temporal arteritis).

Epidemiology—The disease is relatively common, affecting 10 per 100 000 per year in the general population in Europe. Incidence increases with age, and is rare under 50 years; it affects females more than males by 2:1.

Aetiology—An idiopathic disease with some associations with certain types of HLA.

The microscopic appearance of vessels is as follows:
- Thickened nodular vessel wall.
- Necrosis of inner media and gradual replacement with fibrosis.
- Fragmentation of internal elastic lamina.
- Inflammatory cell infiltration: mainly T lymphocytes but also histiocytes and giant cells (hence the name).
- Often complicated by thrombosis.

Clinical features—Patients have ill-defined symptoms of:
- Malaise.
- Tiredness.
- Severe headaches.
- An association with polymyalgia rheumatica.

Investigations characteristically reveal high ESR and hyperglobulinaemia. Diagnosis is made by biopsy of the temporal artery with histological investigation. Management is with corticosteroid therapy to control the disease.

Polyarteritis nodosa

This systemic disease is characterized by inflammatory necrosis of the walls of small and medium-sized arteries. Although the disease is systemic, it causes patchy and focal inflammation with only parts of some arteries being involved.

Epidemiology—A rare disease (about 5–10 per million per year in most populations) but it can occur in all age groups; males more than females by 2:1.

Aetiology—The cause is unknown but the presence of antineutrophil cytoplasmic antibodies suggests an autoimmune pathogenesis. There is also an association with chronic hepatitis B virus antigenaemia.

Pathogenesis—Inflammatory destruction results in the loss of the normal architecture of the vessel wall with necrosis of muscle cells and destruction of the elastic lamina. Healing occurs with fibrous replacement muscular media. Extensive damage to the intima predisposes to thrombosis, which is often followed by vessel occlusion and infarction of target tissue.

Microscopically, the artery wall shows:
- Inflammatory cell infiltration: neutrophils and eosinophils are most numerous.
- Fibrinoid necrosis of segments of artery wall.
- Thrombosis, which is common.

Clinical features include systemic features of inflammation (fever, weight loss, myalgia, and muscle wasting) and the effects of vessel occlusion producing small areas of infarction. Tissues most seriously affected are the kidneys, heart, GI tract, liver, CNS, peripheral nerves, skeletal muscle and skin.

Diagnosis is by:
- Blood: neutrophilia and raised ESR.
- Antineutrophil cytoplasmic antibodies, which are present in most cases.
- Tissue biopsy, usually of a kidney or asymptomatic muscle.

The prognosis depends on the intensity and pattern of organ involvement; 30% of patients develop renal failure and hypertensive complications.

Management is by cyclophosphamide with corticosteroids, which has significantly improved the outcome. Antihypertensive drugs reduce morbidity from hypertensive complications.

Neoplastic vascular disease
Benign
Haemangiomas

Haemangiomas are common developmental malformations composed of dilated vascular spaces derived from blood vessels.

There are three types of haemangioma:
- Capillary haemangiomas (strawberry naevi), which are composed of small, capillary-like vessels.
- Cavernous haemangiomas, which are composed of cavernous, endothelial-lined spaces (vein-like vessels).
- Sclerosing haemangiomas, which are fibrous nodules containing iron pigment produced as a result of fibrosis or sclerosis of a capillary haemangioma.

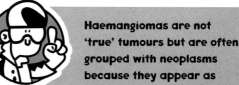

Haemangiomas are not 'true' tumours but are often grouped with neoplasms because they appear as localized tissue masses. They are more accurately described as hamartomas, i.e. non-neoplastic overgrowths of tissue.

Telangiectasias

Dilatations of capillaries are often seen in the elderly, irradiated skin, and liver failure (spider naevi). Vessels are dilated but histologically normal.

Malignant

Kaposi's sarcoma (KS)

This malignant tumour is thought to be derived from endothelial cells; it is rapidly becoming more important and common. There are four patterns of disease:

- Endemic KS (seen in Africa): highly malignant in children (through lymphatic spread) with a more indolent course in adults (through blood spread).
- Classic KS: a rare, low-grade, malignant tumour of the skin that develops in the lower limbs of elderly males; there are blood and lymph node metastases.
- KS in therapeutic immunosuppression, which resembles classic KS.
- Epidemic KS: a highly malignant tumour of the skin seen in patients with AIDS; spreads to lymph nodes and the visceral organs.

Angiosarcoma

A malignant tumour of blood vessel endothelium. This most commonly occurs as a raised bluish-red patch on the face or scalp of elderly people. Progressive enlargement of the tumour is accompanied by ulceration and later metastasis to regional lymph nodes.

DISEASES OF THE VEINS AND LYMPHATICS

Varicose veins

Varicose veins are persistently distended superficial veins in the lower limbs (long and short saphenous veins). They result from incompetent valves which allow the veins to become engorged with blood under the influence of gravity.

Epidemiology—The condition affects 10–20% of the general population at some age. There is an increasing incidence with age, and it is most common above 50. It affects females more than males by 4:1.

See Fig. 7.32 for the predisposing factors of varicose veins.

Anatomy of varicose veins—The superficial and deep venous plexuses of the lower limb are connected by perforating veins (Fig. 7.33).

Pathogenesis—The return of blood from the deep veins is aided by normal contraction of the calf and thigh muscles. If the valves in the perforating veins become incompetent, blood is forced from deep venous plexuses to superficial venous plexuses resulting in increased pressure in the superficial veins; this is a major factor in the development of varicosities.

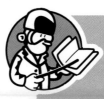

- Define 'vasculitides'.
- Explain the different types of pathogenesis of vasculitides.
- Describe the microscopic appearance of vessels in giant cell arteritis.
- What are the basic features of polyarteritis nodosa?
- Name the different types of haemangiomas.

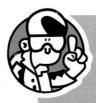

Understanding the anatomy of the superficial veins of the lower limb will enable you to get to grips with the pathogenesis of varicose veins.

Morphological changes

The morphological changes are:

- Increased pressure produces a dilatation of the lumen and an increased tension on vessel walls with compensatory hypertrophy of the muscle and elastic tissues.
- Prolonged increased pressure produces irregular atrophy of muscle and elastic with fibrous replacement leading to stretched, tortuous veins with localized bulging.

Predisposing factors of varicose veins
defective support of vessel wall • familial tendency: in approx. 40% of all cases • gender: significantly increased incidence in females • obesity: adipose tissue = poor venous support; muscle = good venous support • age: degenerative changes in surrounding tissues and decreased activity of muscles →   loss of venous support
increased venous pressure • standing occupations: increased incidence in occupations involving prolonged standing   (venous pressure is greatest on standing) • pregnancy • intravascular thrombosis • tumour masses pressing on veins (e.g. uterine fibroids and ovarian tumours) • garters and other constrictions

Fig. 7.27 Predisposing factors of varicose veins.

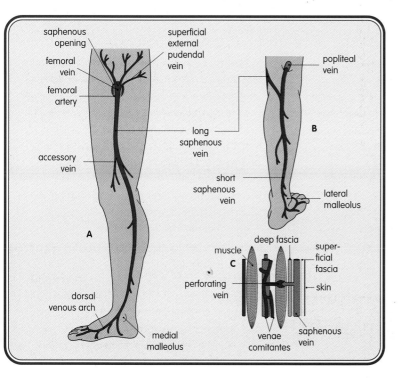

Fig. 7.28 Superficial veins of the right lower limb. (A) Long saphenous vein. (B) Short saphenous vein. (C) 'Venous pump' showing valved perforating veins which link deep and superficial veins.

Sequelae of varicose veins

The sequelae are:

• Oedema (of lower limbs) due to increased hydrostatic pressure.
• Thromboembolism: thrombosis is a frequent complication.
• Dermatitis: varicose dermatitis with pigmentation due to haemosiderin deposition.
• Varicose ulcers: dermatitis may proceed to ulceration, which is very slow to heal.

Thrombophlebitis and phlebothrombosis

Definitions

Thrombophlebitis is thrombosis initiated by inflammation of the vessel wall. Phlebothrombosis is inflammation of the vessel wall secondary to thrombosis of non-inflammatory origin.

A histological differentiation between the two types is in most cases impossible.

Causes

Factors giving rise to stasis:

- Cardiac failure.
- Pregnancy.
- Prolonged bed rest.
- Immobilization.
- Varicose veins.

Factors which cause direct injury or infection of the veins, e.g. trauma or intravenous cannulation.

Affected sites

The most commonly affected sites are:

- Deep leg veins (90% of cases) particularly the lower leg.
- Skull and dural sinuses.
- Portal venous tributaries.
- Pelvic veins.

Presentation

Presentation of both types is similar, with distension of the veins by laminated thrombus. Organization and subsequent recanalization of thrombus may later occur.

Complications

Acute

Acute complications include embolism to the pulmonary arteries or rupture of veins with haemorrhage.

Chronic

Chronic complications are aching pains due to varicose veins, and ulceration.

Management of thrombotic events

Treatment is aimed at preventing the propagation of thrombus. Immediate treatment is by heparin, warfarin, and clot busters (thrombolytic agents) in selected cases.

Long-term treatment is by oral anticoagulants, mobilization, and graduated elastic stockings.

Lymphangitis and lymphoedema

Lymphangitis

This is inflammation of lymphatic channels draining any focus of infection. The channels are dilated and contain inflammatory cells. The condition may result in the spread of the infection in some cases, e.g. in tuberculosis.

Lymphoedema

This is oedema of the tissues due to obstruction of the lymphatics.

Causes of obstructive lymphoedema are:

- Metastatic spread of tumours causing mechanical blockage.
- Surgical removal of nodes.
- Post-irradiation fibrosis.
- Filariases (elephantiases): nematode infection of lymph nodes (commonest culprit is *Wuchereria bancrofti*); transmitted to man by the bite of an infected mosquito.
- Post-inflammatory thrombosis and scarring, e.g. lymphogranuloma venereum.
- Primary lymphatic disorders (rare).

Effects

The effects are:

- Gross swelling.
- Increased predisposition to attacks of lymphangitis and ulceration.
- Severe cases result in thickening of skin and overgrowth of dermal connective tissues leading to elephantiasis.

- Define 'varicose veins'.
- Name the factors that predispose to the development of varicose veins.
- Describe the pathogenesis of varicose veins.
- What is the difference between thrombophlebitis and phlebothrombosis?
- State the main causes of these conditions.
- What are the complications of inflammation and thrombosis of vessel walls?
- Describe the causes of lymphoedema.

8. Pathology of the Respiratory System

The nose and nasopharynx
Inflammatory conditions
Rhinitis

Rhinitis, inflammation of the nasal mucosa, is the most common nasal disorder seen in family practice. The condition may be either acute or chronic.

Acute rhinitis

Aetiology of acute rhinitis is either:

• Infective.
• Allergic.

Infectious rhinitis is usually viral in origin, e.g. the common cold (rhinoviruses, respiratory syncytial virus, para-influenza viruses, coronaviruses) and influenza (influenza virus). Virally induced inflammation of surface epithelial cells is followed by exudation of fluid and mucus from the damaged surface ('runny nose'). Later, submucosal oedema produces swelling which may lead to a partial blockage of the nasal airways.

Allergic rhinitis ('hay fever'): type I (IgE-mediated) hypersensitivity reaction to inhaled materials such as grass and pollens produces a mixed serous–mucous exudate, and submucosal oedema leads to nasal blockage.

Chronic rhinitis

Chronic rhinitis can be caused by either chronic infective inflammation or chronic allergic inflammation and may result in the development of nasal polyps.

Macroscopically, nasal polyps are typically smooth-surfaced, creamy, semi-translucent, ovoid masses.

Microscopically, they have oedematous tissue with scattered infiltrate of chronic inflammatory cells including plasma cells. Eosinophils are often very numerous in allergic polyps.

Sinusitis (inflammation of the sinuses)
Acute sinusitis

The most important type of sinus inflammation is acute maxillary sinusitis (ethmoidal and frontal sinusitis being less common).

Aetiology—Usually secondary to acute rhinitis.

Pathogenesis—In acute rhinitis, there is usually associated inflammation of the sinus linings; swelling of the mucosa around the drainage foramen of the maxillary sinus in the nasal cavity may cause stasis of maxillary sinus secretions. Stasis predisposes to secondary bacterial infection with alteration of the static maxillary fluid from seromucous to purulent.

In severe cases the infection may spread into the ethmoid and frontal sinuses with risk of spread of infection to meninges.

Chronic sinusitis

This condition is characterized by chronically thickened and inflamed mucosa of sinuses, and persistent fluid accumulation.

The condition may arise as a result of:

• Acute sinusitis from failure of drainage of acutely inflamed sinus.
• Chronic inhalation of irritant, e.g. cigarette smoke, industrial exposure.
• Nasal obstruction as a result of a severely deviated nasal septum or from the presence of nasal polyps.

Kartagener's syndrome

This is a syndrome of bronchiectasis, sinusitis and situs inversus (transposition of viscera). Sinusitis is caused by abnormal ciliary function resulting in a failure to clear mucus and bacteria.

Necrotizing lesions
Mucormycotic infections

This fulminant opportunistic fungal infection of the nose is usually the result of immune suppression or prolonged antibiotic therapy. It may be rapidly fatal unless treated promptly with systemic antifungals.

Wegener's granulomatosis

An autoimmune granulomatous vasculitis, this frequently presents with nasal lesions.

Lethal midline granuloma (lymphoma)

This is a condition presenting with progressive ulceration and destruction of the structures in the upper respiratory tract, i.e. the nose, nasopharynx, palate, and sinuses. It is thought to be a form of T cell lymphoma, and characterized histologically by the infiltration of small lymphocytes, plasma cells, blast cells and atypical, large lymphoid cells.

Untreated, death occurs from systemic disease caused by erosion of blood vessels, superadded local infection or the development of pneumonia.

Neoplasms

Nasopharyngeal angiofibroma

This rare benign tumour (also known as juvenile angiofibroma) occurs almost exclusively in males between 10 and 25 years old. The lesions are typically located in the nasopharynx rather than the nose, and during puberty may mimic a malignant tumour in their rapid growth and tendency to erode bone. Ulceration and bleeding are common.

Inverted papilloma

A benign, endophytic (hence 'inverted') tumour of adults, this is associated with human papillomavirus infection. It can be difficult to eradicate and may recur. Malignant transformation occurs in approximately 3%.

Plasmacytomas

This malignant tumour is composed of monoclonal plasma cells. It presents as a soft, haemorrhagic nasal/nasopharyngeal mass, which may progress to disseminated myeloma after many years.

Olfactory neuroblastoma

A rare nasal tumour presenting in the upper part of the nasal cavity, often as a haemorrhagic mass with evidence of bone destruction, it is typically slow growing but may recur after surgical removal. Metastases occur in about 20% of cases.

Nasopharyngeal carcinoma

This is a squamous or anaplastic carcinoma of the nasopharynx (part of pharynx that lies immediately behind the nasal cavities) with characteristic abundant lymphoid tissue in the stroma.

It is strongly associated with Epstein–Barr virus infection, the virus being demonstrable in tumour cells in most cases.

The tumours often remain small and undetected until metastasis to the lymph nodes in the neck has occurred. The vast majority of patients with nasopharyngeal carcinoma have lymph node metastases when they first present.

The prognosis is good with radiation therapy: 80% have a 5-year survival rate for localized disease, and 50% for advanced disease.

The larynx
Inflammatory conditions
Acute laryngitis

This acute inflammation of the larynx may be infective (majority of cases), allergic or irritative.

Infective laryngitis

This typically occurs secondary to either viral or bacterial upper respiratory tract infection involving the nose, sinuses, etc.

Allergic laryngitis

This follows inhalation or ingestion of an allergen.

Irritative laryngitis

This follows ingestion or inhalation of irritant gases or fluids (e.g. ammonia, cigarette smoke) or following irritation by mechanical factors, e.g. endotracheal intubation.

The sequelae are:
- Resolution: infective causes typically resolve without complications.
- Spread of infection may occur throughout the respiratory tract with the development of tracheobronchitis, bronchopneumonia or lung abscesses; it is more common in the elderly or debilitated due to poor cough reflex.
- Airway obstruction: laryngeal oedema can result in a life-threatening narrowing of the airway especially in

children (whose airways are narrower) suffering from *Haemophilus influenzae* epiglottitis or in cases of corrosive chemical ingestion.

Croup

An acute inflammation and obstruction of the respiratory tract involving the larynx, trachea and bronchi, which affects young children (usually aged 6 months to 3 years).

Aetiology—Typically caused by viral infection but secondary bacterial infection can occur.

The condition produces symptoms of laryngitis accompanied by signs of obstruction: harsh difficult breathing (stridor), a rising pulse rate, restlessness and cyanosis.

Treatment is by reassurance and humidification of inspired air which usually reverses the symptoms. In severe cases, the obstruction may require treatment by intubation or tracheostomy.

Chronic laryngitis

This is a chronic inflammation of the larynx, most commonly seen in heavy cigarette smokers. It may lead to a permanent thickening of the laryngeal mucosa and submucosa, particularly where there is associated excess production of keratin ('smoker's keratosis').

Overlying epidermis may also undergo keratotic thickening with dysplastic change in the basal layer; this is a predisposing factor in the development of squamous carcinoma.

Reactive nodules

Polyps

This common benign lesion is associated with upper respiratory tract infection or occurs after vocal abuse, e.g. shouting. It causes hoarseness which will not resolve until the polyp is removed.

Singer's nodules

These are smooth, round, minute nodules located at the nodal point at the junction between the anterior third and posterior two-thirds of the vocal cords. Nodules are especially common in singers and professional voice users, and can alter the character of the voice even when only a few millimetres in diameter. They consist of oedematous connective tissue with submucosal fibrosis covered by squamous epithelium.

Papilloma and papillomatosis

Papilloma

Warty papillomas on the larynx are usually due to infection by the human papillomavirus (HPV 11 and 16). The lesions are usually solitary and confined to the vocal cords. Papilloma is clincially and histologically difficult to distinguish from early verrucous carcinomas (see below).

Juvenile laryngeal papillomatosis

These multiple soft pink papillomas on the vocal cords are largely confined to children. Lesions often extend into other parts of the larynx, sometimes even down the trachea, and have the histological features of florid viral warts. They are typically persistent and recurrent, such that eradication is difficult, often requiring repeated multiple excisions.

Squamous cell carcinoma of the larynx

This accounts for 1–2% of cancers with an incidence of 1–2 per 100 000 per year worldwide. It typically presents after 40 years of age, affecting males more than females (but the incidence is rising in females). The risk factors are smoking, radiation to head and neck, carcinoma *in situ* and keratosis (see above).

The affected sites are:
- Supraglottic region (30%), e.g. epiglottis, false cords and ventricles.
- Glottic region (60%): true vocal cords and anterior and posterior commissures; best prognosis if detected early (early symptom being hoarseness).
- Subglottic region (10%): arising below the true vocal cords and above the first tracheal ring; poor prognosis if late presentation.

Macroscopically, they are ulcerated, diffuse, grey, solid or papillary lesions.

Microscopically, the majority are well-differentiated, keratinizing squamous carcinomas; a minority are poorly differentiated with spindle cells.

Spread can be:
- Local: to adjacent laryngeal structures but often confined by laryngeal cartilages for a considerable time.
- Lymphatic: to regional lymph nodes.
- Haematogenous: occurs late if at all; lungs are the commonest site.

The prognosis depends on location, extent of spread and the presence of lymph node metastasis. Overall prognosis is as follows:

- Glottic tumours—80% (5-year survival).
- Supraglottic tumours—65% (5-year survival).
- Subglottic tumours—40% (5-year survival).

Verrucous carcinoma

This is a variant of laryngeal squamous cell carcinoma, often presenting as a large, warty, papillary tumour with all the clinical features of malignancy. It usually affects one or both of the true vocal cords, the lesions being composed of benign-looking squamous epithelium with hyperkeratosis. However, the tumour is locally destructive and requires surgical removal to prevent fatal obstruction or laryngeal destruction. Metastasis is rare.

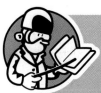

- **What are the causes of acute and chronic rhinitis?**
- **Name the necrotizing lesions that may affect the nose and nasopharynx.**
- **What are the clinical features of nasopharyngeal tumours?**
- **List the causes of acute laryngitis.**
- **Define 'croup'.**
- **Describe the pathology of squamous cell carcinoma of the larynx.**

DISORDERS OF THE LUNGS

Atelectasis

This is a defective expansion and collapse of the lung. It may occur as a result of:

- Obstruction.
- Compression.
- Scarring.
- Surfactant loss.

Obstructive causes

Obstruction of the larger bronchial tubes leads to resorption of air from the lung distal to the obstruction.

Causes of obstruction can be within the lung (retained secretions, inhaled foreign bodies or bronchial cancer) or outside the lung (enlarged lymph nodes as in TB or lung cancer).

Patchy atelectasis describes the pattern of atelectasis associated with chronic obstructive airway diseases.

Compressive causes

Compressive atelectasis is the compression of the lung caused by the accumulation of fluid or air in the pleural cavity.

Scarring

Scarring of the lung may cause contraction of the parenchyma and lung collapse.

Surfactant loss

Surfactant loss can be either developmental or acquired and leads to a generalized failure of lung expansion, termed microatelectasis.

Consequences of atelectasis

The collapse of a lung has important clinical consequences of disturbing respiratory function. Expansion can be aided by physiotherapy and bronchoscopy-mediated removal of the obstructive/compressive cause. However, prolonged atelectasis becomes irreversible.

Chronic obstructive pulmonary disease
Differences between obstructive and restrictive lung diseases
Obstructive lung diseases

Obstructive lung diseases are those diseases in which there is obstruction to the *flow* of air within the lungs, although the lungs themselves may be hyperinflated. If obstruction is long term, then these conditions are collectively known as chronic obstructive pulmonary (or airway) diseases, i.e. COPD.

Restrictive lung diseases

Restrictive lung diseases are those diseases in which there is obstruction to the *expansion* of the lungs (e.g. due to fibrosis or oedema) such that they can only take in a limited amount of air. In these diseases, although the lungs are often underinflated, the rate of air flow is unaffected. These diseases are covered in more detail later under 'Diffuse interstitial diseases' on p. 122.

Both obstructive and restrictive lung diseases can cause significant respiratory impairment with a characteristic pattern of pulmonary function tests (Fig. 8.1).

Chronic obstructive pulmonary diseases (COPD)

There are two main mechanisms by which airflow may be reduced in COPD, causing two different clinical pictures:

- Increased airway resistance, typically by a narrowing of the airways, e.g. chronic bronchitis, bronchiectasis and asthma; results in hypercapnia, hypoxaemia and cyanosis. Patients are often referred to as 'blue bloaters'.
- Decreased outflow pressure due to loss of elastic recoil of the lungs, e.g. emphysema. However, in this case, compensatory hyperventilation leads to relatively normal levels of $Paco_2$ and Pao_2 at rest. Patients are often referred to as 'pink puffers'.

COPDs can be diagnosed with chest X-ray (which may show hyperinflation, flat hemidiaphragms, reduced peripheral vascular markings, and bullae) and lung function tests (Fig. 8.1).

Treatment is by:
- Physiotherapy.
- Bronchodilators (e.g. salbutamol): there is often a reversible element to airway obstruction due to local bronchial irritation causing bronchoconstriction.
- Antibiotics for associated chronic bronchitis.

Note that respiratory centres of patients with COPD are relatively insensitive to CO_2, relying on hypoxic drive to maintain respiratory effort. It is thus dangerous to give these patients supplemental oxygen without careful observation as hypoventilation or apnoea may result.

Emphysema

Emphysema is a permanent dilatation of any part of the air spaces distal to the terminal bronchiole with destruction of tissue but no scarring. It is a common condition with increasing incidence with age, and is more common in males than in females.

The aetiology is unclear but risk factors include cigarette smoking, atmospheric pollution and a family history.

Associations—The majority of cases are seen in conjunction with chronic bronchitis.

Pathogenesis

In normal individuals, extracellular proteases secreted into the lung by inflammatory cells are inhibited by protease-inhibitors (particularly α_1-antitrypsin). In emphysema, these inhibitors are either inactivated (e.g. by smoke) or absent, resulting in continued activity of the proteases with destruction of lung parenchyma (Fig. 8.2). Destruction of respiratory tissue leads to a loss of elastic recoil in the lungs and a decreased area available for gas exchange. About one-third of lung capacity must be destroyed before clinical symptoms of emphysema appear.

Types of emphysema

There are several forms of emphysema, defined by the location of damage in the respiratory acinus (Fig. 8.3):

Characteristic patterns of lung function tests in obstructive and restrictive lung diseases		
	Obstructive lung diseases	**Restrictive lung diseases**
vital capacity (VC)	↓ or normal	↓↓
FEV_1	↓↓	↓
FEV_1/VC ratio	↓	normal or ↑
peak respiratory flow rate (PEFR)	↓	normal

Fig. 8.1 Characteristic patterns of lung function tests in obstructive and restrictive lung diseases.

- Centrilobular: dilatation of the respiratory bronchioles at the centre of acinus. It is most common in men and is closely associated with cigarette smoking. Lesions are most commonly found in the upper lobes.
- Panlobular: dilatation of the terminal alveoli and alveolar ducts, which later affects the respiratory bronchioles, thereby affecting the whole acinus. Typically affects the lower lobes.
- Paraseptal: involves air spaces at the periphery of lobules, typically adjacent to pleura. Typically affects the upper lobes.
- Irregular: irregular involvement of the respiratory acinus, and almost always associated with scarring. It is thought to be caused by the trapping of air caused by fibrosis, and is therefore commonly present around old healed tuberculous scars at the lung apices.

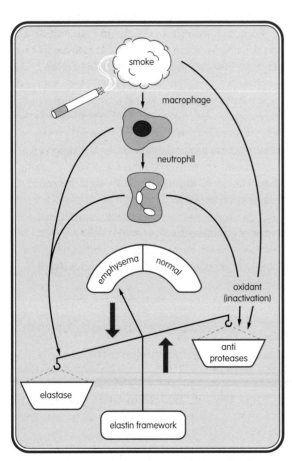

Fig. 8.2 Pathogenesis of emphysema. (Adapted with permission from *The Lungs* by B Corrin, Churchill Livingstone, 1990.)

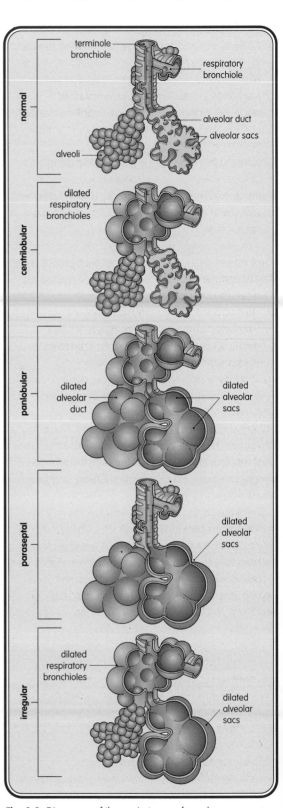

Fig. 8.3 Diagrams of the main types of emphysema.

Clinical features:
- Early stage: rapid respiratory rate enables individuals to maintain blood oxygenation, such that levels of $Paco_2$ and Pao_2 are near normal. Patients are breathless but not cyanosed ('pink puffers'). However, on the slightest exertion patients become increasingly breathless and ultimately hypoxic (type 1 respiratory failure).
- Later stage: despite an increased respiratory rate there is reduced oxygen uptake even at rest. A progressive decline in respiratory function ensues with the development of cyanosis, hypercapnia and cor pulmonale.

The lungs are hyperinflated, the trachea is often descended (i.e. there is decreased distance between the thyroid cartilage and the sternal notch) and the accessory muscles may be hypertrophied. Associated chronic bronchitis may produce cough and sputum. Breath sounds are quiet especially over bullae, often with crepitations or wheezes.

Chronic bronchitis
Chronic bronchitis is defined as a cough productive of sputum on most days for three months of the year for at least two successive years. It typically affects middle-aged men, and most cases are due to cigarette smoking.

Pathogenesis—Constant irritation by cigarette smoke causes chronic inflammation of the respiratory bronchioles (bronchiolitis) and increased mucus secretion.

Hypersecretion of mucus is associated with hypertrophy and hyperplasia of the bronchial mucus-secreting glands. The Reid index gives the ratio of gland to wall thickness in the bronchus, and is significantly increased in cases of chronic bronchitis.

Bronchiolar obstruction must be extensive and widespread to give clinical symptoms. Eventually, extensive mucus plugging leads to the clinical obstructive features of the disease with typical cough and sputum.

Clinical features:
- Early stages: chronic cough with sputum.
- Later stages: disease becomes progressively more severe and is accompanied by hypercapnia, hypoxaemia and cyanosis (often producing 'blue bloaters'). Eventually right heart failure (cor pulmonale) or respiratory failure ensues.

The condition may be complicated by:
- Recurrent low grade bronchial infections caused by bacteria such as *H. influenzae* and *Streptococcus pneumoniae,* or viruses such as respiratory syncytial virus and adenovirus.
- Squamous metaplasia: loss of ciliated cells as a result of squamous metaplasia can further exacerbate the problem.
- Malignancy: persistent injury by smoking may invoke dysplastic changes in metaplastic squamous epithelium, which may ultimately become malignant (squamous cell carcinoma of the bronchus).

Bronchial asthma
An increased irritability of the bronchial tree with paroxysmal narrowing of the airways which may reverse either spontaneously or after treatment.

This is a common disorder, affecting around 10% of children and 5% of adults. Its incidence is thought to be rising, possibly due to environmental atmospheric pollution.

There are several known triggers of asthma:
- Allergy: a large number of allergens can precipitate asthma by inducing an IgE-mediated type I hypersensitivity reaction. Examples include pollen, house dust mites, animal dander, foods, and drugs.
- Infection: respiratory tract infection can trigger bronchoconstriction.
- Occupational exposure: some agents act as allergens, others by direct irritation of the airway.
- Drug induced, e.g. β-antagonists and aspirin.
- Irritant gases, e.g. sulphur dioxide, nitric oxide, ozone in smog.
- Psychological stress can exacerbate attacks.
- Cold air.
- Exercise, especially in combination with cold air.

Asthma is associated with other atopic diseases such as eczema, hay fever and some allergies.

Asthma can be classified into two categories, depending on whether there is an allergic basis to the disease:
- Extrinsic asthma (atopic): early onset asthma triggered by environmental allergens. Individuals often have a family history of allergic

disorders. IgE levels are raised and an immediate type 1 hypersensitivity to the allergen is produced on skin challenge. This is the most common type of asthma.

- Intrinsic asthma (non atopic): a late onset asthma often triggered by infection of the upper respiratory tract. IgE levels are normal, there is no family history of allergic disorders, and skin testing is negative.

However, there is often much overlap between the two types, and many patients do not fit neatly into any one type.

Pathogenesis—In both types of asthma, obstruction is caused by a combination of bronchospasm, oedema and mucus plugging. The exact mechanisms of intrinsic asthma are uncertain, but in the case of extrinsic (atopic) asthma a generalized airway hyperresponsiveness to bronchoconstrictor trigger factors is known to be central to the pathogenesis.

The three phases of extrinsic asthma
- Early (15–20 minutes): a rapid onset bronchoconstriction caused by histamine release from mast cell degranulation. The allergen binds to IgE antibodies on the surface of mast cells causing cross linking of mast cells, resulting in their degranulation (Fig. 8.4).
- Late (4–6 hours): a second wave of bronchoconstriction after recovery from the early phase. Inflammatory mediators released by mast cells during the early phase cause activation of macrophages and chemotaxis of polymorphs and eosinophils into the bronchial mucosa. These cells release inflammatory mediators causing a secondary wave of bronchoconstriction (Fig. 8.5).
- Prolonged hyperreactivity (over days): an exaggerated response of the airway on further re-exposure to the allergen or other bronchoconstrictor trigger factors over ensuing days. It is caused by the persistence of inflammatory cells within the bronchial wall with damage and loss of epithelial cells.

The main structural changes that take place in asthmatic airways are listed below and illustrated in Fig. 8.5:
- Immune cell infiltration: bronchial mucosa is infiltrated by eosinophils, mast cells, lymphoid cells and macrophages.
- Mucosal oedema: extravasation of plasma into submucosal tissues produces a narrowing of the airways.
- Mucus hypersecretion leads to plugging of airways.
- Hypertrophy of bronchial smooth muscle due to recurrent bronchoconstriction.
- Focal necrosis of the airway epithelium, caused by prolonged inflammation.
- Deposition of collagen beneath bronchial epithelium in long-standing cases.
- Sputum contains Charcot–Leyden crystals (derived

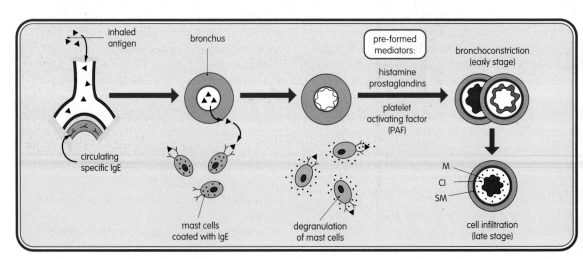

Fig. 8.4 Pathogenesis of the early and late stages of asthma. M = mucus; Cl = cellular infiltration; SM = smooth muscle.

from eosinophil granules) and Curschmann's spirals (composed of mucus plugs from small airways).

Clinical features are as follows:
- Mild disease (majority of cases): acute intermittent episodes of bronchospasm (wheezing, dyspnoea or coughing) are triggered by well-recognized causes.
- Moderate to severe disease (small percentage): increasingly severe and increasingly irreversible asthma in middle or old age (chronic asthma); patients may present with signs of respiratory distress.
- Status asthmaticus: severe, acute disease that does not respond to drug therapy. Air entry may be inadequate to generate any wheeze (the silent chest is an ominous sign) and death may result from acute respiratory insufficiency.

The signs of asthma include widespread, polyphonic, high-pitched wheezes, as the affected airways are of varying size but mostly small calibre. Barrel chest may be seen in cases of chronic asthma.

The main complication is cor pulmonale. Pulmonary vasoconstriction caused by chronic alveolar hypoventilation results in pulmonary hypertension leading to right ventricular hypertrophy.

The disease can usually be successfully controlled by drug therapy:
- β_2-adrenoreceptor agonists, e.g. salbutamol, relax bronchial smooth muscle, acting within minutes.
- Corticosteroids, e.g. beclomethasone. This is the keystone of therapy in moderate to severe asthma, acting over a period of days by decreasing bronchial mucosal inflammations.
- Aminophylline is thought to inhibit phosphodiesterase, thus decreasing bronchoconstriction.
- Anticholinergics may reduce muscle spasm synergistically with β_2-agonists.
- Cromoglycate is useful for prophylaxis in mild asthma, especially in children.

The prognosis is:
- Remission: approximately 50% of cases of childhood asthma resolve spontaneously; remission in adult-onset asthma is less likely.

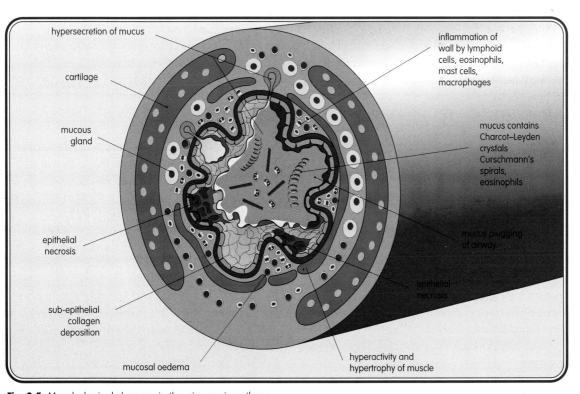

Fig. 8.5 Morphological changes in the airways in asthma.

hypersecretion of mucus

cartilage

mucous gland

epithelial necrosis

sub-epithelial collagen deposition

mucosal oedema

inflammation of wall by lymphoid cells, eosinophils, mast cells, macrophages

mucus contains Charcot–Leyden crystals Curschmann's spirals, eosinophils

mucus plugging of airway

epithelial necrosis

hyperactivity and hypertrophy of muscle

- Mortality: death occurs in approximately 0.2% of asthmatics accounting for about 2000 deaths per year in the UK. Mortality is usually (but not always) preceded by an acute attack and about 50% are more than 65 years old.

Bronchiectasis

This is an irreversible dilatation of the bronchi or their branches. Its causes are:

- Congenital: cystic fibrosis and Kartagener's syndrome (bronchiectasis, dextrocardia and sinusitis).
- Acquired: infection (especially whooping cough, pneumonia or measles in childhood) and obstruction (either by an inhaled foreign body or by a growth).

Widened bronchi are prone to infections, *H. influenzae* and *Pseudomonas aeruginosa* being the most common pathogens. Patients often cough up purulent sputum which may contain blood.

Treatment consists of antibiotics for infections and physiotherapy to drain sputum.

Cystic fibrosis (CF)

A hereditary multisystem disease characterized by the production of abnormally thick mucus, and primarily affecting the lung and pancreas. It is the commonest autosomal recessive disorder affecting 1 in 2500 newborns. Approximately 1 in 25 are heterozygous carriers of the CF gene.

Pathogenesis—The mutated gene has been located to chromosome 7 and encodes for a protein termed the cystic fibrosis transmembrane regulator (CFTR). This protein normally enables the transport of chloride ions across cell membranes. In cystic fibrosis, defective CFTR results in impaired chloride transport, which prevents the release of sodium and water to liquefy mucus. The net result is the production of an extremely thick mucus by the exocrine glands, including the mucus-secreting glands, sweat glands and others.

Viscid mucus may cause obstruction of the following systems:

- Bronchi: abnormally viscid mucus cannot be cleared from the lungs.

- Intestine: causing meconium ileus in newborn babies.
- Pancreas: causing deficiency of the pancreatic enzymes, resulting in malabsorption and failure to thrive.

In the respiratory tract, the bronchi and bronchioles become obstructed by abnormally viscid mucus, which leads to four main problems:

- Infections: obstruction and stagnation of secretions leads to repeated bouts of infection, particularly with *S. aureus* and the mucoid form of *Pseudomonas*.
- Bronchiectasis: a frequent complication (see above).
- Hyperinflation of lungs due to air trapping behind mucin plugs; increased risk of developing pneumothorax.
- Hypoxia, scarring and destruction of the pulmonary vascular bed, leading to pulmonary hypertension and cor pulmonale.

Prognosis—The median age of survival is just over 30 years.

Infections of the lungs

Pneumonia is defined as the consolidation of lung tissue caused by the formation of an intra-alveolar inflammatory exudate as a result of lung infection.

Pneumonia is the fifth most common cause of death in the USA, and is more common in the very young and elderly.

Predisposing factors—Although pneumonia frequently occurs in previously healthy individuals, it is also predisposed by the presence of debility and immobility:

- Suppressed cough reflex, e.g. in coma, anaesthesia, and neuromuscular junction (NMJ) disorders.
- Impaired mucociliary clearance, e.g. through cigarette smoke, irritant gases, viral diseases (such as influenza) and genetic conditions (such as immotile cilia).
- Pulmonary oedema, e.g. due to right-sided cardiac failure.
- Impaired alveolar macrophages: alcohol, cigarette smoke, oxygen toxicity.
- Retention of secretions due to COAD.
- Immunosuppression, e.g. drugs (cytotoxics and immunosuppressives), AIDS, congenital

immunodeficiencies, and leukaemias.

- Drugs: previous course of broad spectrum antibiotics or cytotoxics.
- Instrumentation: endotracheal intubation or mechanical ventilation.
- Prior viral respiratory tract infection.
- Other: prolonged hospitalization, general debility, immobility.

Classification

Pneumonia can be classified according to:

- Microbiology: causative organism may be bacterial, viral, fungal or protozoal.
- Pattern of spread of infection: either lobar or bronchopneumonia.
- Clinical classification: according to circumstances surrounding the development of disease, e.g. community acquired, hospital acquired, disease of immunosuppression, and aspiration pneumonia.

Bacterial pneumonia

This is the commonest type of pneumonia, accounting for 80–90% of cases.

Causative organisms

Knowledge of the circumstances in which a person develops pneumonia is a strong clue as to the likely organism causing the infection (Fig. 8.6).

The clinical features are fever, shortness of breath, cough, and sputum (occasionally with haemoptysis). There are signs of consolidation with bronchial breathing and/or coarse crackles and whispering pectoriloquy.

Bronchopneumonia

Infection is centred on the bronchi but with the extension of the inflammatory exudate into the alveoli, causing a patchy consolidation of the lung (lobular

> **Remember INSPIRATION for the predisposing factors of pneumonia:**
> **I**mmunosuppression
> **N**eurological impairment of the cough reflex
> **S**ecretion retention
> **P**ulmonary oedema
> **I**mpaired mucociliary clearance
> **R**espiratory tract infection (viral)
> **A**ntibiotics and cytotoxics
> **T**racheal instrumentation
> **I**mpaired alveolar macrophages
> **O**ther
> **N**eoplasia

> As a general rule of thumb, community-acquired pneumonia is usually caused by Gram-positive bacteria whereas hospital-acquired pneumonias are mainly due to Gram-negative bacteria.

Common pathogenic bacteria in hospital- and community-acquired pneumonia	
Community-acquired infection	**Hospital-acquired infection**
Streptococcus pneumoniae (>60%) Haemophilus influenzae Legionella pneumophilus Staphylococcus aureus Mycoplasma pneumoniae Chlamydia pneumoniae Chlamydia psittaci	Klebsiella Pseudomonas Escherichia coli Proteus Serratia as well as organisms responsible for community-acquired pneumonia (but much less frequently)

Fig. 8.6 Common pathogenic bacteria in hospital- and community-acquired pneumonia.

distribution). Bronchopneumonia is illustrated in Fig. 8.7.

The condition primarily affects very young, very old or debilitated patients.

The infecting organism depends on whether the infection is hospital or community acquired, but it is quite often of the hospital-acquired variety due to underlying disease.

Pathogenesis—Patients develop retention of secretions which gravitate to dependent parts of the lungs and become infected, hence bronchopneumonia most commonly involves the lower lobes.

Macroscopically, it is usually bilateral with multiple areas of consolidation distributed around bronchi/bronchioles in dependent parts of the lung. Affected areas are firm, airless and have a dark red or grey appearance. Bronchial mucosa is inflamed and pus may be present in the more peripheral bronchi. Patchy collapse is associated with bronchial obstruction. Involvement of the pleura is common with purulent pleuritis.

Microscopically, there is acute inflammation of the bronchi and bronchioles with an acute inflammatory exudate present in the lumina and extending into the peribronchial alveoli.

Complications and sequelae are as follows:

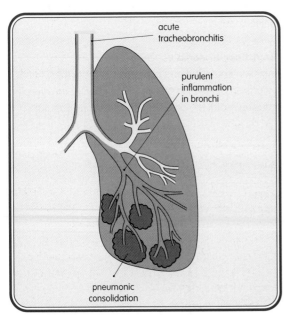

Fig. 8.7 Bronchopneumonia.

- Resolution: complete resolution occurs only if treatment is instituted early, before the onset of structural damage.
- Bronchial damage: imperfect repair of the bronchial mucosa results in scarring of the bronchial wall, with increased predisposition to further infection and to bronchiectasis.
- Lung fibrosis: inflammatory exudate is often not completely absorbed but is organized with residual fibrous scarring.
- Lung abscesses: single or multiple areas of suppuration.
- Empyema: pus in the pleural cavity as a result of extension of infection into pleural cavity.
- Pericarditis: direct extension of infection to the pericardium.
- Death: very common cause of death, particularly as a terminal manifestation of debilitating diseases.

Lobar pneumonia

This is a uniform consolidation of part of a lobe or of the whole lobe caused by infection (Fig. 8.8). The condition often affects otherwise healthy adults, primarily between the ages of 20 and 50 years old. Vagrants and alcoholics who have poor social and medical care are particularly prone to this pattern of pneumonia, which is often caused by *Pneumococcus* or *Klebsiella*.

Pathogenesis—Organisms gain entry to distal air spaces without colonization of bronchi. Infection spreads rapidly through the alveolar spaces and bronchioles, causing acute inflammatory exudation into air spaces.

Macroscopically, the whole lobe becomes consolidated and airless.

Microscopically, the alveoli are filled with an acute inflammatory exudate, which is limited by the pulmonary fissures.

Complications and sequelae are as follows:
- Resolution: most patients recover with their lungs returning to normal structure and function with complete resolution.
- Lung fibrosis: inflammatory exudate is often not completely absorbed but is organized with residual fibrous scarring and permanent lung dysfunction.
- Bacteraemia: bacterial dissemination of organisms can lead to septicaemia with meningitis, arthritis, endocarditis or pyaemic abscesses.

- Lung abscesses: single or multiple areas of suppuration.
- Empyema: pus in the pleural cavity as a result of extension of infection into the pleural cavity.
- Pleural effusion: non-infected effusion is common.
- Death.

Primary atypical pneumonia

This is an inflammation of the alveolar septa by inflammatory cells (acute interstitial pneumonitis) in the absence of any consolidation. Patients develop fever, dry cough and dyspnoea, but there are no signs of consolidation, hence the term 'atypical' pneumonia. It may be caused by several factors including infection by viruses, *Mycoplasma*, and *Chlamydia* and *Rickettsia*.

Viral pneumonia

This is a common cause of pneumonia in early childhood but is much less frequent in healthy adults. The majority of viral lung infections cause an atypical pneumonia, which is typically self-limiting (e.g. cytomegalovirus, measles, or varicella). However, in the immunocompromised host, these infections can prove fatal.

A minority of viruses cause a much more severe pattern of infection. The influenza viruses can cause an acute fulminating pneumonia with pulmonary haemorrhage; the clinical course may be rapidly fatal.

A common complication is secondary infection with pyogenic bacteria, which can transform a mild viral lung infection into a severe suppurative bronchopneumonia; this is particularly common in influenza.

Mycoplasma

Mycoplasma accounts for 15–20% of community-acquired pneumonia. It is more common between 5 and 15 years, but more serious in adults. The organisms cause a low-grade, chronic, atypical pneumonia. It may result in pulmonary fibrosis.

Chlamydia and *Rickettsia*

A number of chlamydial and rickettsial infections may be complicated by the development of pneumonia. Such infections include typhus, psittacosis and Q fever. Fatal cases are rare except in psittacosis.

Pulmonary tuberculosis (TB)

This is a chronic granulomatous infection of the lung caused by *Mycobacterium tuberculosis*. It is uncommon in the UK and other developed countries (at about 7 per 100 000) but extremely common worldwide (up to 500 per 100 000 in parts of Africa). In the UK it mainly affects older people and the immigrant population.

Spread is by various means:
- Inhalation of *M. tuberculosis* in the form of droplets (most common mode).
- Ingestion of food or milk.
- Inoculation of the skin.
- Transplacental spread, i.e. congenital TB.

The predisposing factors are:
- Close contact with infected individuals: increased risk for those living/working in crowded or unhygienic conditions, and for health-care workers.
- Immunosuppression: the very young, very old, immunosuppressive therapy (e.g. corticosteroids, cytotoxics) and other diseases of immunodeficiency, particularly AIDS.
- Malnourishment.
- Other diseases: pre-existing chronic lung disease

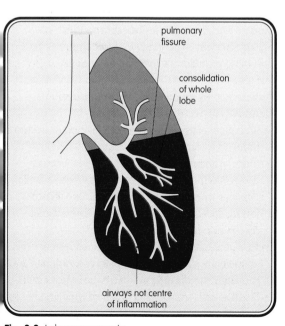

Fig. 8.8 Lobar pneumonia.

pulmonary fissure

consolidation of whole lobe

airways not centre of inflammation

(especially silicosis), diabetes mellitus, and alcoholism.

Pathogenesis—The destructive effects of infection are entirely due to the hypersensitivity reaction of the host directed against bacterial cell wall constituents. The following sequence of events occurs:

1. 0–10 days: mycobacteria excite a transient but marked acute inflammatory response. Neutrophils phagocytose the organisms but are unable to destroy them, as cell walls are resistant to degradation. Instead, engulfed bacteria are drained into local lymph nodes.
2. After 10 days: development of a T cell-mediated immune response (type IV hypersensitivity reaction) to the bacillary cell wall constituents results in cytokine release leading to activation of macrophages. Gradually a chronic inflammatory pattern develops, which is dominated by aggregates of macrophages or granulomas (see Chapter 3) with a central core of necrotic caseous tissue containing viable mycobacteria. Tuberculous granulomas are termed tubercles.

Macroscopically, tubercles appear as pinhead-sized white or greyish foci in the tissues.

Microscopically, tubercles are the histological hallmark of TB infection. A tubercle consists of a central area of amorphous caseous necrosis, surrounded by three cellular layers: an inner layer of activated macrophages including multinucleate macrophages (Langhans' giant cells), a middle layer of lymphocytes, and an outer layer of fibroblastic tissue which merges with surrounding structures and increases in amount with the age of the lesion.

The healing of a tubercle occurs slowly with progressive fibrosis and later calcification. The central necrotic area remains caseous for some time, and mycobacteria may remain viable indefinitely within a healed lesion. Reactivation results in secondary (or post primary) tuberculosis.

TB can be classified into two types, according to the pattern of infection:

- Primary infection: the first encounter with the organism, resulting in the development of a small parenchymal peripheral focus with a large response in draining lymph nodes.
- Secondary infection: reactivation or reinfection of a previously infected individual, resulting in the development of a large, localized, parenchymal reaction but with minimal lymph node involvement.

Primary tuberculosis

The lung is by far the most common site of primary infection. Other sites include the pharynx, larynx, skin and intestine.

Inhaled organisms proliferate in the alveoli at the periphery of the lung, often just beneath the pleura. This primary parenchymal tubercle is termed the Ghon focus. It is often associated with enlarged caseous hilar lymph nodes. The combination of lung and lymph node lesions together constitutes the primary complex or Ghon complex.

Primary tuberculosis will either resolve or progress as shown below.

Resolution

This occurs in the majority of cases. The Ghon focus and caseating granulomas in the lymph nodes heal with fibrosis. The disease does not progress due to the confinement of organisms within a fibrotic shell. However, walled-off bacteria may remain viable within the healed primary complex (latent tuberculosis).

Progression

In patients with poor immunity, the disease is progressive. There is a further spread of mycobacteria with continuing enlargement of the caseating granulomas in the lymph nodes (progressive primary TB). Enlarging nodes spread the infection by eroding into adjacent structures in two ways:

- Bronchus: erosion of an infected lymph node into a bronchus results in tuberculous bronchopneumonia (Fig. 8.9). The bacilli pass down into the bronchi of one lung where infection can then spread into the opposite lung. There is further spread of infection into the bronchioles and alveoli with the development of extensive, confluent, caseating, granulomatous lesions. This condition is known as 'galloping consumption' and is usually rapidly fatal.
- Blood vessel: erosion of an infected lymph node into a blood vessel results in haematogenous spread of mycobacteria to many parts of the body, including

the remainder of the lung, causing miliary tuberculosis (Fig. 8.9).

Secondary tuberculosis

This occurs as a result of the reactivation of quiescent but viable mycobacteria in hosts with weakened immune responses, or as a result of reinfection from the reinhalation of further organisms.

Caseous granulomas typically develop in the apical segments of the lungs, spreading directly and locally but without lymph node lesions. The initiating apical lesion is often called an Assmann focus and is histologically similar to the Ghon focus.

Secondary tuberculosis will either resolve or spread as shown below.

Resolution

Spontaneous healing with fibrosis and calcification occurs, though viable organisms remain without producing any clinical symptoms.

Spread

In adults with poor immune responses, secondary tuberculosis progresses locally with direct extension and continuing caseation. Further spread of mycobacteria produces various types of progressive tuberculosis:

- Apical cavitation fibrocaseous tuberculosis: a direct extension of the infection, and continuing caseation results in the formation of a large caseous mass surrounded by a thin cellular wall. If caseous material is expectorated, a cavity results. The lesion can heal at this stage but may spread further into the bronchi, blood stream or directly into the pleura.
- Tuberculous pneumonia (see above).
- Miliary tuberculosis (see above).

Complications are usually the result of extensive fibrosis involved in healing process:

- Pulmonary fibrosis: lung lesions typically heal with fibrosis, which may be extensive producing localized honeycombing. This is common in relapsing and progressive untreated disease.
- Pleural fibrosis with obliteration of the pleural space.
- Bronchiectasis: scarring of the bronchial walls can cause distal pulmonary collapse, secondary infection and bronchiectasis.

Treatment involves long-term triple therapy with rifampicin, isoniazid, and ethambutol.

Pneumonia in the immunocompromised

The lungs of immunocompromised patients are

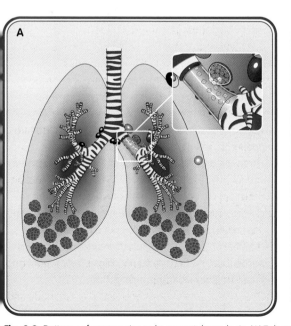
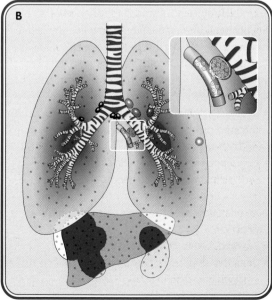

Fig. 8.9 Patterns of progressive pulmonary tuberculosis. (A) Tuberculous bronchopneumonia. (B) Miliary tuberculosis of the lung.

extremely prone to disease by opportunistic infections, i.e. infections caused by micro-organisms that are non-pathogenic to healthy, non-immunocompromised individuals.

Common opportunistic agents include:
- Viruses: cytomegalovirus, varicella-zoster virus, measles (see Primary Atypical Pneumonia, above).
- Fungi: both *Candida* and *Aspergillus* can cause widespread areas of necrosis with the formation of micro-abscesses containing characteristic hyphae; mortality is high.
- Protozoa: *Pneumocystis carinii* pneumonia (PCP) is common in AIDS patients, affecting 30–50% of cases. Alveoli are filled with a fine, foam-like material in which the minute bodies of the organism can be seen. This disease has a 30% mortality rate in AIDS.

Neoplastic diseases of the lungs
Bronchogenic carcinoma
This is the most common cause of death from neoplasia in the UK, affecting 30 000 people per year. Males are affected more than females but with an increasing incidence in women. The peak incidence is between the ages of 40 and 70 years, reflecting the cumulative exposure to several potential causative carcinogens. The UK has the highest incidence of this in the world.

The risk factors include:
- Cigarette smoking: the earlier the age at which smoking starts and the more cigarettes smoked mean an increased risk. Cigarette smoke contains a large number of carcinogens, e.g. polycyclic hydrocarbons. There is a steady decline in risk if smoking stops.
- Occupational factors such as exposure to radioactive material, asbestos, nickel, chromium, iron oxides and coal gas plants.
- Environmental factors such as radon (a natural radioactive gas in certain geographic areas).

There are four main histological types of lung carcinoma:
- Squamous cell carcinoma—50%.
- Small cell anaplastic carcinoma ('oat cell carcinoma')—20%.
- Adenocarcinoma (including bronchioalveolar carcinoma—20%.

- Large cell anaplastic carcinoma—10%.
A small proportion of tumours are mixed adeno-carcinoma/squamous carcinoma.

Tumours may be central (all types) or peripheral (mainly adenocarcinomas):
- Central or hilar tumours (70%) arise in relation to the main bronchi extending into the bronchial lumen and invading the adjacent lung.
- Peripheral tumours (30%) arise in peripheral airways or alveoli, often occurring in relation to scars and frequently extending to the pleural surface.

The route of spread is as follows:
- Local: central tumours invade locally either through the bronchial wall into the surrounding lung, or along the outside of the bronchi (peribronchial spread) to distant parts of the lung. Direct extension into pleura and adjacent mediastinal structures is a feature of advanced disease.
- Lymphatic spread: carcinomas spread to the ipsilateral and contralateral peribronchial and hilar lymph nodes. Compression of adjacent tissues by infiltrated nodes may then cause symptoms.
- Transcoelomic spread: tumour cells may seed within the pleural cavity, causing a malignant pleural effusion.
- Haematogenous spread to the brain, bone, liver and adrenal glands.

Histological types
Squamous cell carcinoma
This is the most common type of lung cancer thought to be derived from metaplastic squamous epithelium, which develops to line the main bronchi as a result of exposure to agents such as cigarette smoke.

Tumours are typically central and close to the carina, frequently presenting with features related to bronchial obstruction. Compared with other types, they are relatively slow growing and may be resectable.

Histologically, the tumours show a range of differentiation from well-differentiated lesions producing lots of keratin, through to poorly differentiated lesions with only a few keratin-producing cells.

Small cell (oat cell) anaplastic carcinoma
Highly malignant tumours arise from the bronchial

epithelium, but exhibit differentiation into neuroendocrine cells containing neurosecretory granules.

Due to the neuroendocrine type, this form of cancer is often associated with ectopic hormone production.

Macroscopically, these tumours are usually centrally located and are associated with a rapid rate of growth. Metastases are usually present at time of diagnosis.

Microscopically, the cells are round to oval and have little cytoplasm. The nuclei are thought to resemble oat grains, hence the alternative name. In certain situations there can be diagnostic confusion with tumour of lymphoid cells.

Large cell anaplastic carcinoma
This poorly differentiated tumour is thought to be of either squamous or adenocarcinoma origin. Lesions may be central or peripheral and are composed of large cells with nuclear pleomorphism and frequent giant cell forms. They have a poor prognosis and are frequently widely disseminated at the time of diagnosis.

Adenocarcinoma
A tumour derived from glandular cells, such as mucous goblet cells, Clara cells or type II pneumocytes. A proportion of adenocarcinomas are thought to originate in areas of pre-existing lung scarring (scar cancers). Adenocarcinoma has the slowest rate of growth, and differs from other types of lung cancer because it has an equal sex incidence, is not thought to be associated with cigarette smoking, and characteristically develops as a peripheral tumour.

There are four main histological patterns:
- Acinar: prominent gland-like spaces lined by columnar epithelium.
- Papillary: fronds of tumour on thin septa.
- Solid carcinoma with mucin production: poorly differentiated lesions.
- Bronchioalveolar carcinoma (see below).

Clinical features of lung cancer
There are no early symptoms of lung cancer; it is usual for a lesion to have been growing for many years before clinical presentation. The presenting symptoms of lung cancer are outlined in Fig. 8.10 and can be classified into:
- Pulmonary symptoms: most common types of presenting symptom.
- Metastatic symptoms: metastatic spread is present

in 70% of patients at presentation, and 30% of patients present with symptoms caused by metastatic disease.
- Local symptoms: local spread within the thorax can cause several clinical syndromes.
- Non-metastatic extrapulmonary syndromes: lung cancer frequently causes systemic syndromes which are not associated metastatic effects and may rarely be a presenting feature of disease.

Diagnosis is through clinical features (see above), imaging (chest X-ray and CT scans) and histological confirmation of the following:
- Sputum cytology.
- Cytology of pleural effusion.
- Percutaneous needle aspiration under image guidance: cytological preparation obtained.
- Bronchoscopy and biopsy: small tumour biopsy obtained.

Prognosis and staging—Histological types and stage of lung cancer determine the outcome and its likely response to treatment. Survival is better for early stage disease, except for small cell carcinoma.

The staging system used for lung cancer is shown in Fig. 8.11.

Treatment
Surgical intervention
Tumours are classified as either operable or inoperable according to the stage of the disease; only 10% of all lung tumours are considered operable at diagnosis. The key elements that offer a reasonable prospect of success with surgery include the following features:
- The tumour must be within a lobar bronchus or at least 2 cm distal to the carina.
- No direct extension to the chest wall, diaphragm or pericardium.
- No involvement of the heart great vessels, trachea, oesophagus or vertebrae.
- No malignant pleural effusion.
- No contralateral nodal involvement.
- No distant metastases.

Of those patients who undergo tumour surgery, only 20% have successful resection of the tumour.

Clinicopathological features of lung cancer	
Cause	**Clinical features**
pulmonary involvement	cough (80%): infection distal to airway blocked by tumour haemoptysis (70%): ulceration of tumour in bronchus dyspnoea (60%): local extension of tumour chest pain (40%): involvement of pleura and/or chest wall wheeze (15%): narrowing of airways systemic features: weight loss, anorexia and malaise
local spread	Horner's syndrome (see Chapter 6, pp. XX–XX): local invasion of cervical sympathetic ganglion hoarseness: spread to the left hilar region may cause recurrent laryngeal nerve palsy pain in T1 dermatome and wasting of intrinsic hand muscles: caused by brachial neuritis as a result of direct invasion of plexus by apical tumours pericarditis: due to direct tumour invasion
metastatic spread	pathological fracture CNS symptoms (brain metastasis) hepatomegaly or jaundice (liver metastasis)
Non-metastatic extrapulmonary syndromes	
endocrine disturbances	inappropriate ADH secretion: by small cell carcinoma and characterized by low sodium and plasma osmolality with high urine osmolality ectopic ACTH secretion: caused by small cell carcinoma and associated with Cushing's syndrome hypercalcaemia: caused by secretion of parathormone-related peptide by a squamous cell carcinoma
neurological syndromes	peripheral sensory motor neuropathy cerebellar degeneration causing ataxia proximal myopathy dermatomyositis Lambert–Eaton myaesthenic syndrome: associated with small cell tumours
hypertrophic pulmonary osteoarthropathy (HPOA)	finger clubbing swelling of wrists and ankles with periosteal new bone formation (seen in 2–3% of squamous cell carcinomas and adenocarcinomas)

Fig. 8.10 Clinicopathological features of lung cancer.

TNM staging of lung cancer		
Stage	**TNM group**	**Clinical**
stage I	T1 N0 M0 T1 N1 M0	tumour <3 cm; distal to origin of lobar bronchus (T1) with (N1) or without (N0) spread to ipsilateral hilar nodes no metastases (M0)
stage II	T2 N0 M0 T2 N1 M0	tumour >3 cm, 2 cm distal to the carina, which invades visceral pleural (T2) with (N1) or without (N0) spread to ipsilateral hilar nodes no metastases (M0)
stage III	all T3/T4 cases all N3 cases all M1 cases	all tumours involving the carina; involving mediastinal structures (T3/T4) all tumours with spread to contralateral nodes (N3) all cases of metastases (M1)

Fig. 8.11 TNM staging of lung cancer.

Radiotherapy and chemotherapy

Tumours are grouped into two categories according to differences in prognosis and response to radio- and chemotherapy.

Small cell lung carcinoma (SCLC)

This is very sensitive to radiotherapy and chemotherapy but the disease is usually extensive at diagnosis such that survival is still poor despite local control of tumour. Treatment offers good palliation of pain, cough and dyspnoea. Radiotherapy and combination chemotherapy cause complete local response in 30% of cases with a median survival of 11 months (as compared to three months if untreated), and a one year survival of 45%.

Non-small cell lung carcinoma (NSCLC)

Inoperable cases may be treated with radiotherapy depending on clinical circumstances. The role of chemotherapy is limited. Overall prognosis is poor with only 50% two year survival without spread, 10% with spread.

See Fig. 8.12 for a summary of histological types of lung cancers.

Bronchioalveolar carcinoma

This is a special type of adenocarcinoma derived from alveolar or bronchial epithelial cells (Clara cells and type II pneumocytes). There are two types:

- Multifocal diffuse infiltrative tumours: replace areas of lung in a manner resembling pneumonic consolidation. Cells are tall, columnar, have few mitoses and secrete mucin.
- Single, grey masses of tumour up to 10 cm in diameter. Cells are cuboidal with hyperchromatic nuclei and mitoses, and form papillary structures; there is often no mucin secretion. In the absence of metastases, this subtype has a better prognosis than other forms of lung cancer.

Metastatic lung disease

Secondary cancers of the lung are more common than primary cancers. Tumours can arise in any location, except the brain, but most are in the kidney, breast, testis and gastrointestinal tract. Route of spread to the lung is most commonly via the blood or lymphatics. Usually, discrete nodules are seen scattered throughout both lungs.

Occasionally, the lymphatics may be diffusely involved, leading to an appearance of lymphangitis

Summary of histological types of lung cancers				
	Small cell	**Squamous**	**Large cell**	**Adenocarcinoma**
relative incidence	10%	50%	10%	20%
gender differences	males > females	males > females	males > females	males = females
associated with cigarette smoking	yes	yes	yes	no
site	centrally located	centrally located	centrally located	peripherally located; often originating in areas of pre-existing lung scarring
non-metastatic symptoms	ADH secretion ectopic ACTH secretion Lambert–Eaton myaesthenic syndrome	hypercalcaemia HPOA	–	HPOA
rate of growth	fast; metastases usually present at diagnosis	slow growing; metastasizes late	fast	slowest growing

Fig. 8.12 Summary of histological types of lung cancers.

carcinomatosa. In this condition, the blockage of lymphatics causes severe breathlessness due to the failure of removal of interstitial fluid from the lung parenchyma. This condition is rapidly fatal.

Carcinoid tumours

These are neuroendocrine tumours of the lungs, representing about 5% of all pulmonary neoplasms. The majority of tumours are benign, although a minority have the potential for local recurrence or metastasis (atypical pulmonary neuroendocrine tumours).

In contrast to intestinal carcinoid tumours, most pulmonary lesions do not secrete 5-hydroxytryptamine.

Bronchial hamartomas

These common benign lesions composed of tissue are normally encountered in the lung. Most are 1–3 cm in diameter and largely consist of cartilage, being firm and glistening white in appearance (often termed chondromas). Other elements are bronchial epithelium, fat and muscle. Bronchial hamartomas are asymptomatic and are mainly discovered at post mortem examination.

Miscellaneous mesenchymal tumours

These tumours can be either benign, (e.g. neurofibromas, lipomas, etc., or malignant (sarcomas are extremely rare in the lung).

Diffuse interstitial diseases

Interstitial lung diseases are a group of non-infectious, non-malignant disorders in which there is inflammation of the alveolar walls with a thickening of the interstitium between the alveoli, usually with fibrosis.

This is also known as alveolitis and often loosely referred to as pulmonary fibrosis.

Disorders can be classified into acute and chronic interstitial diseases as shown in Fig. 8.13.

Chronic pulmonary fibrosis

A progressive diffuse fibrosis of the lung interstitium occurring as a result of chronic interstitial disease.

Causes of chronic interstitial disease are listed in Fig. 8.13 and can be classified into three aetiological groups:

- Idiopathic, e.g. sarcoidosis and cryptogenic fibrosing alveolitis.
- Dust inhalation: inorganic dust (pneumoconioses, i.e.

coal miner's pneumoconiosis, silicosis, asbestosis) and organic dust (extrinsic allergic alveolitis, e.g. farmer's lung or bird fancier's lung).
- Iatrogenic: drugs (e.g. nitrofurantoin, amiodarone and anticancer drugs—methotrexate, cyclophosphamide and bleomycin) and radiation (see p. 129).

The initiating mechanism of interstitial inflammation depends on the aetiology, but in all cases there is ultimately:

- Neutrophil migration: inflammatory process results in the migration of large numbers of neutrophils, with the release of toxic-free radicals and tissue-damaging proteolytic enzymes into the alveoli.
- Enlargement and desquamation of the flat type I alveolar cells through which gases normally diffuse.
- Replacement of type I pneumocytes by thicker surfactant producing type II cells and bronchiolar cells that have migrated down from the bronchioles.
- Accumulation of fibroblasts within the interstitium and increased production of collagen.

Macroscopically, the lung is converted into a mass of cystic airspaces separated by areas of dense collagenous scarring. This characteristic appearance is termed 'honeycomb lung' as the cut surface is said to resemble a honeycomb.

Acute and chronic interstitial diseases of the lung	
acute	adult respiratory distress syndrome (ARDS) drug and toxin reactions acute radiation pneumonitis diffuse intrapulmonary haemorrhage
chronic	pneumoconiosis idiopathic fibrosing alveolitis sarcoidosis extrinsic allergic alveolitis diffuse malignancies connective tissue disease, e.g. rheumatoid disease, scleroderma drug-induced pulmonary fibrosis chronic pulmonary oedema, e.g. as in mitral stenosis with raised pulmonary venous pressure chronic radiation pneumonitis rare disorders, e.g. alveolar proteinosis, histiocytosis

Fig. 8.13 Acute and chronic interstitial diseases of the lung.

Microscopically, the cystic spaces are lined by flattened or cuboidal epithelium. Walls (interstitium) are irregular, thick and fibrous and contain hypertrophic muscle. Muscular arteries show muscle hypertrophy and fibrosis, and specific changes of underlying disease may also be present.

The clinical feature of the early stage is a slowly increasing respiratory insufficiency due to reduced lung capacity and residual volume, reduced compliance, and reduced diffusion capacity.

The characteristic signs are dyspnoea, cough and finger clubbing.

In end stage disease, fibrosis of the alveolar walls greatly reduces the pulmonary capillary network, leading to right ventricular hypertrophy and the development of pulmonary hypertension with eventual right heart failure (cor pulmonale). Death results from a combination of respiratory and cardiac failure.

Diagnosis is based on the following investigations:
- History (including occupation and hobbies) and clinical features.
- Lung function tests: restrictive pattern of lung function tests (refer to Fig. 8.1).
- Chest X-ray.
- Bronchioalveolar lavage.
- Lung biopsy.

The pneumoconioses

This is a group of interstitial lung diseases resulting from chronic exposure to inorganic dust. The three most common types of pneumoconioses are coalworker's pneumoconiosis, silicosis, and asbestosis.

In the normal lung, inhaled dust is coughed out, or ingested by macrophages. However, if the dust is toxic to macrophages there is local inflammation, secretion of cytokines and stimulation of fibrosis. The end result is a restrictive pattern of respiratory dysfunction.

Coalworker's pneumoconiosis (CWP)

This interstitial lung disease is caused by inhaling coal dust. It has four types of pathology:
- Simple CWP.
- Complicated CWP.
- Progressive massive fibrosis.
- Caplan's syndrome.

Simple coalworker's pneumoconiosis (macular CWP)
This condition is not associated with any clinically significant impairment of respiratory function, despite the following pathological changes:
- Focal aggregates of dust-laden macrophages in the lymph nodes and in small macules within the lung. Lymph nodes are enlarged, firm and contain pigment-laden macrophages and fibrosis. Macules are 2–5 mm in diameter, and most common in the upper lobes, subpleurally and in the peribronchial regions.
- No significant scarring.
- Diagnosed on chest X-ray by the presence of small nodules in the lung fields.
- At autopsy, the nodules are not palpable and do not exceed 10 mm.

Complicated coalworker's pneumoconiosis (nodular CWP)
This is similar to simple CWP but the lesions are nodular and associated with some scarring. Adjacent areas show signs of emphysema, and the nodules are usually palpable at autopsy.

Progressive massive fibrosis (PMF)
Patients have severe respiratory impairment with a mixed restrictive and obstructive pattern. The condition is relentlessly progressive and may present long after active exposure to coal dust. Pathologically, the condition is characterized by large nodules with the following characteristics:
- Greater than 10 mm in diameter with significant scarring.
- Most common in the upper lobes or in the mid-zonal region.
- Often have a central necrotic area.
- Often surrounded by emphysema.

Caplan's syndrome
This condition occurs in pneumoconiosis in association with rheumatoid disease, where the nodules appear large, carbon-pigmented, and rheumatoid. It is rarely symptomatic but may be mistaken on X-ray for PMF lesions or tumour.

Silicosis

An interstitial lung disease, this is caused by the inhalation of quartz-containing dust (quartz being silicon dioxide), which is abundant in stone and sand.

It is associated with occupations involving slate

mining, stone masonry, foundry and pottery work, tunnelling, quarrying, and coal mining through granite rocks.

Pathogenesis—Silicates are toxic to macrophages, which stimulate cytokine generation precipitating inflammation with fibrosis and nodule formation, thus:
- Short heavy doses produce acute silicoses with pulmonary oedema and alveolar exudation.
- Prolonged exposure produces formation of multiple fibrous nodules composed of collagen in the lungs. Nodules expand and cause extensive destruction of lung tissue. Histologically, silica particles can be seen in nodules using polarized light.

Tuberculosis is a common complication of silicosis (silicotuberculosis). This is thought to be due to impaired local defences as a consequence of accumulated silica in macrophages.

Asbestosis

This interstitial lung disease is caused by the inhalation of asbestos, a fibrous silicate mineral that was widely used between 1890 and 1970. It is associated with occupations involving asbestos mining/processing, the building industry, insulating and fire resistant material, and shipyard and ship's engine room work.

There are two main forms of asbestos:
- Serpentine asbestos (including white asbestos): this is the most common form; fibres persist in the lung for a limited time.
- Amphibole asbestos (including blue and brown asbestos): fibres persist in the lung for many years and are the main cause of malignant mesothelioma.

Risk of disease depends on the duration and intensity of exposure, and the type of asbestos (short fibres are less pathogenic).

The characteristics of asbestosis are:
- There is usually a latent period of 25 years before clinical symptoms become evident.
- Interstitial fibrosis is maximal at lung bases, and asbestos bodies may be seen histologically.
- The disease progresses with an increasing restrictive defect associated with interstitial fibrosis.
- Pulmonary hypertension and cor pulmonale develop in the late stages.

Diagnosis is made on the bases of occupational exposure, changes on chest radiograph (linear shadows in the lung bases), and a pattern of restrictive defect on lung function testing.

Other pulmonary diseases caused by asbestos include the following:
- Pleural plaques.
- Pleural fibrosis.
- Mesothelioma.
- Lung carcinoma.

Sarcoidosis

Sarcoidosis is a multisystem disease of unknown aetiology characterized by the presence of histiocytic and giant cell granulomatous inflammatory reaction primarily affecting the lymph nodes and lungs.

Its prevalence is 10 per 100 000 cases in the UK but this disease shows a geographical variation, being higher in Ireland, Sweden, and the black population of New York, but rare in Asians.

Maximum incidence lies between 30 and 40 years of age, affecting females more than males.

Other affected sites are the skin, eyes, liver, spleen, nervous system, phalanges, parotid glands and (rarely) the heart.

The aetiopathogenesis is unknown but thought to involve the type IV hypersensitivity reaction. The disease seems to be less common in smokers.

Histology shows non-caseating histiocytic granulomas in the lung interstitium. Patients with lung involvement present with slowly progressive dyspnoea and cough and are found to have lung shadowing on chest radiograph with enlargement of the hilar lymph nodes.

Diagnosis—Subcutaneous injection of sarcoid tissue homogenate induces granulomas in affected patients (the Kveim test).

Prognosis—Approximately 70% of patients recover with steroid therapy, and 35% show progression to interstitial fibrosis and development of honeycomb lung.

Idiopathic pulmonary fibrosis (cryptogenic fibrosing alveolitis)

This chronic fibrosis of the lung interstitium as a result of interstitial pneumonitis has no apparent cause. It is an uncommon disease that mostly occurs between 45 and 65 years of age, with equal incidence between males and females.

The aetiopathogenesis is unknown.

There is interstitial fibrosis with type II pneumocyte hyperplasia, which may progress to honeycomb lung. The condition presents with insidious onset of dyspnoea and tachycardia. There is usually a progression to respiratory failure within five years.

Diffuse pulmonary haemorrhagic syndromes
Goodpasture's syndrome
In this autoimmune disorder, complement causes severe damage as a result of the binding of autoantibodies to basement membranes of the alveoli (producing haemoptysis as a result of pulmonary alveolar haemorrhage) and the glomeruli (producing haematuria due to glomerulonephritis) (see 'Diseases of the glomerulus' in Chapter 10).

Idiopathic pulmonary haemosiderosis
A rare condition of unknown aetiology characterized by recurrent episodes of haemoptysis, cough and dyspnoea which is most often seen in children. There is evidence of diffuse alveolar damage with type II pneumocyte hyperplasia.

Rheumatoid disease
The lungs and pleura are affected in about 10–15% of patients with rheumatoid disease (see p. 287).

Extrinsic allergic alveolitis
This immune-mediated interstitial granulomatous inflammation is caused by inhaling organic dusts. The most common types are farmer's lung (caused by inhalation of fungal spores present in mouldy hay) and pigeon fancier's lung (caused by inhalation of avian protein antigen in bird droppings).

The pathogenesis is a combination of type III (immune-complex deposition) and type IV (cell-mediated delayed) hypersensitivity reactions to the inhaled antigen, resulting in diffuse interstitial fibrosis which is most marked in the upper lobes. The condition is progressive resulting in honeycomb lung and respiratory failure.

Diseases of vascular origin
Pulmonary congestion and oedema
Pulmonary oedema is defined as an increase in extravascular fluid in the alveolar walls (pulmonary interstitium), which, if severe, subsequently affects the alveolar spaces.

Pathogenesis—Normally, a balance exists between hydrostatic pressure forcing fluid out of the capillaries and colloid osmotic (oncotic) pressure preventing such a loss, such that only a small amount of fluid passes into the interstitium. This fluid is drained from the lung via lymphatic channels.

In pulmonary oedema, the amount of fluid passing into the lungs exceeds the lymphatic drainage capacity such that there is an accumulation of fluid within the interstitium. This increases the stiffness of the lungs, giving rise to a subjective sensation of dyspnoea.

Macroscopically, the lungs are heavy and congested. In fatal cases, fluid flows from the cut surfaces, and can often be seen in the large airways.

Microscopically, the interstitium is wider, the capillaries are congested and the alveoli are filled with proteinaceous fluid.

Clinical features of hypoxic respiratory failure may result due to a combination of ventilation/perfusion imbalance caused by fluid in the alveoli, and airway narrowing from accumulation of peribronchial fluid.

Pulmonary oedema can result from:
- Altered haemodynamic forces: increased hydrostatic pressure; decreased oncotic pressure.
- Injury to the alveolar capillary wall.
- Blockage of lymphatic drainage.

Haemodynamic pulmonary oedema
Pathogenesis of haemodynamic oedema is described in Chapter 3.

Increased capillary hydrostatic pressure
This is the commonest cause of pulmonary oedema, and may be the result of:
- Left ventricular heart failure: e.g. due to cases of myocardial infarction, aortic valve disease, mitral regurgitation and tachyarrhythmias.
- Pulmonary venous hypertension, e.g. due to mitral stenosis.
- Constrictive pericarditis or pericardial effusions.
- Fluid overload: excess infusion of crystalloid solutes.

In chronic left heart failure, prolonged increased hydrostatic pressure can lead to rupture of capillaries with leakage of red cells into the interstitium and alveoli. Macrophages of the interstitium and alveoli phagocytose haemoglobin and accumulate iron pigment. These cells are often termed 'heart failure cells'.

Decreased plasma osmotic pressure
This is seen in hypoproteinaemia. Aetiology is:
- Malnutrition.
- Nephrotic syndrome.
- Hepatic failure.
- Intravenous infusion of hypotonic solutes.

Pulmonary oedema due to alveolar capillary injury
Diffuse alveolar damage causes an increased permeability of alveolar capillary membrane leading to pulmonary oedema, haemorrhage, cell necrosis and hyaline membrane formation. This types of damage is seen in adult respiratory distress syndrome (see below).

Blockage of lymphatic drainage
Lymphatic obstruction prevents drainage of fluid to lymphatic channels. Obstruction may be caused by tumour emboli in lymphangitis carcinomatosa.

Adult respiratory distress syndrome (ARDS)
An acute restrictive lung disease characterized by pulmonary exudation and oedema with widespread systemic metabolic derangements.

Many conditions predispose to ARDS, most commonly systemic sepsis and severe trauma. The causes are listed in Fig. 8.14.

Causes of ARDS	
Cause	**Clinical features**
blood-borne	major trauma, especially associated with raised intracranial pressure septicaemia major burns disseminated intravascular coagulation massive blood transfusion amniotic fluid embolism acute pancreatitis cardiac surgery with bypass antitumour chemotherapy paraquat poisoning
air-borne	pulmonary aspiration of gastric contents inhalation of toxic fumes or smoke near drowning pneumonia from many causes requiring ventilation

Fig. 8.14 Causes of ARDS.

The exact pathogenesis is unknown in many cases, but events that take place in the lung in ARDS are termed diffuse alveolar damage and occur in two phases, namely an acute exudative phase (destruction of alveolar lining cells) and a late organization phase (cell proliferation and fibrosis).

In severe cases of ARDS, cytokines liberated from the lung vascular bed can enter the systemic circulation and may cause systemic endothelial activation with neutrophil activation leading to multi-organ failure.

Acute exudative phase
A damaging stimulus causes a massive insult to the alveolar capillary walls, which results in the following events:
- Necrosis of type 1 alveolar epithelium.
- Exudation of fibrin and fluid into the alveolar spaces forming hyaline membrane.
- Microthrombosis in the alveolar capillaries.
- Adherence and activation of neutrophils with release of neutrophilic enzymes.
- Haemorrhage into the alveoli.

Late organization phase
Here, the lungs are congested and ventilation is impaired. Organization involves:
- Regeneration of type 2 pneumocytes.
- Proliferation of fibroblasts with fibrous organization of hyaline membrane.
- Collagenous scarring results in interstitial fibrosis or fibrous obliteration of the alveolar spaces.

Fig. 8.15 shows the main events and outcomes in ARDS.

Following the damaging stimulus there is a latent period of 4–24 hours before symptoms develop; dyspnoea develops before changes are visible on chest radiographs. ARDS develops progressively over a period of 24–48 hours.

A clinical diagnosis of ARDS depends on:
- Presence of a condition known to precipitate ARDS (listed in Fig. 8.14).
- Refractory hypoxaemia (Pao_2 < 8.0 kPa on >40% O_2).
- Radiographic evidence of evolving diffuse pulmonary shadowing.
- Clinical signs of developing restrictive disease.

Treatment is with continuous positive airway pressure ventilation and intensive support of cardiac circulatory and renal functions.

Mortality for ARDS is about 70%. Patients usually die from systemic inflammatory response syndrome with multi-organ failure. Of those who survive, 20% have some permanent lung dysfunction due to the organization of exudate and persisting restrictive defect.

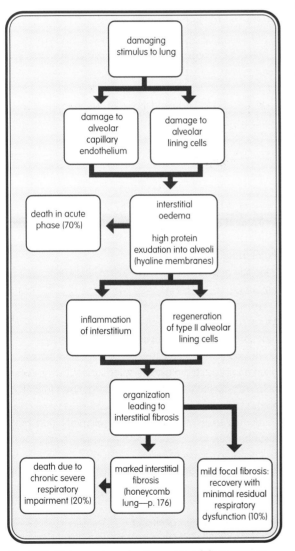

Fig. 8.15 Main events and outcomes in adult respiratory distress syndrome.

Embolism, haemorrhage and infarction
Pulmonary embolism (PE)
This is the occlusion of a pulmonary artery, most commonly by thromboemboli originating in the systemic veins (Fig. 8.16). The condition accounts for 1% of all hospital deaths, but rising to 30% in patients with severe burns or trauma.

The vast majority of cases are caused by emboli arising from thrombosis of the deep leg veins (calf, popliteal, femoral and iliac veins). Conditions predisposing to leg vein thrombosis are outlined in Chapter 7, p. 102.

The consequences of PE are pulmonary hypertension (which puts a strain on the right side of the heart) and infarction of the lung (which occurs in only about 10% of cases of PE, as dual circulation protects against ischaemic necrosis).

Clinical features of PE
The effect of PE depends on the extent of the pulmonary vasculature blockage and the time scale involved:
- Massive PE (5% of cases) is a sudden blockage of more than 60% of the pulmonary vasculature, resulting in electromechanical dissociation of the heart, i.e. the heart continues to beat but there is no output as pulmonary vascular resistance is too high. This results in cardiovascular collapse and rapid death.
- Major PE (10% of cases) is a blockage of the middle-sized pulmonary arteries. These patients commonly experience breathlessness. Lung infarction develops in about 10% of such cases, and it can lead to haemoptysis and, if adjacent to the pleura, pleuritic chest pain. If untreated, patients may develop a subsequent massive thromboembolism.
- Minor PE (85% of cases) is a blockage of the small peripheral vessels by small emboli. Patients may be asymptomatic or may experience breathlessness and pleuritic chest pain as a result of small infarcts. As with major pulmonary embolism, patients may develop a subsequent massive thromboembolism if untreated.
- Recurrent minor pulmonary embolism (minority) is a blockage of the many small peripheral arteries over a period of many months by recurrent small emboli.

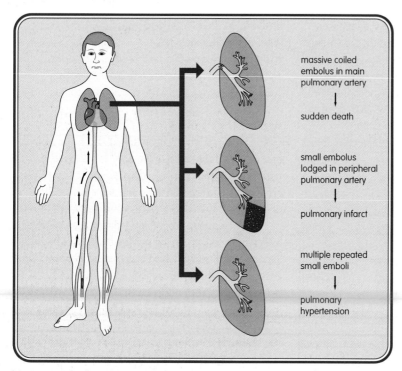

massive coiled
embolus in main
pulmonary artery

↓

sudden death

small embolus
lodged in peripheral
pulmonary artery

↓

pulmonary infarct

multiple repeated
small emboli

↓

pulmonary
hypertension

Fig. 8.16 Pulmonary thromboembolism. (Adapted with permission from *General and Systematic Pathology*, 2nd edn, by J.C.E. Underwood, Churchill Livingstone, 1996.)

The condition can lead to the obliteration of the vascular bed with the development of pulmonary hypertension and right heart strain.

Prevention and treatment
Pulmonary thromboembolism is the most common preventable cause of death in hospital patients. Prevention involves:
- Mobilizing early following surgery.
- Antiembolic stocking.
- Heparin prophylaxis.

Treatment is with oxygen, analgesia and anticoagulation therapy (heparin, warfarin).

Non-thrombotic emboli
These are rare, but include:
- Fat, following a bone fracture.
- Amniotic fluid during labour.
- Air (post trauma or post surgery).
- Decompression sickness, e.g. in deep sea divers ('the bends'). Rapid decompression releases nitrogen bubbles which cause problems in the CNS and bones, and can produce functional obstruction of the pulmonary vessels.

- Foreign bodies.
- Tumour embolism: renal or bronchial cell carcinoma.

Pulmonary infarction
Infarction of lung tissue is usually associated with embolism.

The lower lobes are involved in 75% of cases. Macroscopically, pulmonary infarcts are typically haemorrhagic (because of blood entering from the bronchial circulation) and wedge shaped, and there is often an associated pleural reaction which causes chest pain. With time, the infarct becomes organized to form a fibrous scar.

Microscopically, there is extravasation of blood into necrotic lung.

Common sequelae include:
- Pulmonary dysfunction due to the loss of lung tissue.
- Pulmonary vascular obstruction leading to cor pulmonale.
- Pleurisy and pleural effusion.
- Healing, with fibrous scar.
- Septic infarction due to either a primary septic embolism or secondary infection leading to abscess formation.

Pulmonary hypertension and vascular sclerosis

This is increased arterial pressure of the lung vasculature, the main causes of which were listed in Fig. 7.14, the most important being:

- Chronic obstructive airways disease.
- Interstitial fibrosis of the lungs.
- Chronic pulmonary venous congestion.

Pulmonary hypertension causes irreversible structural changes to:

- Pulmonary vasculature: medial hypertrophy of the muscular arteries (increased smooth muscle) and pulmonary veins (arterialization); occlusion of the pulmonary arteries caused by intimal proliferation.
- Lungs: interstitial fibrosis.
- Right side of the heart: increased workload of the right side of the heart causes ultimate development of right heart failure (cor pulmonale).

The clinical effects are breathlessness and the symptoms and signs of right-sided cardiac failure.

Diseases of iatrogenic origin

Drug-induced lung disease

There are many drugs available on the market that have pulmonary side effects. A few examples are given below.

Chronic pulmonary fibrosis can be caused by cancer drugs and amiodarone.

Asthma can by induced by aspirin (though the mechanism is unknown) and certain β-blockers (by bronchoconstriction caused by an antagonistic effect on β_2-receptors of bronchial smooth muscle).

Complication of radiotherapy

Acute radiation pneumonitis

Excessive exposure to radiation causes diffuse alveolar damage, and is an established cause of ARDS.

Chronic radiation pneumonitis

Less severe exposure occurring over a longer period of time results in progressive pulmonary fibrosis with the typical restrictive defect of pulmonary function.

Lung transplants

Heart–lung transplants are usually carried out for cardiac problems associated with pulmonary vascular hypertension.

Single lung transplants may be carried out for cystic fibrosis or pulmonary fibrosis. To avoid rejection, all transplant patients require immunosuppression for life.

- Explain the differences between obstructive and restrictive lung diseases, and describe the characteristic patterns of lung function tests.
- Describe the pathogenesis and morphological features of extrinsic (atopic) asthma.
- Define 'pneumonia' and explain the difference between the broncho- and lobar types.
- Describe the histological types of carcinoma of the bronchus.
- Name the acute and chronic interstitial lung diseases.
- Describe the morphological features of chronic pulmonary fibrosis.
- What are the three most common types of pneumoconiosis?

DISORDERS OF THE PLEURA

Inflammatory pleural effusions

Serofibrinous pleuritis

This acute inflammation of the pleura is accompanied by an accumulation of high protein fluid (>30 g protein/L; exudate) containing fibrinogen/fibrin between the pleural surfaces.

The condition is commonly due to infection, infarction or tumour.

Pathogenesis—Effusion is the result of movement of fluid through damaged vessel walls.

Effusion is typically unilateral, with the pleural surface covered by a fibrinous exudate. The fluid consists of a straw-coloured fibrinous fluid containing mesothelial cells, lymphocytes and polymorphs. In neoplastic diseases, malignant cells can also be identified within pleural fluid.

Common sequelae include:
- Atelectasis: compression of the lungs causes pulmonary collapse and respiratory impairment.
- Adhesions: formation of fibrous adhesions between the visceral and parietal pleura.
- Fibrosis: obliteration of the pleural space by fibrosis, which is common in long-standing effusions.
- Empyema (see below).

Suppurative pleuritis (empyema)
This is an acute inflammation of the pleura with accumulation of pus in the pleural cavity. Typically caused by pulmonary infection (e.g. pneumonia, tuberculosis, lung abscess), it can also result as a complication of thoracic surgery or penetrating chest wall injury.

Common sequelae include septicaemia (haematogenous spread of infection to other organs) and atelectasis (lung collapse as a result of compression).

Haemorrhagic pleuritis
This acute inflammation of the pleura with the accumulation of a blood-stained exudate, is often caused by tumour or pulmonary infarcts.

Non-inflammatory pleural effusions
Hydrothorax
This collection of low protein fluid (<30 g protein/L; transudate) is due to the movement of excess fluid through normal vessel walls. Common causes are:
- Cardiac failure (most common): increased hydrostatic pressure in pulmonary hypertension.
- Hypoalbuminaemia: decreased oncotic pressure.
- Vena caval obstruction: decreased oncotic pressure.

Effusions are usually bilateral, and the pleural surface appears normal. Fluid is straw-coloured and contains occasional lymphocytes and mesothelial cells.

 **The difference between 'transudate' and 'exudate', and the conditions that cause these types of pleural effusions, are common questions in examinations.**

The condition can cause pulmonary collapse (compression of the lungs causing respiratory impairment) or may resolve completely (resorption of fluid on correction of the cause with no structural alterations).

Haemothorax
Bleeding into the chest, which is most commonly the result of:
- Trauma, especially with rib fractures.
- Surgery.
- Pulmonary infarction.
- Spontaneous rupture of diseased arteries, e.g. atheromatous and dissecting aortic aneurysm.

If blood remains within the pleural cavity, the result is organization and pleural fibrosis.

Chylothorax
The accumulation of chyle within the pleural cavity, caused by a leakage of chyle from the thoracic duct, is typically the result of malignant infiltration, surgery or trauma.

Pneumothorax
This is the presence of air in the pleural cavity, the causes are described in Fig. 8.17.

Causes of pneumothorax		
Cause	**Type**	**Clinical features**
spontaneous	primary	idiopathic rupture of pulmonary 'bleb'; most common in thin young males
	secondary	COPD: emphysema, chronic bronchitis and asthma pneumonia cystic fibrosis whooping cough pleural malignancy
traumatic	chest injury	penetrating chest wounds rib fractures oesophageal rupture
	iatrogenic	subclavian cannulation positive pressure artificial ventilation pleural aspiration oesophageal perforation during endoscopy lung biopsy

Fig. 8.17 Causes of pneumothorax.

Spontaneous pneumothorax can be either primary (of unknown cause occurring in otherwise healthy individuals) or secondary (i.e. secondary to lung disease).

Traumatic pneumothorax is a result of chest injury or is iatrogenic.

Complications of pneumothorax include:

- Atelectasis: lung collapse due to compression of the underlying lung.
- Tension pneumothorax: progressive increase in air pressure within the pleural cavity, causing massive collapse of the affected lung, mediastinal shift and compression of the contralateral lung producing life-threatening respiratory insufficiency. The condition occurs as a result of a valve-like mechanism at the point at which air enters the pleural cavity such that air enters the cavity in inspiration but does not escape in expiration.

Neoplasms of the pleura

Pleural fibroma

This is a benign tumour of submesothelial connective tissue. The causes are unknown but there is no association with asbestos. The tumour is well-circumscribed, localized and attached to the pleural surface by a pedicle. Histologically, it is composed of fibroblast-like cells with abundant collagen fibres.

Metastatic neoplasms

These are the commonest pleural tumours, most frequently arising from the lungs or breast, but can arise from any malignant tumour. They are usually associated with a high-protein exudate (see above).

Malignant mesothelioma

This primary neoplasm of the pleura is extremely rare, except following asbestos exposure, and usually presents after a latent period of up to 50 years.

Macroscopically, the tumours are highly malignant and spread locally around the pleural cavity and pericardium. However, haematogenous/lymphatic metastasis is rare.

Microscopically, mesotheliomas have spindle cells and glandular patterns.

Clinical features include chest pain and breathlessness, and there is commonly recurrent or persistent pleural effusions.

Prognosis—Death is usually within ten months of diagnosis.

- Explain the differences between serofibrinous pleuritis and hydrothorax.
- Name the common causes of an exudative pleural effusion.
- Name the common causes of a transudate pleural effusion.
- Classify the causes of pneumothorax.
- What is a tension pneumothorax?
- Describe the neoplasms that can affect the pleura.

9. Pathology of the Gastrointestinal System

DISORDERS OF THE UPPER GASTROINTESTINAL TRACT

The mouth and oropharynx
Congenital abnormalities
Cleft palate and cleft (hare-) lip
These are the commonest major congenital malformations of the mouth and frequently occur together as a result of the same process, namely a failure of fusion of during the embryonic period.

Prevalence:
- Cleft lip with or without cleft palate occurs in approximately 1 in 1000 births (males more than females).
- Cleft palate with or without cleft lip occurs in approximately 1 in 2500 births (females more than males).

Aetiology—A few cases are associated with a chromosomal abnormality (e.g. trisomy 13 or 18) but in the majority of cases no teratogenic factor can be identified.

Morphology:
- Cleft lip: may be unilateral or bilateral, involving the lip only or extending upwards and backwards to include the floor of the nose and the alveolar ridge (Fig. 9.1).
- Cleft palate: considerable variation, from a small

defect in the soft palate (bifid uvula) which causes little disability to a complete separation of the hard palate combined with a cleft lip (Fig. 9.2).

The effects are an abnormal facial appearance, defective speech, and feeding difficulty with extensive lesions (child is unable to suck).

Management is by artificial feeding, with plastic surgery recommended between 1 and 2 years of age.

Infections and inflammation
Non-infective stomatitis
Aphthous ulcers
These are tiny, painful, shallow ulcers on a background of red mucosa typically occurring on the lips, tongue or

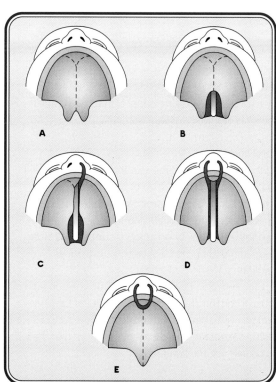

Fig. 9.2 Different types of cleft palate. (A) Cleft uvula. (B) Cleft soft and hard palate. (C) Total unilateral cleft palate and cleft lip. (D) Total bilateral cleft palate and cleft lip. (E) Bilateral cleft lip and jaw.

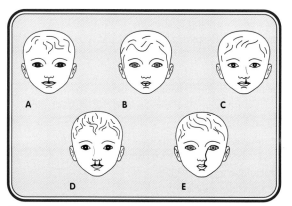

Fig. 9.1 Different types of cleft lip. (A) Median cleft upper lip. (B) Median cleft lower lip. (C) Unilateral cleft lip. (D) Bilateral cleft lip. (E) Oblique facial cleft.

buccal mucosa. The ulcer crater is covered by a creamy exudate composed of fibrin and inflammatory cells, mainly neutrophils.

Aetiology and pathogenesis are unknown. These ulcers are associated with Crohn's disease, coeliac disease, and Behçet's syndrome, but also occur in 20% of the normal population.

Aphthous ulcers are extremely common (commonest oral ulcers), recurrent (but usually of short duration), and occur singly or in groups.

Rarely, large ulcers (up to 3 cm across) occur, sometimes persisting for several weeks before healing with fibrosis.

Infective stomatitis
The majority of infections of the lips and buccal cavity are due to either viruses or fungi. The most common conditions are described below.

Herpes simplex virus
Viral infections of the lips and mouth usually manifest as large blisters or crops of small painful vesicles, which eventually erode to form shallow tender ulcers.

Infection of the mouth with herpes simplex virus (HSV) is known as herpetic stomatitis.

Blisters develop on the gingiva and palate, which eventually rupture leaving shallow ulcers. Severe herpetic stomatitis is important in immunosuppressed patients, particularly those with AIDS.

Oral candidiasis
This is an infection of the mouth with *Canidida albicans* (also known as 'oral thrush'). It is common in infants but less common in adults unless there are predisposing factors such as diabetes mellitus, or an immunosuppressed state (e.g. immunosuppressive therapy, advanced malignancy or HIV infection).

The condition develops as white patches on palatal, buccal and tongue surfaces composed of tangled fungal hyphae mixed with acute inflammatory cells and some desquamated epithelium. Underlying epithelium is acutely inflamed and red.

Glossitis
This inflammation of the tongue either arises as a result of infective stomatitis (see above) or else is due to a deficiency of nutritional factors, especially niacin, riboflavin, folic acid and vitamin B_{12}:

- Acute deficiency: tongue is red, raw and painful because of atrophy of papillae.
- Chronic deficiency: tongue appears moist and unduly clean.

Oral manifestation of systemic disease
Many oral pathologies are manifestations of systemic diseases. Examples include aphthous ulcers occurring in Crohn's and coeliac disease, and angular cheilitis/glossitis in iron-deficiency anaemia.

Neoplastic disease
Precancerous and benign
Leukoplakia (keratosis)
This premalignant epithelial dysplasia may precede the development of carcinoma. The condition is characterized by white, firm, smooth patches (hyperkeratosis) beginning at the side of the tongue and later spreading over the dorsum. In the early stages the tongue is not painful but later the patches are split by fissures with resultant tenderness.

This condition can also affect the oral mucosa, but is less typical.

Erythroplakia (erythroplasia)
Less common than leukoplakia, this is characterized by the presence of red velvety patches of epithelial atrophy and pronounced dysplasia. It is seen mainly in elderly males on the buccal mucosa or the palate.

Malignant
Squamous cell carcinoma
This is the commonest tumour of the mouth, and is derived from lining epithelium. It may arise in pre-existing dysplasia. It affects 2 per 100 000 in the UK, affecting men more than women by about 2:1. The risk factors are:
- Smoking: direct relationship between number of cigarettes smoked per day and risk of developing oral cancer.
- Alcohol: moderate intake = decreased risk, excessive intake = increased risk.
- Nutritional deficiencies.
- Candidal infection.
- Viral infections.

Macroscopically, there are raised nodular lesions and central ulceration with hard raised edges.

Microscopically, the tumour is typically well-differentiated and keratinizing.

The sites are:
- Lips (most common): usually recognized early and amenable to surgery.
- Tongue: typically occurring on lateral border of anterior two-thirds.
- Cheek or floor of mouth (less common in the UK): generally asymptomatic, resulting in extensive local invasion making surgical removal difficult.

Prognosis—May infiltrate locally and metastasize to regional lymph nodes in the neck. Five year survival is about 50%.

The oesophagus
Congenital abnormalities
Oesophageal atresia
The upper end of the oesophagus is intact but ends in a blind pouch. Oesophageal atresia affects 1 per 4000 live births, and more than 85% of cases are associated with the tracheo-oesophageal fistula (Fig. 9.3).

Oesophageal atresia with the tracheo-oesophageal fistula
The lower oesophagus is normal at the gastro-oesophageal junction, but tapers proximally and communicates with the trachea. The cause is deviation of the tracheo-oesophageal septum in a posterior direction.

The effects are:
- Fetus: inability to swallow amniotic fluid results in polyhydramnios, the accumulation of an excessive amount of amniotic fluid.
- Neonate: initially appears healthy, but swallowed fluid returns through nose and mouth and respiratory distress occurs.

Surgical repair of oesophageal atresia now results in survival rates of more than 85%.

Oesophageal stenosis
There is a narrowing of the lumen of the oesophagus, usually occurring in the distal third either as a web or as a long segment of oesophagus with a threadlike lumen. The causes are:
- Incomplete recanalization of oesophagus during development.
- Failure of blood vessels to develop in affected area → atrophy of a segment of its wall.

Webs and rings
These localized constrictions of the oesophagus are due to mucosal folds or muscular contractions.

In Plummer–Vinson or Paterson–Brown–Kelly syndrome, upper oesophageal webs are associated with dysphagia in patients with iron-deficiency anaemia, cheilosis and glossitis. This is a rare but important condition because of an association with the development of postcricoid and oral carcinoma.

Inflammation of the oesophagus (oesophagitis)
Reflux oesophagitis
Inflammation of the oesophagus caused by reflux of gastric acid into its lower part is the commonest oesophageal abnormality. The condition affects 3–4% of the general population, can occur at any age (but with increased incidence over the age of 55 years) and affects males more than females.

See Fig. 9.4 for a table of the predisposing factors of reflux oesophagitis.

Its symptom is a burning pain in the centre of the lower chest or hypochondrium commonly known as 'heartburn'.

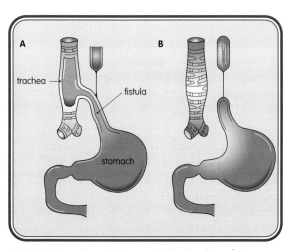

Fig. 9.3 Oesophageal atresia. (A) Blind ending of oesophagus with fistula formed between lower part and trachea. (B) Oesophageal atresia with no fistulous communication. Very rare.

The complications are:

- Peptic ulceration of lower oesophagus: development of small ulcers which become chronic with fibrosis.
- Lower oesophageal stricture: chronic peptic ulceration causes progressive fibrous thickening of the lower oesophagus wall producing difficulty in swallowing.
- Barrett's oesophagus (also termed columnar epithelial-line oesophagus): persistent oesophageal reflux causes metaplasia of lower oesophageal mucosa, the squamous epithelium being replaced by glandular epithelium composed of tall columnar cells. Metaplasia of oesophagus predisposes to the development of adenocarcinoma.

Relevant investigations include endoscopy and 24 hour intraluminal pH monitoring.

Management is by:

- Lifestyle alterations: stop smoking, decrease alcohol intake.
- Drug therapy: antacids, alginates, mucosa-protective agents, prokinetics, H$_2$-receptor antagonists, proton pump inhibitors.
- Surgery: vagotomy, repair of hiatal defect or fundal plication.

Other less common causes of oesophagitis are:

- Infective agents: *Candida albicans*, herpes simplex and cytomegalovirus are an important cause of acute oesophagitis in the immunosuppressed.
- Physical agents: irradiation or ingestion of caustic agents.
- Skin diseases, e.g. pemphigus, epidermolysis bullosa and Behçet's syndrome may cause oesophageal ulceration with extensive separation of epithelium from submucosa producing blistering followed by erosion.

Lesions associated with motor dysfunction
Achalasia

Achalasia is a condition in which muscular contraction of the oesophagus and relaxation at its lower end are not coordinated, leading to retention of the food bolus. This may occur at any age but is mainly seen in middle-aged individuals. The cause is unknown but reduced numbers of ganglion cells in the muscle plexus have been noted in long-standing cases.

The consequences are:

- Difficulty in swallowing (dysphagia): increasing slowly over years.
- Regurgitation of undigested food.
- Occasional severe chest pain caused by oesophageal spasm.
- Megaoesophagus: oesophageal distension occurs over a period of time.
- Increased predisposition to development of carcinoma of the oesophagus.

Chagas' disease

Infection by *Trypanosoma cruzi* causes a condition similar to achalasia with destruction of the myenteric plexus. It is common in South America.

Others
Hiatus hernia

This is a common condition in which the upper part of the stomach herniates through the diaphragmatic oesophageal opening (hiatus) into the thoracic cavity.

The incidence is 5 per 1000 in the UK, but it is 50–100 times less common in Asia and Africa.

The causes are:

- Congenital (rare): short oesophagus.
- Acquired (majority): a consequence of increased intra-abdominal pressure and loss of diaphragmatic muscular tone with ageing.

There are two types (Fig. 9.5):

- Sliding hiatus hernia (90%): stomach herniates through oesophageal diaphragmatic hiatus.
- Rolling (paraoesophageal) hiatus hernia (10%): stomach protrudes through a separate defect alongside the oesophagus.

Predisposing factors of reflux oesophagitis	
factors that increase intra-abdominal pressure	over-eating pregnancy poor posture
factors that render the lower oesophageal sphincter lax or incompetent	hiatus hernia smoking alcohol ingestion

Fig. 9.4 Predisposing factors of reflux oesophagitis.

The complications are reflux oesophagitis and peptic ulceration in the intrathoracic part of the stomach and the lower oesophagus.

Diverticula

Oesophageal diverticula are outpouchings of one or more layers of the oesophageal wall. They can develop by either:

- Pulsion: pressure from within the oesophagus creates a diverticulum. This is common immediately above sphincters.
- Traction: external forces pull on the wall, usually from adherent inflammatory lesions, classically tuberculous lymph nodes. This is common near the midpoint of the oesophagus.

The site may be either:

- Immediately above the upper oesophageal sphincter (Zenker's diverticulum).
- Near the midpoint of the oesophagus (traction diverticulum).
- Immediately above the lower oesophageal sphincter (epiphrenic diverticulum).

The complications are dysphagia (where the diverticula frequently become permanently distended with retained food and cause difficulties in swallowing) and an increased risk of oesophageal perforation on endoscopy.

Lacerations

Oesophageal perforation is rare, but may be caused by:

- Traumatic rupture: usually associated with vomiting.
- Impaction of a sharp foreign body.
- Intubation of strictures.

'Mallory–Weiss tear' is an oesophageal laceration as a result of vomiting. A classical symptom is vomiting of clear fluid (pretearing), followed by vomiting of blood (post-tearing).

Oesophageal varices

These are varicosed, dilated submucosal veins in the oesophagus.

The condition is caused by portal hypertension (most commonly associated with cirrhosis of the liver).

Pathogenesis—Oesophageal veins normally drain into both systemic and portal venous systems.

Increased pressure in the portal venous system (e.g. as a result of severe diffuse long-standing liver disease) causes dilatation of the oesophageal veins to form oesophageal varices, which often protrude into the lumen.

Rupture of the varices or ulceration of overlying mucosa can produce a torrential haemorrhage into the oesophagus and stomach, often precipitating vomiting of blood.

Management

There are three stages:

1. Local measures to control bleeding.
2. Reduction of portal venous pressure.
3. Prevention of recurrent bleeding.

Local measures to control bleeding are:

- Sclerotherapy: injection of varices with an irritant

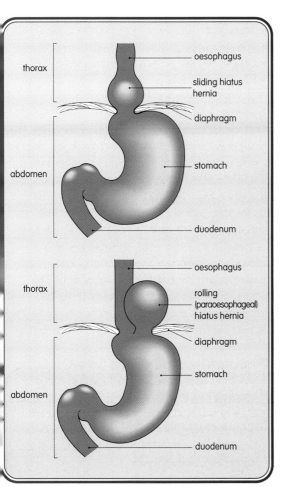

Fig. 9.5 Types of hiatus hernia. (A) Sliding hiatus hernia. (B) Rolling hiatus hernia.

solution which causes thrombophlebitis (see Chapter 7) resulting in obliteration of varices by thrombosis and subsequent scarring. This is the most important initial treatment.

- Balloon tamponade: two balloons exert pressure in fundus of stomach and in the lower oesophagus. Pressure on the varices prevents bleeding, and allows time for the use of more definitive therapy.
- Transjugular intrahepatic portasystemic stent shunting (TIPSS): stent is placed between the hepatic and portal veins thus providing a portasystemic shunt to reduce portal pressure.
- Oesophageal transection: transection of the varices with stapling gun.

Reduction of portal venous pressure can be achieved with drugs, e.g. vasopressin and somatostatin.

Prevention of recurrent bleeding can be achieved with:
- Sclerotherapy.
- Banding: varices are sucked into an endoscope accessory and occluded with a tight rubber band. Occluded varix subsequently sloughs with variceal obliteration. Fewer side effects than sclerotherapy.
- TIPSS.
- Propanolol: reduces portal venous pressure in portal hypertension.

Neoplastic disease
Barrett's oesophagus
Definition—Metaplastic replacement of normal squamous oesophageal epithelium with glandular epithelium.

The condition is caused by persistent oesophageal reflux; approximately 10% of these patients will develop Barrett's oesophagus.

Barrett's oesophagus predisposes to the development of adenocarcinoma. Metaplastic glandular epithelium can progress to epithelial dysplasia and then to frank adenocarcinoma.

Benign neoplastic disease
Benign tumours of the oesophagus are rare. The majority are leiomyomas derived from the smooth muscle of muscularis propria, the minority being derived from nerves, i.e. schwannomas and neurofibromas.

Barrett's oesophagus is a classic example of metaplasia and is the best example to quote in an examination.

Malignant neoplastic disease
The most common malignant tumours of the oesophagus are squamous carcinomas and adenocarcinomas. Incidence is 5–10 per 100 000 per year in the UK. Risk factors are:
- Smoking/alcohol.
- Dietary (tannic acid, food colourings).
- Barrett's oesophagus.
- Corrosives.
- Achalasia.
- Iron-deficiency anaemia.
- Genetic: tylosis.
- Infection: bacterial, fungi, viruses (HPV).

Squamous cell carcinomas
These are more common than adenocarcinomas. They mostly develop in men who are heavy alcohol drinkers or heavy smokers, and may be preceded by an epithelial dysplastic change. They usually present late when the tumour is large enough to compromise oesophageal lumen and cause dysphagia. They are most common in the middle and lower oesophagus.

Adenocarcinomas
These mainly occur in the lower oesophagus. The majority arise in areas of epithelial metaplasia (Barrett's oesophagus) but some are primary carcinomas of the stomach that have infiltrated the lower oesophagus.

Clinical features of oesophageal tumours
- Common: dysphagia, anorexia, weight loss, anaemia (acute or chronic).
- Rare: hoarse voice (involvement of larynx or left recurrent laryngeal nerve palsy), supraclavicular lymphadenopathy, tracheo-oesophageal fistula, aorto-oesophageal fistula.

Investigations are:
- Chest X-ray: mediastinal mass, pulmonary metastases, pleural effusion.

- Barium swallow.
- Upper GI endoscopy: proximal extent of tumour, biopsy, dilatation.
- CT/MRI: check other organs for metastases.
- Endoscopic ultrasound: good for staging disease.
- Respiratory function tests: prognostic for resection.

Management:
- Palliative: usually for treatment of dysphagia (intubation, dilatation, bypass, laser treatment).
- Curative: surgery or radiotherapy.

The prognosis is poor for both types of malignant oesophageal tumours, that for squamous carcinoma being slightly better than adenocarcinoma because it is more responsive to radiotherapy.

Survival post treatment—30% at 1 year, 20% at 2 years, 5% at 5 years.

- **Name the common developmental abnormalities of the mouth, and state their prevalence.**
- **What are aphthous ulcers?**
- **Describe the neoplastic lesions that may arise in the mouth.**
- **Outline three congenital anomalies of the oesophagus.**
- **Describe the features of reflux oesophagitis.**
- **What is Barrett's oesophagus?**

DISORDERS OF THE STOMACH

Congenital abnormalities
Diaphragmatic hernias
These are described in the previous section (pp. 136–137).

Pyloric stenosis
Marked narrowing of the pylorus (gastric outflow tract) causes obstruction to the passage of food such that the stomach becomes markedly distended and the stomach's contents are expelled with considerable force. The disorder can be congenital or acquired.

Congenitally, it is a common anomaly, affecting 4 per 1000 live births, males more than females by 5:1. Hypertrophy of pyloric circular and longitudinal muscle layers causes projectile vomiting.

Acquired causes are:
- Fibrous stricture from a duodenal ulcer.
- Oedema from pyloric channel or duodenal ulcer.
- Carcinoma of stomach antrum.
- Adult hypertrophic pyloric stenosis.

Symptoms are mainly nausea and vomiting. Signs include wasting, dehydration and a succussion splash which may be elicited 4 hours or more after the last meal or drink.

Inflammation
Acute gastritis
This superficial acute inflammation of the gastric mucosa is typically caused by ingested chemicals, the most common being alcohol, aspirin and NSAIDs such as indomethacin.

Acute erosive gastritis
Focal loss of the superficial gastric epithelium causes dyspepsia with vomiting and occasionally, if the erosions are numerous, haematemesis may occur.
Causes are:
- NSAIDs.
- Heavy acute alcohol ingestion.
- Severe stress or shock (e.g. after major trauma or burns).
- Hypotension: acute hypoxia of surface epithelium.

Chronic gastritis
Chronic inflammation of the gastric mucosa is a common condition. It increases with age to over 50% in persons over 50 years old, and is more common in developed countries.

The condition is present in over 90% of patients with duodenal ulceration, in about 70% of those with gastric ulceration, and it is also common in those with gastric cancer.

There are three aetiological types of classification:
- Infectious: *Helicobacter pylori*-associated gastritis.
- Immune: pernicious anaemia and atrophic gastritis without pernicious anaemia.
- Reactive: post gastrectomy or adjacent to erosions/ulcers.

139

Helicobacter-associated gastritis

This is the most common form of chronic gastritis accounting for more than 90% of cases, and may arise at any age. The pyloric antrum is the most severely affected area, but damage is also seen in the fundus.

Pathogenesis is as follows:
- Colonization: *Helicobacter pylori* colonizes epithelial surface beneath thin layer of mucus.
- Urease production: bacterium produces enzyme 'urease' which breaks down urea to give CO_2 and NH_3, the latter providing protection from the acid secretions of the stomach.
- Immune response: presence of organism results in an immune response → epithelial damage.
- Persistence of infection: once established infection may persist for years.

The morphological features are:
- Mucin depletion leading to damage to the underlying epithelium.
- Atrophy of gastric glands.
- Mixed acute and chronic inflammatory cell reaction in lamina propria and superficial epithelium.
- Intestinal metaplasia: normal gastric epithelium is replaced by a type similar to that of small intestine.

The tests available for diagnosis of *H. pylori* infection are listed in Fig. 9.6.

Autoimmune chronic gastritis

This organ-specific autoimmune disease associated with pernicious anaemia is generally seen in elderly patients with the development of severe atrophy of the mucosa (atrophic gastritis). It particularly affects the body of the stomach.

Antibodies are of two types:
- Antibodies against gastric parietal cells (90%): associated with decreased hydrochloric acid production (hypochlorhydria).
- Antibodies against intrinsic factor (60%) → failure of absorption of dietary vitamin B_{12} → interference with normal erythropoiesis in bone marrow → megaloblastic macrocytic anaemia (pernicious anaemia).

The most common form is atrophic gastritis with achlorhydria but without pernicious anaemia. In this condition antibodies of both types are often present, but there is a residual ability to absorb vitamin B_{12}. However, patients may develop pernicious anaemia with time.

The morphological features are:
- Loss of specialized cells.
- Fibrosis.
- Infiltrate of plasma cells and lymphocytes.
- Intestinal metaplasia.

Reactive gastritis (reflux gastritis)

In this pattern of mucosal injury the dominant feature is epithelial change with minimal inflammatory cell infiltrates. The causes are threefold:
- Idiopathic: majority of cases.
- Reflux of alkaline bile-containing duodenal fluid into lower part of stomach. This may be caused by

Test for diagnosis of *Helicobacter pylori* infection		
Type	**Test**	**Diagnosis**
non-invasive	urea breath test	radiolabelled urea is administered; urease produced by *H. pylori* → radioactive CO_2, which can be detected on the breath
	serology	antibodies to *H. pylori* can be detected in serum
invasive	histology	organisms can be seen in biopsy material
	culture	can be cultured from biopsy material
	CLO (*Campylobacter*-like organism) test	biopsy added to test kit containing urea. If urease present, NH_3 produced causes change in colour of indicator

Fig. 9.6 Diagnosis of *Helicobacter pylori* infection.

motility disturbances (e.g. due to gallstones or cholecystectomy) or pyloric incompetence (as a result of previous surgery to pylori area).
- Drugs: NSAIDs may cause direct damage to the mucus layer.

Peptic ulcers are a common topic in examinations.

Morphological features are:
- Epithelial desquamation.
- Foveolar hyperplasia.
- Vasodilatation.
- Mucosal oedema.

Complications of chronic gastritis
Regardless of cause, all forms of chronic gastritis can cause intestinal metaplasia (producing an increased predisposition to undergo dysplastic change with eventual transformation into carcinoma), and peptic ulcerations caused by damage to the gastric lining by acidic gastric secretions.

Gastric ulceration
Peptic ulcers
These are ulcers of the oesophagus, stomach or duodenum caused by damage to the epithelial lining by gastric secretions, particularly acid.

It is estimated that about 10% of the Western population experience peptic ulceration at some time. Ulcers usually develop in adulthood and have a natural history of repeated healing and relapse over many years.

Sites are:
- Lower oesophagus (due to gastric reflux).
- Stomach: most common on distal lesser curve.
- Duodenum: commonest site of peptic ulceration.
- Gastroenterostomy sites.

Aetiology is probably multifactorial. Ulcers are commonly associated with H. pylori, NSAIDs, and stress. Less commonly, they may be associated with acid hypersecretion (e.g. gastrinoma), infection, duodenal obstruction/disruption and vascular insufficiency, or radiation induced.

Other factors, such as chronic gastritis, smoking and genetic predisposition, are also believed to play a role in the pathogenesis, although the mechanisms are poorly understood.

Pathogenesis—Upper GI mucosa is normally protected by either squamous epithelium (oesophagus) or an acid-resisting mucus barrier containing

neutralizing bicarbonate ions. Peptic ulceration occurs when the aggressive action of acid and pepsin is not opposed by adequate mucosal protective mechanisms:
- Oesophageal ulceration: most important cause is reflux of acid gastric secretion on to the unprotected oesophageal mucosa.
- Duodenal ulceration: most important factor is hypersecretion of acid by the stomach.
- Gastric ulceration: predisposing factors include regurgitated bile in pyloric incompetence and surface epithelial damage by H. pylori infection or by non-steroidal, anti-inflammatory agents.

Macroscopically, peptic ulcers are typically 1–2 cm in diameter (but can be much larger) with sharply defined borders surrounding the ulcer crater.

Microscopically, the ulcer crater usually penetrates into the muscularis propria of the stomach and has four histological zones, namely:
- Superficial layer of fibrin and inflammatory exudate.
- Fibrinoid necrosis.
- Granulation tissue.
- Fibrosis.

Complete healing of the ulcer leads to fibrous replacement of muscle with regrowth of epithelium over the scar. Clinical features include epigastric pain (alleviated by antacids), nausea and heartburn (oesophageal ulcers).

Complications and sequelae are as follows:
- Healing, which usually occurs slowly but can be hastened by acid-inhibiting agents or mucosal protectants.
- Haemorrhage: a common cause of upper GI bleeding.
- Adherence and erosion: ulcer penetrates full thickness of the stomach or duodenal wall, adhering and eroding into underlying tissue, particularly the pancreas or liver.

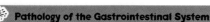
- Perforation: ulcer perforates, leading to peritonitis.
- Fibrous strictures: seen in peptic ulcers of the oesophagus; fibrous thickening caused by healing leads to scarring of oesophagus and obstruction. In the stomach, ulcers may cause pyloric stenosis.
- Malignant change (rare).

Management is by:
- Lifestyle alterations: stop smoking, decrease alcohol intake.
- Medical: eradication of *H. pylori* (antibiotics), acid suppression (antacids, proton pump inhibitors, H_2 receptor antagonists, etc.).
- Surgery: partial gastrectomy, vagotomy.

Acute gastric ulcer
Acute peptic ulcers usually develop from areas of erosive gastritis and are predisposed by the same conditions as erosive gastritis. In contrast to chronic ulcers, they are generally multiple and shallow with minimal surrounding inflammation or fibrosis.

Acute ulcers may heal without scarring, or may progress to chronicity.

Hypertrophic gastropathy
Ménétrier's disease
This rare disease of unknown cause is characterized by gross hyperplasia of gastric pits, atrophy of glands and a marked overall increase in mucosal thickness. It is associated with hypoalbuminaemia as a result of gastric protein loss via superficial ulcerations.

Hypertrophic hypersecretory gastropathy
An extremely rare condition, this is characterized by acid hypersecretion and gastric protein loss.

Zollinger–Ellison syndrome
This syndrome of gastric hypersecretion, multiple peptic ulcers and diarrhoea is caused by the gastrin secreting tumour (gastrinoma) of the pancreatic G cells (see Chapter 11).

Neoplastic disease
Benign
Benign gastric polyps are rare compared to the incidence of malignant tumours of the stomach. The types are:
- Hyperplastic polyps: commonest polyp of stomach formed by regeneration of mucosa often at the edge of an ulcer.
- Adenomatous polyps: true benign tumours of the surface epithelium ranging up to 5 cm in size. Very rare but carry a risk of malignant change.
- Fundal polyps: cystic glandular lesions seen mainly in women.
- Harmartomatous polyps: occur in Peutz–Jeghers syndrome (hereditary condition of multiple polyps in small intestine associated with pigmented areas around lips, inside mouth and on palms and soles).

Other benign tumours of the stomach are derived from mesenchymal tissues, the most common being leiomyomas. These appear as mucosal or intramural nodules and are usually asymptomatic.

Malignant
Gastric adenocarcinomas
The vast majority of gastric carcinomas are adenocarcinomas derived from mucus-secreting epithelial cells. They affect 20–40 people per 100 000 per year, and are typically seen in patients after the age of 30, the incidence rising greatly after the age of 50 years. Males are affected more than females by 3:2.

They are common in the Far East and certain parts of South America and Scandinavia, but less so in western Europe and North America.

The sites are:
- Pylorus (60%): often produce symptoms of obstruction to gastric outlet.
- Fundus (20–30%): typically a fungating, ulcerating mass.
- Cardia (5–20%): may produce dysphagia.

Unlike chronic peptic ulcers of the stomach, they are not confined to the lesser curvature.

Aetiology is unknown but dietary factors are suggested to account for geographical variation, e.g. ingestion of smoked and salted preserved foods. Other risk factors include:
- Chronic gastritis and intestinal metaplasia.
- Gastric adenomatous polyps.
- Postgastrectomy patients with persisting gastric inflammation.
- Gastric cancer families (rare).
- *H. pylori* infection: prevalence of *H. pylori* infection frequently runs parallel with the incidence of gastric cancer, and patients with antibodies to the bacterium have a higher risk of gastric cancer.

The sequence of events in the development of gastric carcinomas is as follows:

normal mucosa → chronic gastritis → intestinal metaplasia → dysplasia → intramucosal carcinoma (early gastric cancer) → invasive carcinoma

Gastric cancers are classified as either early or advanced according to the extent of their spread through the stomach wall.

Early gastric cancer
This is confined to the mucosa and/or submucosa regardless of whether spread has occurred to regional lymph nodes. It is associated with a good prognosis.
   The cancer is further divided into three types according to macroscopical appearance (Fig. 9.7).

Advanced gastric tumours
These extend into or beyond the main muscle coats, and are associated with a poor prognosis. They are further divided into three types macroscopically (Fig. 9.8):

- Polypoid: protrudes into stomach lumen and presents early due to a feeling of gastric discomfort and bleeding of protrusion when traumatized. Usually amenable to surgical excision and has the best prognosis.
- Ulcerating (commonest type): similar to benign peptic ulcers but with raised edge, necrotic shaggy base, and an absence of the radiation folds seen in benign peptic ulcers.
- Diffuse infiltrative pattern (linitus plastica): presents late and has worst prognosis. Tumour spreads extensively within mucosa and submucosa producing a shrunken, inexpansible, rigid stomach. Symptoms are usually non specific; loss of appetite and vomiting due to small capacity of stomach and its inability to distend under a food load. Surface ulceration is not a prominent feature and so haematemesis is not common until late stages. Metastatic spread to lymph nodes and liver is usually present at time of clinical presentation.

Other gastric tumours
Other forms of malignancy are rare in the stomach, but include lymphomas (see Chapter 14), carcinoid tumours (p. 181), and secondary tumours from other sites.

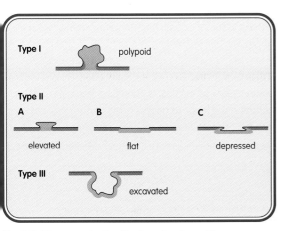

Fig. 9.7 Macroscopic classification of early gastric cancers: type I polypoid; type II is further divided into (A) elevated, (B) flat, and (C) depressed; type III excavated.

Comparison of the types of advanced gastric carcinomas			
	Polypoid	**Ulcerative**	**Diffuse infiltrative**
incidence	common	very common	rare
haemorrhage	yes	yes	not until late stage
prognosis	good	intermediate	poor
involvement	focal	focal	diffuse

Fig. 9.8 Comparison of the types of advanced gastric carcinomas.

143

- State the causes of pyloric stenosis.
- Describe the three main patterns of chronic gastritis.
- Name the sites that may be affected by peptic ulcers.
- Explain the pathogenesis and list the complications of peptic ulcers.
- Describe the classification of gastric adenocarcinomas.
- Describe the pathologies associated with *Helicobacter pylori* infection.

GENERAL ASPECTS OF HEPATIC DAMAGE

Patterns of hepatic injury

Following hepatic injury, the liver has a limited set of responses:

- Necrosis.
- Inflammation.
- Regeneration.
- Fibrosis.

All pathological processes of the liver result in one or more of the above reactions.

Necrosis

Acute hepatocellular injury can result in variable forms of necrosis. The underlying type of necrosis depends on aetiology.

Coagulative necrosis

This is typically a result of ischaemia (see Chapter 3).

Councilman bodies

During the death of individual liver cells (by apoptosis), single, dead hepatocytes form brightly eosinophilic, shrunken structures known as Councilman bodies.

Hydropic degeneration

This is the ballooning of individual hepatocytes generally as a result of viral hepatitis. It is a mild change but may progress to necrosis.

Focal necrosis

Necrosis of small groups of hepatocytes, occurs in acute viral- or drug-induced hepatitis.

Zonal necrosis

Necrosis confined to certain zones is seen with certain diseases, e.g. centrilobular area (zone 3) is affected in paracetamol toxicity (Fig. 9.9).

Massive necrosis

Necrosis of the majority of hepatocytes. Occurs with fulminant hepatic damage and is seen in some cases of viral- and toxin-induced damage.

Piecemeal necrosis

Liver cells at the interface between parenchyma and fibrous tissue are destroyed, together with lymphocytic or plasma cell infiltrate.

Inflammation

Inflammation of the liver is known as hepatitis, and is a common response to a wide array of damage, e.g. viral infection, autoimmune disorders, drugs and toxins.

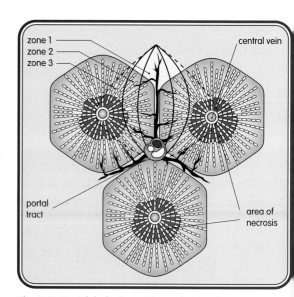

Fig. 9.9 Centrilobular (zone 3) zonal necrosis.

Regeneration

Under normal circumstances there is very little liver cell proliferation. However, following hepatic injury, liver cell regeneration occurs to restore liver function; this is a crucial phenomenon for recovery for patients with fulminant or subfulminant liver failure.

Fibrosis

Repeated chronic damage to the liver can result in fibrosis. Growth factors produced as part of inflammatory response are thought to stimulate proliferation and differentiation of mesenchymal cells (the normally inconspicuous fat-storing cells of Ito located in the space of Disse) into collagen-secreting fibroblasts.

Development of fibrosis is an important complication of several liver diseases and is one of the characteristic features of cirrhosis.

Cirrhosis

An irreversible condition in which the liver's normal architecture is diffusely replaced by nodules of regenerated liver cells separated by bands of collagenous fibrosis. Cirrhosis represents the end-stage of many processes. It involves:

- Long-standing destruction of liver cells.
- Chronic inflammation that stimulates fibrosis.
- Regeneration of hepatocytes to cause nodules.

Macroscopically, the liver is tawny and characteristically knobbly (due to nodules). On a cut surface, parenchyma is replaced by nodules of regenerated hepatocytes separated by fine fibrosis.

Microscopically, the nodules of hepatocytes are separated by bands of collagenous tissue. Bile ducts and portal vessels run in the fibrous septa.

Cirrhosis can be classified either according to the size of regenerative nodules (Fig. 9.10) or according to its aetiology (Fig. 9.11). However, an aetiological classification is most useful in determining prognosis and treatment. The clinical features of cirrhosis are illustrated in Fig. 9.12.

Consequences are:

- Liver failure: reduced hepatocyte function (decreased synthesis of proteins, failure of detoxification).
- Portal hypertension and its complications (see below): a result of impeded blood flow through liver.

- Reduced immune competence → increased susceptibility to infection.
- Increased risk of development of hepatocellular carcinoma.
- Increased risk of development of portal vein thrombosis.

Portal hypertension, ascites and splenomegaly
Portal hypertension

This is a continued elevation in portal venous pressure, normal portal venous pressure being 7 mmHg. Causes of portal hypertension can be classified according to whether the site of obstruction to flow is:

- Prehepatic: blockage of vessels before the hepatic sinusoids.

Classification according to nodular size	
Type	**Nodule size**
micronodular	≤3 mm
macronodular	3 mm–2 cm
mixed micro- and macronodular	mixture of small and large

Fig. 9.10 Classification according to nodular size.

Classification according to incidence in the Western world	
common	alcoholic liver disease cryptogenic (no cause found) chronic hepatitis caused by hepatitis B and C viruses
uncommon	autoimmune chronic hepatitis primary biliary cirrhosis chronic biliary obstruction (biliary cirrhosis) cystic fibrosis
treatable but rare	haemochromatosis Wilson's disease
rare	α_1-antitrypsin deficiency galactosaemia glycogenosis type IV tyrosinaemia

Fig. 9.11 Classification according to incidence in the Western world.

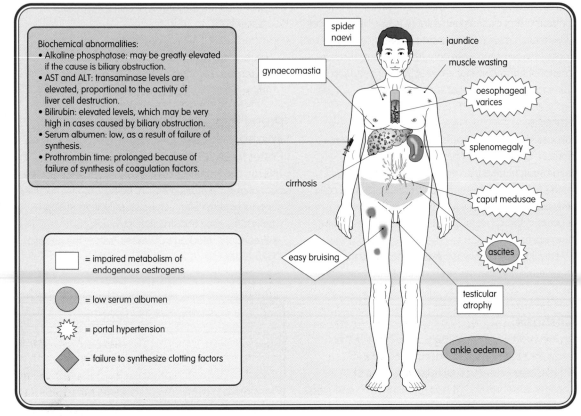

Biochemical abnormalities:
- Alkaline phosphatase: may be greatly elevated if the cause is biliary obstruction.
- AST and ALT: transaminase levels are elevated, proportional to the activity of liver cell destruction.
- Bilirubin: elevated levels, which may be very high in cases caused by biliary obstruction.
- Serum albumen: low, as a result of failure of synthesis.
- Prothrombin time: prolonged because of failure of synthesis of coagulation factors.

= impaired metabolism of endogenous oestrogens

= low serum albumen

= portal hypertension

= failure to synthesize clotting factors

spider naevi
jaundice
gynaecomastia
muscle wasting
oesophageal varices
splenomegaly
cirrhosis
caput medusae
easy bruising
ascites
testicular atrophy
ankle oedema

Fig. 9.12 Clinical signs of cirrhosis.

- Hepatic: blockage in the hepatic sinusoids.
- Posthepatic: blockage in the central veins, hepatic veins or vena cava.

See Fig. 9.13 for a table of the causes of portal hypertension.

Complications—Portal hypertension causes back-pressure in the portal vascular bed leading to splenomegaly, ascites, and varicose venous channels.

Classification of portal hypertension	
prehepatic	portal vein thrombosis
hepatic	cirrhosis idiopathic portal hypertension hepatic fibrosis: caused by schistosomiasis (important cause in endemic areas) polycystic disease of the liver
posthepatic	disease of hepatic veins and branches

Fig. 9.13 Classification of portal hypertension.

New varicose venous channels open up between the portal venous system and systemic venous system. Main sites are the lower oesophagus—oesophageal varices (see pp. 137–138) which may cause bleeding, the umbilicus (channels are called caput medusae), and the anus (rectal varices).

The causes and effects of portal hypertension are shown in Fig. 9.14.

Ascites

Ascites is the accumulation of fluid in the peritoneal cavity.
Causes are:
- Peritonitis.
- Malignancy in the peritoneal cavity.
- Hypoproteinaemia.
- Portal hypertension.

Main causes of portal hypertension are:
- Cirrhosis of the liver (most common).
- Portal vein thrombosis.
- Hepatic vein thrombosis (Budd–Chiari syndrome).

Pathogenesis of ascites in cirrhosis—Increased transudation of fluid in ascites occurs as a result of:

- ↑ Hydrostatic pressure in portal veins.
- ↓ Plasma oncotic pressure (due to lowered albumin synthesis by damaged liver cells).

Fig. 9.15 is a table describing the types of ascites.

Clinical features are abdominal distension with fullness in the flanks, shifting dullness on percussion, and fluid thrill.

Management is by:

- Restricted Na⁺ intake.
- Diuretic drugs, e.g. spironolactone.
- Paracentesis: drainage of 3–5 litres over 1–2 hours is used for immediate relief. Drainage to dryness must be supported by giving colloid (e.g. plasma) as required.
- LeVeen shunt: long tube with one-way valve running subcutaneously from peritoneum to internal jugular vein in neck. Allows ascitic fluid to pass directly into systemic circulation. Complications of infection, thrombosis and pulmonary oedema limit its use.
- TIPSS (see p. 138): relieves portal hypertension.

Prognosis—Only 10–20% of patients survive 5 years from its appearance.

Portosystemic shunts

Venous communications that link portal and systemic venous systems become enlarged in portal hypertension. The four sites of portal–systemic anastomosis are:

- Lower third of the oesophagus: left gastric vein (portal tributary) anastomoses with oesophageal veins (systemic tributary).
- Halfway down the anal canal: superior rectal veins (portal tributary) draining upper half of anal canal anastomose with middle and inferior rectal veins (systemic tributaries).
- Paraumbilical veins: connect left branch of portal vein with superficial veins of anterior abdominal wall (systemic tributaries).
- Veins of ascending colon, descending colon, duodenum, pancreas and liver (portal tributaries) anastomose with renal, lumbar, and phrenic veins (systemic tributaries).

Pathogenesis—Under normal conditions, portal venous blood traverses the liver and drains into the inferior vena cava of systemic venous circulation by way of the hepatic veins. In portal hypertension, this direct route is blocked and the portal venous blood is forced through smaller communications that exist between the portal and systemic systems.

Anastomotic channels become dilated resulting in the development of varicose venous channels, namely:

- Oesophageal varices (see pp. 137–138): may cause bleeding.
- Caput medusae: distension of paraumbilical veins.
- Haemorrhoids.

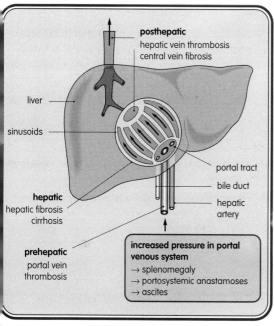

Fig. 9.14 Causes and effects of portal hypertension.

Types of ascites	
Transudate low protein fluid (<11 dg/l)	**Exudate** high protein fluid (>11 dg/l)

cirrhosis
constrictive pericarditis
cardiac failure
hypoalbuminaemia,
  e.g. nephrotic syndrome
	malignancy
	peritonitis
	pancreatitis
	Budd–Chiari syndrome
	hypothyroidism
	lymphatic obstruction
	  (chylous ascites)

Fig. 9.15 Types of ascites.

Splenomegaly

Increased pressure in the portal vein is transmitted to the splenic vein resulting in splenomegaly (see Chapter 14).

Jaundice and cholestasis

Jaundice

This presents as a yellowing of the skin or sclerae, indicating excess bilirubin in the blood.

The biochemical definition of jaundice is an increase in the plasma bilirubin level above the normal level of about 18–24 µmol/L (i.e. 1.2 mg/dL).

Clinical jaundice is when levels of bilirubin are above 50 µmol/L (i.e. 2.5 mg/dL), manifesting as a yellow discoloration of the sclerae and skin.

The metabolism of bilirubin is illustrated in Fig. 9.16.

Cholestasis

Failure of bile flow caused by the obstruction of either small (intrahepatic) or large (extrahepatic) bile ducts results in jaundice due to conjugated hyperbilirubinaemia.

Jaundice can be classified according to aetiology (Fig. 9.17) or according to chemical analysis of the bilirubin in the blood (Fig. 9.18).

Unconjugated versus conjugated hyperbilirubinaemia

Unconjugated

Excess bilirubin is not water soluble and cannot be excreted in urine. Urine is therefore of normal colour but faeces may be slightly darker due to increased excretion of fat-soluble bilirubin into bile. Unconjugated hyperbilirubinaemia is not associated with itching.

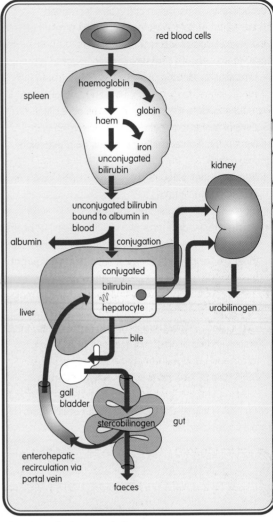

Fig. 9.16 Bilirubin metabolism.

Causes of jaundice	
Cause	**Clinical consequence**
prehepatic causes	haemolysis (commonest cause)
intrahepatic causes	hereditary enzyme defects, e.g. Dubin–Johnson, Rotor's, Gilbert's and Crigler–Najjar syndromes drugs causing intrahepatic cholestasis pregnancy-associated cholestasis hepatocellular damage, e.g. alcohol, virus hepatitis
posthepatic (obstructive) causes	large duct obstruction as a result of: • gallstones • strictures caused by inflammation or fibrosis • extrahepatic biliary atresia • compression by extrinsic masses, e.g. carcinoma of the pancreas, enlarged lymph nodes

Fig. 9.17 Causes of jaundice.

Conjugated

Excess bilirubin is conjugated to form bilirubin-glucuronate, which is water soluble. The features of conjugated hyperbilirubinaemia are:

- Pale stools: bilirubin conjugate is not excreted into the intestine but accumulates in the liver either as a result of biliary obstruction (cholestasis) or as a result of its impaired excretion into bile (rare).
- Dark urine: conjugated bilirubin (water soluble) accumulates in the liver and is excreted in the urine.
- Pruritus: conjugated bilirubin is deposited in the skin, causing severe itching.

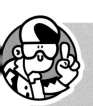

Two important points to note about jaundice:
- **Liver disease is not the only cause of jaundice; there are other causes, e.g. haemolysis.**
- **Many patients with significant liver disease are not jaundiced.**

Hepatic failure
Hepatic encephalopathy

A neuropsychiatric syndrome caused by liver disease, this occurs most often in patients with cirrhosis but is also seen in more acute form in fulminant hepatic failure. Pathogenesis is:

- Liver failure: liver is unable to remove exogenous/endogenous compounds from the circulation. Neurotoxins accumulate and mimic the action of endogenous neurotransmitters.
- Shunting: in portal hypertension, there is shunting of portal blood past the liver directly into the systemic circulation.

The overall effect is a biochemical disturbance of brain function. The condition is reversible and rarely shows marked pathological changes in the brain.

Hepatorenal syndrome

Renal failure secondary to liver failure occurs in advanced cirrhosis, and almost always in conjunction with ascites.

The kidneys themselves are normal. Renal failure is thought to result from altered systemic blood flow including diminished renal flow.

Classification of jaundice according to chemical composition of bilirubin			
Type	**Cause**	**Example**	**Features**
unconjugated hyperbilirubinaemia	prehepatic	haemolysis	urine: normal faeces: dark
	intrahepatic	impaired bilirubin uptake (Gilbert's syndrome) impaired bilirubin conjugation Crigler–Najjar syndrome drugs, e.g. rifampicin	increased risk of pigment gallstones no itching (excess urobilinogen with haemolysis)
conjugated hyperbilirubinaemia	intrahepatic non-cholestatic	impaired bilirubin excretion into bile: • Dubin–Johnson syndrome • Rotor's syndrome	urine: dark faeces: pale itching
	intrahepatic cholestatic	small bile duct obstruction: • acute/chronic hepatitis • cirrhosis • intrahepatic tumours • pregnancy-associated cholestasis • sclerosing cholangitis • intrahepatic biliary atresia	urine: dark faeces: pale itching
	posthepatic	large bile duct obstruction	urine: dark faeces: pale itching

Fig. 9.18 Classification of jaundice according to chemical composition of bilirubin.

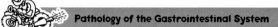

Prognosis—Recovery depends on improvement of liver function but in chronic liver disease this seldom occurs.

Liver transplantation
Liver transplantation is, necessarily, a treatment for liver failure for which there is no other medical therapy.

Conditions for which liver transplantation is most commonly performed
These are shown in decreasing order of frequency.

Chronic liver disease (end-stage)
The conditions are:
- Primary biliary cirrhosis.
- Primary sclerosing cholangitis.
- Alcoholic liver disease.
- Metabolic liver disease.

Fulminant hepatic failure
Examples of this include disease due to non-A or non-B hepatitis, or idiosyncratic drug reactions.

Hepatic tumours
Transplantation is only considered in the absence of extrahepatic malignancy.
   Signs of end-stage liver disease:
- Sustained or increased jaundice (bilirubin more than 100 µmol/L).
- Ascites not responding readily to medical therapy.

- Describe the responses of the liver to hepatic injury.
- Define 'cirrhosis' and list the most common causes.
- State the causes of portal hypertension.
- What are the main causes of ascites?
- Describe the aetiology and pathogenesis of hyperbilirubinaemia.
- What is hepatic encephalopathy and how does it arise?

- Malnutrition.
- Hypoalbuminaemia (<30 g/L).

Risks involved are:
- Rejection: immunosuppressives used to lower risk.
- Sepsis: prophylactic antibiotic therapy.
- Poor biliary drainage due to biliary strictures of leaks.

Prognosis is very good and improving. One year survival is 75–85%.

DISORDERS OF THE LIVER AND BILIARY TRACT

Congenital errors of metabolism
Haemochromatosis
This condition is caused by excessive deposition of iron in tissues. There are two types: primary haemochromatosis (also known as hereditary haemochromatosis) and secondary haemochromatosis (also called haemosiderosis).

Primary haemochromatosis
This inherited autosomal recessive trait leads to excessive absorption of iron from the gut. Its prevalence is thought to be quite high, affecting up to 1% of the population in some areas. At least 90% of patients are male, probably because females are protected by iron loss in menstruation and pregnancy.

Secondary haemochromatosis
This condition results from excessive iron accumulation caused by other primary diseases (e.g. alcoholism) and by repeated blood transfusions for diseases with abnormalities of red cell formation, particularly thalassaemia.

Effects of iron accumulation
Iron accumulates as haemosiderin in many tissues including the liver, pancreas, pituitary, heart and skin. Affected tissues appear rusty brown due to haemosiderin in cells, as follows:
- In the liver: hepatocyte necrosis (possibly from generation of free radicals), ultimately resulting in cirrhosis often with hepatomegaly.
- In the heart: infiltration of cardiac muscle can cause cardiomyopathy with heart failure.

The term 'bronzed diabetes' is often used to describe haemochromatosis due to the combination of diabetes and hyperpigmentation.

- In the pancreas: damage to pancreatic islets may result in diabetes mellitus.
- In the skin: leaden grey pigmentation of skin due to excess melanin, especially in exposed parts—axillae, groins and genitalia.

Diagnosis—In the blood there is a high saturation of transferrin, and high serum iron and ferritin levels; in the liver, biopsy shows heavy iron deposition and hepatic fibrosis, which may have progressed to cirrhosis.

Management:
- Reduction of dietary ferritin.
- Weekly venesection (bleedings) of 500 mL until serum iron is normal.
- Therapy for cirrhosis and diabetes mellitus.

Wilson's disease

This autosomal recessive disorder of copper metabolism results in chronic destructive liver disease.

Normally, dietary copper is taken up by the liver, complexed to ceruloplasmin (a copper-binding protein) and then the whole complex is secreted into the plasma. Circulating ceruloplasmin is subsequently recycled by the liver, with any remaining associated copper being re-excreted into the bile.

In Wilson's disease, a mutation in a copper transport ATPase gene results in failure of the liver to secrete the copper–ceruloplasmin complex into the plasma. The copper complex accumulates within the hepatocytes, and on saturation of ceruloplasmin, free copper overspills into the blood and is deposited in the brain and cornea.

The effects of this are:
- In the liver: chronic hepatitis, which progresses to cirrhosis.
- In the brain: psychiatric disorders, abnormal eye movements, and movement disorders resembling Parkinson's disease.

- In the eye: development of greenish-brown discoloration around cornea (Kayser–Fleischer rings).

Diagnosis—Low levels of serum ceruloplasmin in the blood; confirm by liver biopsy.

Management is by copper chelators, e.g. penicillamine.

α_1-antitrypsin deficiency

Affected individuals with this inherited condition fail to produce the normal active extracellular protease inhibitor α_1-antitrypsin.

Pathogenesis—α_1-antitrypsin is normally produced and secreted by the liver to inhibit the activity of protease enzymes. Mutations in the genes encoding the inhibitor prevent their secretion such that protease enzymes are not inhibited.

In heterozygotes, there is an increased risk of lung damage, especially emphysema in smokers. Homozygotes develop emphysema and liver disease (cholestatic jaundice in the neonate, and chronic hepatitis and cirrhoses).

Others

Reye's syndrome

This rare syndrome is characterized by acute encephalopathy with cerebral oedema as a result of sudden severe impairment of hepatic function (fulminant hepatic failure). It occurs primarily in children and adolescents following an infectious illness such as influenza or chickenpox which has often been treated with aspirin.

Neonatal hepatitis

This clinical condition with many causes presents as neonatal jaundice.

Main causes are:
- Idiopathic (50% of cases).
- α_1-antitrypsin deficiency (30% of cases).
- Viral hepatitis.
- Hepatitis due to toxoplasma, rubella, cytomegalovirus or herpes simplex (i.e. TORCH group).
- Metabolic causes, e.g. galactosaemia or hereditary fructose intolerance.
- Extrahepatic biliary atresia.
- Congenital hepatic fibrosis.

Prognosis—Children with neonatal hepatitis generally recover. However, cases associated with biliary atresia require a surgical bile drainage operation.

Infectious and inflammatory disease
Viral hepatitis

This viral infection is a common cause of acute hepatitis. The main so-called hepatitis viruses are a group of hepatotrophic viruses. Although all cause a primary hepatitis, they are unrelated and belong to different viral types.

Clinical features are similar in all forms of acute hepatitis regardless of aetiology.

Symptoms are nausea, anorexia, low-grade pyrexia and general malaise. Signs are hepatomegaly with tenderness, and jaundice one week after onset of symptoms, peaking at about 10 days.

Investigations—Raised serum levels of conjugated bilirubin, aspartate transaminase and alanine transaminase.

Hepatitis A

This RNA virus of the picorna group is prevalent in tropical countries, but uncommon in developed countries.

It is the commonest travel related illness in the UK!

Transmission is via the faecal–oral route, e.g. from:
- Nurseries or institutions where hygiene levels are inadequate (person to person via hand-to-hand contact).
- Recreational activities in waters contaminated by sewage outfalls.
- Ingestion of sewage-contaminated shellfish.
- (Sexual) oral–anal contact.

Its time course is illustrated in Fig. 9.19.

Prognosis—The majority of patients recover fully with recovery of abnormal liver function tests. However, a small minority (1–3 per 1000) develop fulminant hepatic failure with a mortality rate of 85%.

Disease never causes chronic hepatitis and infection confers subsequent immunity. A vaccine is available for long-term immunity.

Hepatitis B

A DNA virus of the Hepadna group. It can integrate into host DNA.

Transmission can be:
- Blood borne: blood transfusions, IV drug abusers, tattooing, acupuncture.
- Sexual: sexual intercourse.
- Vertical: transmission from mother to child; perinatal (transplacental), postnatal (breast milk).

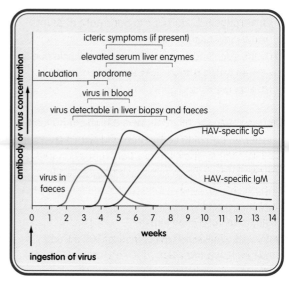

Fig. 9.19 Course of infection in hepatitis A.

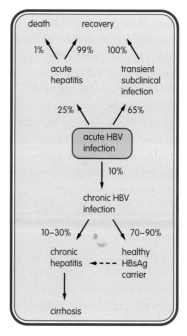

Fig. 9.20 Diagram summarizing possible courses of infection. (Adapted with permission from *Clinical Medicine*, 3rd edn, by P. Kumar and M. Clarke, Baillière Tindall, 1994.)

There are five clinical patterns of infection (Fig. 9.20):

- Asymptomatic infection (65%): subclinical infection but may progress to chronic hepatitis or patient may become a carrier.
- Acute self-limiting hepatitis (25%): patients develop jaundice, malaise and anorexia, but majority recover (about 1% mortality) and have lifelong immunity.
- Fulminant acute hepatitis (rare) causing massive necrosis of liver cells.
- Chronic hepatitis (5–10% of cases): may progress to cirrhosis or may recover to become asymptomatic carrier.
- Asymptomatic carrier state: may later develop chronic hepatitis.

The time course for hepatitis B is illustrated in Fig. 9.21.

Complications are cirrhosis (as a result of chronic hepatitis) and hepatocellular carcinoma, as carriers of hepatitis B are 200 times more likely to get liver cancer (typically 20–30 years post infection) than non carriers.

Treatment is with large doses of α/β interferon for carriers. Vaccination is available, but up to 10% of normal individuals fail to produce protective antihepatitis B antibodies.

Hepatitis C, D and E
Hepatitis C
This RNA viral infection was formerly known as non-A non-B hepatitis.

Transmission is as for hepatitis B. (Hepatitis C is the commonest cause of transfusion-associated hepatitis.)

Infection is asymptomatic in 10–35% of cases although it may progress to the carrier state. However, the majority of patients develop acute hepatitis (in 65–90% of cases).

Chronic hepatitis develops in 50–75% of those infected, following a relapsing and remitting course.

Treatment is with α-interferon and ribavirin.

Hepatitis D
An RNA virus that can only cause infection in the presence of hepatitis B virus, transmission is as for hepatitis B virus. Both viruses may be acquired simultaneously or hepatitis D may be acquired later as a superinfection.

The virus increases the severity of chronic hepatitis and may predispose to the development of fulminant hepatitis.

Hepatitis E
An RNA virus with a transmission as for hepatitis A, infection by hepatitis E is clinically similar to hepatitis A infection.

Other viruses
Non-hepatotrophic viruses may also cause hepatitis. Examples include group B arbovirus (yellow fever), Epstein–Barr virus and cytomegalovirus.

Autoimmune hepatitis
This chronic form of hepatitis is also known as lupoid hepatitis. It has a prevalence of about 4 per 10 000, and typically occurs in women (70%) between the ages of 20 and 40 years.

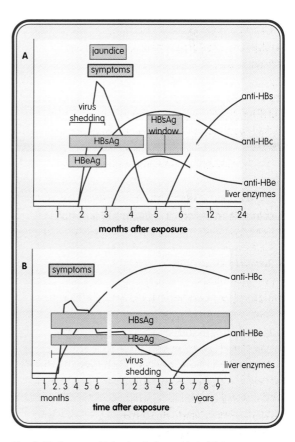

Fig. 9.21 Course of infection in hepatitis B. (A) Acute hepatitis. (B) Chronic hepatitis. (HBsAg, hepatitis B surface antigen; HBeAg, hepatitis B e antigen; anti-HBs, antibody to HBsAg; anti-HBc, antibody to hepatitis B core antigen; anti-HBe, antibody to HBeAg.) HBsAg window is time point where neither HBsAg nor anti-HBs can be detected because of immune complex formation.

Aetiology is unknown, and, despite the name, no immune mechanism has been proven. However, the condition is associated with hyperglobulinaemia, autoantibodies (antismooth muscle antibodies and antinuclear antibodies) in the serum and with other autoimmune disorders such as thyroiditis, arthritis and Sjögren's syndrome (dry eyes and mouth).

Clinically, there is insidious onset of anorexia, malaise and fatigue accompanied by abdominal distension and mild jaundice (with dark urine and itching).

Complications are cirrhosis, liver cell failure and hepatocellular carcinoma.

Investigations:
- Liver function tests: hyperbilirubinaemia, moderately raised transaminase levels, slight elevation of alkaline phosphatase.
- Full blood count: ESR is typically elevated, and there may be normochromic anaemia.
- Serology: presence of antinuclear antibodies, antismooth muscle antibodies.

The disease may run a relapsing and remitting course, but progresses inexorably to cirrhosis.

Treatment is with corticosteroids and azathioprine which can slow the progression of the disease.

Prognosis—Patients who do not respond to treatment will almost always progress to cirrhosis. Also many patients develop cirrhosis despite having a response to treatment. If end-stage liver disease develops, liver transplantation is an effective procedure.

Fulminant hepatitis

This rare syndrome of hepatic encephalopathy results from sudden severe impairment of hepatic function.

Aetiology—Any cause of acute liver damage if sufficiently severe such as:
- Viral infections (commonest cause), e.g. hepatitis B.
- Postviral infections, e.g. Reye's syndrome.
- Drugs, e.g. paracetamol overdose.
- Poisons, e.g. carbon tetrachloride.
- Non-viral infections, e.g. *Leptospira, Toxoplasma gondii, Coxiella burnetii.*
- Metabolic: Wilson's disease, pregnancy.
- Ischaemic: shock, severe cardiac failure, Budd–Chiari syndrome.

The pathogenesis of hepatic encephalopathy has already been described, see p. 149.

Fulminant hepatitis is distinguished from hepatic encephalopathy occurring as a result of deterioration in chronic liver disease by its occurrence within 8 weeks of onset of the precipitating illness, in the absence of evidence of pre-existing liver disease.

Clinical features are:
- Cerebral disturbance (mental changes progressing from confusion to stupor and coma).
- Weakness, vomiting and nausea.
- Rapidly developing jaundice.
- Asterixis: flapping tremor.
- Ascites and oedema.

The liver may enlarge initially but later becomes impalpable; disappearance of hepatic dullness on percussion indicates shrinkage and a bad prognosis.

Complications:
- Cerebral oedema: may cause intracranial hypertension.
- Respiratory failure: as a result of both cerebral oedema and pulmonary oedema.
- General vasodilatation: hypotension and hypothermia.
- Infection.
- Coagulation disorders.
- Necrotic cirrhosis.
- Pancreatitis.
- Renal failure: deterioration parallels that of liver failure.
- Metabolic: hypoglycaemia, hypokalaemia, hypocalcaemia, hypomagnesaemia, acid–base disturbance.

There is no specific treatment. Management is by close observation in a high dependency or intensive care unit so that complications can be corrected promptly.

Prognosis:
- 66% of patients with minor signs survive.
- Only 10% of patients with coma survive.
- Those who recover from fulminant hepatic failure usually regain normal hepatic structure and function.

Postnecrotic cirrhosis

This rapidly developing cirrhosis follows extensive necrosis, e.g. postfulminant hepatitis.

Liver abscess

This localized collection of pus within the liver is walled off and surrounded by damaged and inflamed liver tissue. Liver abscesses are rare but important as they are inevitably fatal if untreated.

Pyogenic abscesses

The most common organisms are *Escherichia coli*, various streptococci, and other enterobacteria.

Mode of infection:

- Blood borne: via portal vein (mesenteric infections) or hepatic artery (bacteraemia).
- Ascending spread from colonization of biliary tract (most common): almost always predisposed by biliary obstruction.
- Penetrating trauma.

Clinical features:

- Symptoms: fever, malaise, rigors and weight loss, pain in right upper quadrant sometimes with radiation to right shoulder (may be pleuritic).
- Signs: hepatomegaly in 50% of patients, mild jaundice.

Investigations include liver imaging, and needle aspiration at ultrasound examination to confirm diagnosis and provide pus for culture.

Management is by antibiotics and drainage of the abscess.

Prognosis—The mortality of liver abscesses is 20–40%, usually through failure to make the diagnosis.

Amoebic abscess

The most common organism is *Entamoeba histolytica*, which is transmitted from bowel to liver via blood. The disease is rare in the UK but common worldwide and must be considered in patients travelling from endemic areas such as Africa, Asia and South America.

Alcohol, drugs and toxins

Alcoholic liver disease

Alcohol abuse is the most common cause of liver disease in Western countries, and women are more prone to alcohol-induced liver damage than men.

Alcohol is metabolized almost exclusively in the liver, and liver damage is related to daily alcohol intake. Toxicity of ethanol is probably due to generation of its metabolic breakdown product, acetaldehyde.

Its effects are fatty liver, acute hepatitis, and cirrhosis.

Fatty liver (hepatic steatosis)

This is the most common lesion of alcoholic liver disease. The condition is characterized by the accumulation of fat globules within the cytoplasm of hepatocytes, and is reversible on cessation of alcohol ingestion.

Metabolism of ethanol takes precedence over metabolism of fat, so that fat accumulates in the liver cells. The condition reflects severe metabolic derangement and may affect a few or almost all hepatocytes.

Alcoholic hepatitis

This is acute hepatitis with focal necrosis of liver cells. At high concentrations, alcohol causes toxic injury to hepatocytes, evoking an inflammatory reaction, which is reversible on abstinence. However, continued alcohol consumption causes the development of fibrosis around central veins. The result is hepatic fibrosis that may progress to cirrhosis.

The illness resembles acute viral hepatitis (see pp. 152–153) and liver function tests show raised levels of transaminases and γ-glutamyl transpeptidase.

Alcoholic cirrhosis

Irreversible architectural disturbance occurs as a result of sustained alcoholic liver injury.

Normal liver architecture is diffusely replaced by nodules of regenerated liver cells separated by bands of collagenous fibrosis. This may develop after episodes of acute alcoholic hepatitis or may be insidious in its onset presenting only as end-stage liver disease.

It affects fewer than 10% of patients suffering from chronic alcoholism.

Drugs and toxins

The liver is the main organ of drug metabolism and consequently drugs are a common cause of liver disease. Hepatotoxic drugs may be divided into two main groups: intrinsic hepatotoxins and idiosyncratic hepatotoxins.

Intrinsic hepatotoxins

These have dose-dependent, predictable toxic effects. They are responsible for a high incidence of toxic damage to the liver via either direct toxicity of an unmetabolized drug or normal hepatic conversion to toxic metabolite.

Idiosyncratic hepatotoxins

These have non-dose-dependent, unpredictable toxic effects. They cause liver disease in a small percentage of exposed individuals as a result of hypersensitivity (drug-mediated autoimmunity) or abnormal drug metabolism.

Circulatory disorders of the liver

Overview

Vascular disorders of the liver (Fig. 9.22) can be classified into one of three categories depending on their pathogenetic mechanisms:

- Obstruction to outflow: hepatic vein obstruction.
- Lobular compromise.
- Obstruction to inflow: obstruction of portal vein or hepatic artery occlusion.

Diseases causing obstruction to outflow (hepatic vein obstruction)

Veno-occlusive disease

There is widespread occlusion of central hepatic veins.

Budd–Chiari syndrome

In this rare condition, obstruction occurs in the larger hepatic veins, and sometimes the inferior vena cava.

Cardiac disease

Right-sided cardiac failure causes congestion of the inferior vena cava which results in obstruction of hepatic vein outflow, hence hepatic damage.

Clinical manifestations depend on the cause and speed with which obstruction develops, but congestive hepatomegaly and ascites are features in all patients.

Diseases resulting in lobular compromise

Cirrhosis

Distortion and destruction of the hepatic vascular architecture causes sinusoid occlusion.

Non-cirrhotic fibrosis

Fibrotic damage to the liver does not amount to a true cirrhosis:

- Infective: schistosomiasis.
- Drugs: alcohol, hypervitaminosis A, vinyl chloride, arsenic.
- Congenital: congenital hepatic fibrosis and infantile polycystic disease.
- Nodular regenerative hyperplasia.

Systemic circulatory disturbances

Shock from any source causes severe hypoperfusion, resulting in zonal necrosis.

Diseases resulting in obstruction to inflow

Extrahepatic

Portal vein obstruction

The predisposing factors are:

- Portal vein thrombosis (due to local sepsis, polycythaemia rubra vera, pre-existing sinusoidal portal hypertension due to cirrhosis).
- Extrinsic compression of portal vein.
- Congenital stenosis.

Hepatic artery occlusion

This occlusion can be caused by:

- Thrombosis secondary to intrinsic disease of hepatic arteries (e.g. polyarteritis nodosa or arteriolar sclerosis).
- Embolism: infective endocarditis.
- Accidental ligation.

Intrahepatic

Occlusion of intrahepatic portal vein branches causes areas of venous infarction which are seen as congested zones with a wedge-shaped pattern. Such zones are also termed red infarcts or Zahn's infarcts.

Liver infarction

True infarction of the liver is rare because of its dual blood supply and rich anastomosis of blood flow through the sinusoids. However, hepatic blood flow may be compromised in the following conditions:

- Surgical trauma or accidental ligation of hepatic artery.
- Therapeutic arterial embolization of the liver or therapeutic hepatic arterial ligation (performed to treat isolated neoplastic masses).
- Bacterial endocarditis: embolism.
- Eclampsia.
- Polyarteritis nodosa.

Portal vein obstruction

Obstruction of the portal vein results in portal hypertension and its associated complications (see p. 148). The causes may be thrombotic or non thrombotic.

Thrombotic conditions (those that predispose to portal vein thrombosis) are:

- Inflammatory: thrombophlebitis and intra-abdominal sepsis (e.g. appendicitis, cholecystitis, pancreatitis).
- Neoplastic: hepatocellular carcinoma, metastatic liver tumours and haematological malignancies (e.g. polycythaemia rubra vera, essential thrombocytosis, myelofibrosis).
- Cirrhosis: leads to portal hypertension and stasis.
- Splenic vein thrombosis by propagation.

Non thrombotic conditions are external compression (e.g. by tumour masses) and cirrhosis.

Passive congestion

Congestive cardiac failure causes venous outflow obstruction in the liver due to back pressure transmitted as described below:

inferior vena cava → hepatic vein → central veins → centrilobular congestion

Centrilobular sinusoids are dilated by blood, and the centrilobular hepatocytes undergo atrophy and necrosis (centrilobular noecrosis) and give rise to the appearance of what is described as a 'nutmeg liver' (chronic passive venous congestion).

The condition is common in tricuspid valve incompetence when the liver is pulsatile.

Arterial hypotension may complicate right-sided cardiac failure causing necrosis of the centrilobular hepatocytes with elevation of serum transaminase levels.

Budd–Chiari syndrome

This rare condition is caused by occlusion of the main hepatic vein or (more rarely) the intrahepatic vena cava (Fig. 9.23).

Obstruction of the hepatic vein causes severe hepatic congestion with atrophy and/or necrosis of liver cells in affected areas. Fibrous scarring eventually occurs in areas of hepatocyte necrosis. True cirrhosis supervenes in a minority of cases.

Clinical manifestations—Patients develop severe acute disease with:

- Painful hepatomegaly.

Vascular disorders of the liver	
Cause	**Example**
outflow (hepatic vein) obstruction	veno-occlusive disease Budd–Chiari syndrome right-sided cardiac failure
lobular compromise	cirrhosis non-cirrhotic fibrosis: • infective, e.g. schistosomiasis • drugs, e.g. alcohol, hypervitaminosis A, vinyl chloride, arsenic • congenital, e.g. congenital hepatic fibrosis, infantile polycystic disease • nodular regenerative hyperplasia

inflow obstruction	systemic circulatory disturbances, e.g. shock
	
	extrahepatic
	• portal vein obstruction:
	  portal vein thrombosis
	  extrinsic compression of portal vein
	  congenital stenosis
	• hepatic artery occlusion:
	  hepatic artery thrombosis
	  embolism, e.g. infective endocarditis
	  accidental ligation
	intrahepatic
	• occlusion of intrahepatic portal vein branches

Fig. 9.22 Vascular disorders of the liver.

Aetiology of Budd–Chiari syndrome	
idiopathic	underlying cause cannot be found in more than half of cases
thrombotic causes	haematological diseases, for example: • primary proliferative polycythaemia • paroxysmal nocturnal haemoglobinuria • deficiencies of antithrombin III, proteins C and S pregnancy/oral contraceptives
local compression of hepatic vein (rare)	obstruction due to tumours, e.g. liver, kidneys or adrenals congenital venous webs inferior vena caval stenosis

Fig. 9.23 Aetiology of Budd–Chiari syndrome.

- Acute portal hypertension.
- Rapid development of ascites.
- Jaundice.

Death results, unless therapeutic portosystemic vascular anastomosis is performed.

Veno-occlusive disease

This condition is caused by widespread occlusion of central hepatic veins leading to clinical features similar to those of Budd–Chiari syndrome (see above).

Causes are hepatic irradiation, cytotoxic drugs, and the ingestion of plants containing toxic alkaloids (common in Jamaica and certain areas of Africa in those who drink herbal teas).

Pathogenesis is unclear but involves fibrosis around central veins ultimately resulting in obliteration of vein lumen.

Clinical features, investigations and management of veno-occlusive disease are similar to those of Budd–Chiari syndrome.

Hepatic disease in pregnancy
Pre-eclampsia and eclampsia
Pre-eclampsia

This is high blood pressure (more than 140/90 mmHg) developing during pregnancy in a woman whose blood pressure was previously normal. It occurs in about 10% of pregnancies.

HELLP syndrome

This syndrome of haemolysis, elevated liver tests and low platelets in the blood occurs in approximately 10% of all women with pre-eclampsia. The liver may be destroyed by the development of disseminated intravascular coagulation (see Chapter 14). Irregular areas of necrosis occur as a result of fibrin thrombi deposition in adjacent portal vessels.

- Mild cases: liver function remains normal, although liver blood tests may be abnormal.
- Severe cases: large parts of the liver may be damaged or destroyed leading to symptoms similar to severe viral hepatitis.
- Extremely severe cases: life-threatening haemorrhage into parts of the liver or abdomen may occur.

This disease resolves immediately after delivery, and the liver generally heals itself within days to weeks.

However, whilst disease is ongoing, the mother is at risk of complications of liver damage and bleeding, and the baby is at risk of premature delivery or stillbirth.

Eclampsia

This is the occurrence of one or more convulsions not caused by other conditions such as epilepsy or cerebral haemorrhage in a woman with pre-eclampsia. It is associated with severe epigastric pain, nausea and vomiting, and severe hepatic damage. Fetal and maternal death may occur.

Liver histology shows fibrin deposition and ischaemic necrosis.

Acute fatty liver of pregnancy

This serious but rare condition presents in the third trimester with symptoms of fulminant hepatitis (jaundice, vomiting, abdominal pain and possibly coma), affecting 1 in 4000 pregnancies.

Aetiopathogenesis is unknown but is characterized by widespread centrilobular microvesicular fatty change in hepatocytes.

Untreated cases are associated with a high maternal and fetal mortality. Early recognition of the condition and treatment by Caesarean section have greatly improved the outlook.

Intrahepatic cholestasis of pregnancy

Cholestasis occurring as a result of intrahepatic causes appears in the second or third trimester, lasts for the duration of the pregnancy and resolves within 2–4 weeks of delivery.

Aetiology of the syndrome is uncertain but it is probably caused by an inherited susceptibility of a patient's liver cells to oestrogens. The condition is sometimes precipitated by oral contraceptives.

Symptoms are pruritus (almost always starts in third trimester and remits within about 2 weeks of delivery) and jaundice (occurs in about half of the patients).

The fetus remains unharmed but the condition tends to recur in subsequent pregnancies.

Neoplasia of the liver
Benign tumours
Hepatic adenomas

These typically affect premenopausal women, and are predisposed by oestrogen-containing oral contraceptives.

The macroscopic appearance is of well-circumscribed nodules up to 20 cm in size.

The microscopic appearance closely resembles that of a normal liver, except that no portal structures are seen.

Complications—The majority of lesions are asymptomatic, but may cause problems if they rupture, leading to intra-abdominal bleeding.

Bile duct adenomas
Very common lesions composed of abnormal bile ducts in a collagenous stroma these appear as small white nodules, often beneath the liver capsule. They may be mistaken for metastatic tumour deposits at laparotomy.

Haemangioma
These are common hamartomas composed of abnormal vascular channels in a collagenous stroma. They are found at autopsy in 2–5% of the population, typically seen beneath the capsule as a dark lesion (usually 2–3 cm in size).

Malignant
Primary
Hepatocellular carcinoma
Carcinoma of hepatocytes is the commonest primary tumour of the liver. Uncommon in the UK (affects about 1 per 100 000) it is up to 100 times more common in parts of Africa and the Far East, probably because of the higher incidence of hepatitis B and contaminating mycotoxins. Males are affected more than females by 8:1.

Predisposing factors are cirrhosis (independent of cause), hepatitis B infection with chronic carrier state, and mycotoxins contaminating food (e.g. aflatoxins produced by the fungus *Aspergillus flavus* which frequently contaminates stored nuts and grains in tropical countries).

Prognosis is very poor with median survival of under 6 months from diagnosis.

Cholangiocarcinoma
This is an adenocarcinoma arising from the intrahepatic bile duct epithelium. It accounts for 5–10% of all cases of primary liver tumours.

Predisposing factors:
- Chronic inflammatory disease of intrahepatic biliary tree, particularly sclerosing cholangitis.
- Disease caused by liver flukes.

Lesions are associated with a very poor prognosis; most patients do not survive more than 6 months from diagnosis.

Angiosarcomas
These highly malignant tumours are derived from vascular endothelium, and characterized by multifocal haemorrhagic nodules within the liver. The tumours are rare unless there has been exposure to:
- Thorotrast (a radiological contrast agent used until the 1950s).
- Vinyl chloride monomer (used in plastics industry to make PVC).
- Arsenic (administered in the past in certain tonics).
- Anabolic steroids.

Secondary tumours
The majority of malignant liver tumours are metastatic. The most common primary carcinomas, which metastasize to the liver, are of the lung, breast, colon and stomach.

Many other tumours also spread to the liver (lymphomas, melanomas, leukaemias, etc.) but they are numerically less frequent.

Mode of spread is via the blood stream, through the portal vein (tumours of the GI tract) and the systemic circulation (other tumours).

Clinically, the liver is enlarged, feeling hard and craggy on palpation.

Small deposits of tumour have little clinical effect. However, extensive metastases cause compression of the intrahepatic bile ducts leading to obstructive jaundice.

Disorders of the biliary tree
Disorders associated with biliary cirrhosis
Biliary cirrhosis is the result of the long-standing obstruction of bile ducts leading to the development of obstructive jaundice, liver cell necrosis and fibrosis with regenerative nodules. The main causes:
- Primary biliary cirrhosis: intrahepatic bile duct destruction of unknown aetiology.
- Secondary biliary cirrhosis: unrelieved obstruction of the main extrahepatic bile ducts.
- Sclerosing cholangitis: inflammation and fibrosis of bile ducts.

Biliary obstruction causes oedema and expansion of

intrahepatic portal tracts with portal tract fibrosis. Bile droplets develop in biliary canaliculi, which may rupture and cause death of adjacent hepatocytes (so-called 'bile infarct'). Over a long period of time, liver cell death, regeneration and fibrosis result in cirrhosis.

Primary biliary cirrhosis

This cirrhosis occurs as a result of a chronic destruction of intrahepatic bile ducts. (Also known as chronic destructive non-suppurative cholangitis.) It affects 5 per 100 000 in the UK, typically among the middle-aged population. Females are affected more than males by 10:1.

Aetiology is unknown but thought to involve immune phenomena (antimitochondrial antibodies in more than 90% of cases).

It is often associated with other autoimmune diseases, e.g. RA, thyroiditis, SLE, scleroderma and Sjögren's syndrome (dry eyes and mouth).

Pathogenesis is progressive, chronic, granulomatous, inflammatory damage with fibrosis which spreads from portal tracts to the liver parenchyma. The condition eventually leads to cirrhosis and its complications over a period of about 10 years.

There are four stages:

1. Florid bile-duct inflammation with granulomata.
2. Ductular proliferation (periportal).
3. Scarring (bridging fibrosis).
4. Cirrhosis.

Clinical features in the early stages are tiredness, fatigue and arthralgia, with pruritus and mild jaundice. In the late stages, patients develop true cirrhosis with features of:

- Jaundice.
- Pruritus with excoriation.
- Hepatosplenomegaly.
- Malabsorption (weight loss, osteomalacia, osteoporosis).
- Xanthelasma and possible xanthomata.
- Other complications of liver failure.

Investigations are:

- Blood: liver function tests show features of cholestasis (raised alkaline phosphatase, cholesterol and bile acids); demonstration of antimitochondrial antibodies.
- Liver biopsy showing compatible histology.
- ERCP shows patent and non-dilated biliary tree (rules out obstructive causes of cirrhosis).

Management—No specific therapy is available. Treatment with drugs is ineffective and liver transplantation is often necessary.

Secondary biliary cirrhosis

This occurs as a result of prolonged mechanical obstruction to bile flow in large ducts outside the liver or within the porta hepatis. Causes are:

- Gallstones: impacted in common bile duct.
- Tumours, e.g. carcinoma of bile duct, carcinoma of pancreas.
- Strictures: usually following surgery.
- Congenital diseases: choledochal cyst, extrahepatic biliary atresia.
- Parasitic obstruction (rare).

Histological features—Bile pigment accumulates in hepatocytes, in dilated biliary canaliculi and in Kupffer cells. Prolonged obstruction causes:

- Extravasation of bile from dilated canaliculi with development of characteristic 'bile infarcts'.
- Extravasation of bile from small intrahepatic bile ducts with development of characteristic portal tract lesions 'bile lakes'.
- Eventual development of cirrhosis.

Complications are cholangitis (inflammation of the bile ducts, usually as a result of superimposed infection) and those of cirrhosis (p. 145).

Primary sclerosing cholangitis

Chronic inflammation and fibrosis of bile ducts with stricture formation causes progressive obstructive jaundice. The condition affects 1 per 100 000 with peak incidence between 25 and 40 years, males more so than females. Aetiology is unknown.

There is a strong association with ulcerative colitis, as follows:

- 60% of patients with primary sclerosing cholangitis have ulcerative colitis.
- 5% of patients with ulcerative colitis develop primary sclerosing cholangitis.

This disease is not associated with immunological features of primary biliary cirrhosis.

The effects are:

- Large intra- and extrahepatic bile ducts: development of fibrous strictures with segmental dilatation causing the 'beaded' appearance on ERCP.
- Medium-sized ducts, and ducts in portal tracts: inflammation with concentric fibrosis around ducts.
- Small bile ducts in portal tracts: replaced by collagenous scarring (vanishing bile ducts).

Clinical features—Patients develop cholestatic jaundice (pale stools, dark urine and itching of the skin) with progression to cirrhosis over a period of about 10 years. There is an increased risk of developing cholangiocarcinomas.

Fig. 9.24 shows a summary of disorders associated with biliary cirrhosis.

Diseases of the gallbladder
Gallstones

Gallstones (stones formed in the gallbladder) are the most common cause of disease affecting the biliary tree. They occur in 10% of all adults in the UK, females more often than males by 2.5:1; and 30% of the women are over 65. The number of stones per patient has varied from one to 26 000.

However, despite the high incidence of gallstones, only about 1% of total patients with gallstones develop complications.

There are two types of gallstone: cholesterol stones (80% of all stones), and pigment stones (20% of all stones). Both types also contain calcium salts, e.g. bilirubinate, carbonate, phosphate and palmitate.

Cholesterol stones

Here, the major constituent of the stone is, of course, cholesterol.

Pathogenesis:

- Hypersecretion of cholesterol (most common mechanism).
- Decreased secretion of bile salts, due to either defective bile synthesis or excessive intestinal loss of bile salts.
- Abnormal gallbladder function.

Risk factors for cholesterol stones are shown in Fig. 9.25.

	Summary of disorders associated with biliary cirrhosis		
	Primary biliary cirrhosis	**Secondary biliary cirrhosis**	**Primary sclerosing cholangitis**
prevalence	5 per 100 000	?	1 per 100 000
sex association	females > males by 10:1; typically affecting middle-aged population	?	males > females with peak incidence between 25 and 40 years
aetiology	unknown, probably autoimmune	gallstones tumours strictures congenital diseases parasitic obstruction (rare)	unknown
bile duct changes	progressive chronic granulomatous inflammatory damage with fibrosis eventual cirrhosis	development of bile infarcts and bile lakes bile duct hyperplasia eventual cirrhosis	narrowing and obliteration of intra- and extrahepatic bile ducts eventual cirrhosis
Lab findings			
liver function tests	features of cholestasis (increased alkaline phosphatase, cholesterol and bile acids)	same	same
sera	antimitochondrial antibodies	–	–
ERCP	patent and non-dilated biliary tree	dilation of large ducts	fibrous strictures with segmental dilatation → 'beaded' appearance

Fig. 9.24 Summary of disorders associated with biliary cirrhosis.

Bile pigment stones

Here, the major constituent of the stones is bile pigment (calcium bilirubinate). They are typically found in patients with chronic haemolysis due to increased bilirubin production, hence pigment stones are typically black. In the Western world, the most common causes of pigment stones are hereditary spherocytosis and sickle cell disease.

In the Far East, brown pigment stones are related to biliary parasites.

Gallstones may be asymptomatic (80% have no symptoms), symptomatic (pain and other symptoms) or complicated.

Characteristics of pain are:
- Sites are the epigastrium (80%); right upper quadrant (20%); left upper quadrant, lower chest (rare).
- Radiation is to the back.
- Nature: severe gripping pain with varying intensity (biliary colic). Resolves when stone falls back into gallbladder or passes into common bile duct.
- Onset is sudden.
- Duration of about 2 hours.
- Aggravating factors are associated with eating, typically coming on about 30 minutes after food ingestion.

Complications include:
- Cholecystitis: inflammation of gallbladder caused by impaction of stone in neck of gallbladder or cystic duct.
- Jaundice: impaction of stone in common bile duct (choledolithiasis), leading to biliary obstruction.
- Cholangitis: inflammation of bile duct usually as a result of biliary obstruction complicated with bacterial infection.
- Pancreatitis: impaction of stone distal to opening of pancreatic duct.

Investigations are:
- Abdominal X-ray: stones are calcified in 10–20%.
- ERCP.
- Percutaneous transhepatic angiogram.
- Ultrasound (most useful).

Management is by:
- Surgery (cholecystectomy).
- Bile acids (chenodeoxycholic or ursodeoxycholic): prevents formation of new stones but cannot dissolve pre-existing ones.
- Lithotripsy: useful for those patients unsuitable for surgery.

Cholecystitis

This is inflammation of the gallbladder. Aetiology is almost always associated with gallstones. There are two types, acute and chronic.

Acute cholecystitis

This acute inflammation of the gallbladder is precipitated by the chemical effects of concentrated static bile within. It is typically due to obstruction of gallbladder outflow by gallstones, and may be exacerbated by secondary infection with enteric organisms such as *E. coli*.

In severe cases, the lumen distends with pus causing increased risk of perforation and peritonitis.

Empyema is an inflamed gallbladder greatly distended with pus.

Chronic cholecystitis

Invariably associated with gallstones, the gallbladder wall is thickened and rigid from fibrosis, with variable chronic inflammatory infiltration of the mucosa and submucosa. The thickened wall may contain sinuses (Aschoff–Rokitansky sinuses).

Risk factors for cholesterol stones	
age	↑ cholesterol secretion
female	↑ cholesterol secretion
pregnancy	↑ cholesterol secretion ↓ bile secretion impaired gall bladder motility
obesity	↑ cholesterol secretion
rapid weight loss	↑ cholesterol secretion
racial	↑ cholesterol secretion
gall bladder stasis brief fast parenteral therapy spinal cord injury	impaired gall bladder motility

Fig. 9.25 Risk factors for cholesterol stones.

Hartmann's pouch is a pathological dilatation in the neck of the gallbladder formed by increased intraluminal pressure or stone.

Mucocele
This is sterile obstruction of the neck by a gallstone. A lack of inflammation permits the gallbladder to distend.

Carcinoma of the gallbladder
This is usually an adenocarcinoma, invariably associated with gallstones and chronic cholecystitis. Most cases are seen in women over the age of 70 years. Poor prognosis due to liver invasion.

Pathogenesis
Duct obstruction
Impaction of a gallstone distal to the site of union of a common bile duct and pancreatic duct results in:
- Reflux of bile up pancreatic duct → toxic injury to pancreatic acini.
- Increased intraductal pressure → enzymatic leakage from pancreatic ducts.

Note: chronic alcohol ingestion may also produce increased intraductal pressure due to production of a protein-rich pancreatic fluid, which can form solid plugs in smaller pancreatic ducts

- Describe two congenital errors of metabolism that affect the normal functioning of the liver.
- Compare the pathologies of hepatitis A, B and C.
- Outline the complications of fulminant hepatitis.
- Describe the pathogenesis of alcoholic liver disease.
- Classify the vascular disorders of the liver.
- What is Budd–Chiari syndrome? Describe its aetiology.
- Define 'biliary cirrhosis' and name the disorders associated with this condition.
- Summarize the complications of gallstones.

A useful mnemonic for memorizing the causes of pancreatitis is GET SMASH'D, i.e. Gallstones, Ethanol, Trauma, Shock, Mumps, Autoimmune (PAN), Scorpion bites (rare in the UK!), Hyperlipidaemia (also hypercalcaemia and hypothermia), Drugs.

DISORDERS OF THE EXOCRINE PANCREAS

Pancreatitis
Acute pancreatitis
This acute inflammation of the pancreas is caused by destructive effect of enzymes released from pancreatic acini. It affects 5–10 per 100 000 per year in Western communities. By far the most common causes of acute pancreatitis are gallstones (50% of cases) and alcohol ingestion (20%). These and other causes are classified in Fig. 9.26.

Causes of acute pancreatitis	
Cause	Example
mechanical obstruction of pancreatic ducts	gallstones trauma postoperative
metabolic/toxic causes	alcohol drugs, e.g. corticosteroids, thiazide diuretics, azathioprine hypercalcaemia hyperlipidaemia
vascular/poor perfusion	shock atherosclerosis hypothermia polyarteritis nodosa (PAN)
infections	mumps

Fig. 9.26 Causes of acute pancreatitis.

Direct acinar injury

Less common causes of pancreatitis, e.g. viruses, drugs, trauma, etc., may result from direct acinar damage. The three patterns of pancreatic necrosis are:

- Periductal necrosis: necrosis of acinar cells adjacent to ducts. Typically caused by duct obstruction, particularly associated with gallstones and alcohol.
- Perilobular necrosis: necrosis of the periphery of lobules. Caused by poor vascular perfusion of their zone as a result of shock and hypothermia.
- Panlobular necrosis: necrosis affects all portions of the pancreatic lobule. May be due to spread from initial periductal perilobular necrosis or may be panlobular from the start.

Irrespective of the cause of pancreatitis, acinar damage leads to the liberation of lytic enzymes (proteases and lipases) causing necrosis of normal tissue. A vicious circle of events is begun in which enzymatic release results in further acinar damage etc.:

- Lipases $\rightarrow$ fat necrosis. Causes discoloration of skin around abdominal wall (Cullen's or Grey Turner's sign).
- Proteases $\rightarrow$ destruction of pancreatic parenchyma. Endocrine destruction results in hyperglycaemia.
- Elastase and other enzymes $\rightarrow$ vascular damage with haemorrhage into pancreas or peritoneum. Extensive haemorrhage is known as acute haemorrhagic pancreatitis.

Clinical features are:

- Symptoms: severe central abdominal pain of sudden onset, often radiating into back. Nausea and vomiting.
- Signs: tachycardia, fever, jaundice, shock, ileus, rigid abdomen, discoloration around the umbilicus (Cullen's sign) or in the flanks (Grey Turner's sign).

Complications may be local affecting the pancreas and GI or systemic.

Pancreatic complications are:

- Pancreatic pseudocyst: conversion of necrotic pancreas into a cyst filled with serosanguinous fluid.
- Abscess formation: infection of necrotic pancreatic tissue.
- Chronic pancreatitis: however, most cases of chronic pancreatitis are not preceded by acute episodes.

GI complications are:

- Haemorrhage: gastric and duodenal erosions.
- Intestinal ileus: paralysis of ileum due to local inflammation caused by pancreatic enzymes.
- Duodenal obstruction: compression of duodenum by pancreatic mass.

Systemic complications are:

- Peritonitis.
- Shock: due to trapping of litres of extracellular fluid in the gut, peritoneum and retroperitoneum; or due to haemorrhage.
- Adult respiratory distress syndrome (ARDS).
- Renal failure as a result of shock.
- Diabetes mellitus: destruction of endocrine pancreas.
- Subcutaneous fat necrosis: release of pancreatic lipases.

Investigations are:

- Full blood count: neutrophil leukocytosis.
- Blood sugar: hyperglycaemia in severe disease.
- Liver function tests: $\uparrow$ bilirubin, $\uparrow$ alkaline phosphatase, $\downarrow$ albumen.
- Serum amylase: greatly elevated.

Management is by physiological support and treatment of:

- Shock: intravenous saline, plasma, or whole blood.
- Respiratory failure: endotracheal intubation and positive pressure ventilation.
- Pain: analgesia (pethidine and prochloperazine).

Prognosis—Mortality is about 20% (negligible in mild cases, but up to 50% in cases with a severe haemorrhagic pancreatitis).

Death may be from shock, renal failure, sepsis or respiratory failure with contributory factors being protease-induced activation of complement, kinin, and the fibrinolytic and coagulation cascades.

Chronic pancreatitis

This is chronic inflammation and fibrosis of the pancreas with a relapsing and remitting course.

It is a relatively rare disease but with increasing incidence due to the increasing incidence of alcoholism. Typically occurs between the ages of 35 and 45 years; males more so than females.

Aetiology—The main causes of chronic pancreatitis are outlined in Fig. 9.27.

Pathogenesis is thought to be similar to the mechanisms involved in acute pancreatitis. However, there is permanent impairment of function.

Morphological features:
- Chronic inflammation.
- Fibrous scarring.
- Loss of pancreatic parenchymal elements.
- Duct strictures with formation of intrapancreatic calculi (stones).

Clinical features are:
- Recurrent bouts of severe abdominal pain.
- Malabsorption (due to reduced lipase and protease secretion): steatorrhoea (fat in faeces); creatorrhoea (undigested meat in faeces).
- Diabetes mellitus (destruction of pancreatic parenchyma).

Episodes of acute pancreatitis may complicate chronic pancreatitis.

Relevant investigations include imaging and function tests.

Imaging is by plain radiograph (for calcification of the pancreas), ultrasound and CT, and ERCP.

Function tests are:
- Secretin/CCK/stimulation test.
- Glucose tolerance test.
- Five day stool collection for fat excretion.
- Liver function tests.

Management is by:
- Abstinence from alcohol.
- Pancrax: pancreatic extract with or without antacids to prevent inactivation by gastric acid.
- Supplementation of fat soluble vitamins.
- Diet and insulin for diabetics.
- Surgery for pseudocysts and biliary obstruction.

Pseudocysts

A collection of fluid and necrotic inflammatory debris is localized either within the pancreas itself or more commonly in the adjacent tissue, particularly the lesser sac. They are not 'true' cysts (as they have no epithelial lining) but are surrounded by a zone of inflammatory granulation tissue, and communicate into the pancreatic duct system. They occur in both acute and chronic forms of pancreatitis.

Neoplasms of the pancreas
Cystic tumours

These benign, well-circumscribed masses are composed of multiple cystic cavities lined by either serous or mucin-secreting epithelium.

Carcinoma of the pancreas

This common tumour accounts for 3–5% of cancer deaths in the UK. It is typically seen in patients over 60 years of age, but occasionally in younger people, and more often in males than females.

Associations include cigarette smoking, alcohol, a diet high in fat and carbohydrate, and diabetes in women.

Macroscopic appearance—Gritty, grey, hard nodules invading adjacent gland and local structures.

The tumour arises with different frequencies in different part of the pancreas: 60% in the head, 10% in the body, 10% in the tail; and 20% of pancreatic cancers exhibit a diffuse pattern.

Carcinoma in the head of the pancreas tends to present early with obstructive jaundice. As a result, tumours are on average smaller at diagnosis than in other sites

Main causes of chronic pancreatitis		
	Cause	**Pathogenesis**
common	chronic alcoholism (majority of cases)	protein plugs form in ducts and become calculi; ducts are obstructed, inflamed and scarred
	biliary tract disease	gallstones or anatomical abnormalities of pancreatic ducts
	idiopathic chronic pancreatitis	pathogenesis uncertain
rare	cystic fibrosis	protein plugs in ducts
	familial pancreatitis	autosomal dominant
	tropical pancreatitis	uncertain cause; prevalent in India and Africa

Fig. 9.27 Main causes of chronic pancreatitis.

Microscopic appearance—Lesions are typically moderately differentiated adenocarcinomas composed of glandular spaces in a fibrous stroma.

Routes of spread:

- Local leads to obstructive jaundice, or invasion of the duodenum.
- Lymphatic: to adjacent lymph nodes.
- Blood: to the liver.

Clinical features are:

- Weight loss, anorexia and chronic persistent pain in epigastrium radiating to the back.
- Obstructive jaundice with painless palpable dilatation of gallbladder (Courvoisier's sign).
- Migratory thrombophlebitis: development of multiple thromboses in superficial and deep leg veins (Trousseau's syndrome).

Management is by:

- Curative resection (Whipple's procedure): rarely possible due to extensive disease.
- Palliative surgery: often performed to bypass obstruction of the bile duct (relieving jaundice) and obstruction of the duodenum.

Prognosis is extremely poor, 90% of patients dying within 6 months of diagnosis.

- Describe the aetiology and pathogenesis of acute pancreatitis.
- List the complications of acute pancreatitis.
- State the causes of chronic pancreatitis.
- What are pancreatic pseudocysts?
- Name the risk factors associated with development of carcinoma of the pancreas.
- What is the prognosis for pancreatic carcinoma?

DISORDERS OF THE INTESTINE

Congenital abnormalities
Meckel's diverticulum

Diverticulum (outpouching) of the ileum is caused by persistence of part of the yolk stalk. This arises as a result of incomplete regression of the yolk stalk (vitello-intestinal duct) during the embryonic period, such that a tubular diverticulum is present in the ileum.

Meckel's diverticulum occurs in 2% of the population,

Rule of 2s for Meckel's diverticulum:
- **Prevalence: 2% of the population.**
- **Site: 2 feet from the ileocaecal junction.**
- **Length: 2 inches.**

and in males more than females by about 3:1.

Macroscopically, it is 2 inches (5 cm) long and located 2 feet (61 cm) from the ileocaecal junction.

Microscopically, there is a muscular wall and a lining like that of small bowel epithelium, often mixed with gastric acid-secreting epithelium or heterotopic pancreatic tissue.

Complications—The majority of these diverticula are asymptomatic; however, the following complications may develop in a very small minority, typically before the age of 10 years:

- Volvulus: may cause problems by acting as the apex of a volvulus if tethered to the umbilicus by a fibrous cord.
- Inflammation: similar to that seen in acute appendicitis.
- Peptic ulceration: may develop if acid secreting epithelium is present.
- Intussusception.

Congenital aganglionic megacolon (Hirschsprung's disease)

This congenital condition is characterized by dilatation of the colon due to the absence of the normal myenteric plexus distal to dilatation. It occurs in 1 per 5000 live births.

This condition always involves the rectum and may be present in continuity for a variable distance along the bowel. Some cases involve only short segments of rectum, others the rectosigmoid segment, and in rare cases there may be total colonic or total intestinal aganglionosis.

Macroscopically, there is a narrowing of an abnormally innervated bowel segment, and dilatation and muscular hypertrophy of a proximal bowel segment.

Microscopically, there is an absence of normal myenteric and submucosal plexus ganglion cells, and hypertrophy of nerve fibres within submucosa and muscularis mucosae, with extension of abnormal axons up into lamina propria.

Clinical features—The disease usually presents in early childhood with symptoms of colonic obstruction, i.e. constipation, abdominal distension, and vomiting.

Diagnosis—Radiological examination with small amounts of barium demonstrates a small, empty rectum, a narrowed segment above, and wide dilatation of the colon full of retained faeces. A biopsy of the rectal mucosa will confirm the diagnosis.

Treatment is by excision of the abnormal segment of colon and rectum.

Note that megacolon can also be a result of acquired disease. However, acquired megacolon differs macroscopically from Hirschsprung's disease in that there is no narrowed segment, dilatation extends down to the anus, and the rectum is full of faeces.

Causes of acquired megacolon:
- Psychogenic megacolon: disregard for the urge to defecate.
- Prolonged laxative abuse: degeneration of myenteric plexus.
- Smooth muscle disorders: degeneration of colonic smooth muscle, e.g. scleroderma.
- Chagas' disease: infection by *Trypanosoma cruzi* with destruction of myenteric plexus. Common in South America.
- Obstruction, e.g. in the case of a polypoid colorectal carcinoma.
- Toxic megacolon: complication of ulcerative colitis (see below).

Atresia and stenosis

'Atresia' results in complete intestinal obstruction, whereas 'stenosis' (narrowing) results in incomplete obstruction. These defects are most common in the duodenum and small intestine; rare in the colon.

They are probably caused by infarction of fetal bowel as a result of impairment of its blood supply due to fetal vascular accident, e.g. an excessively mobile loop of intestine may become twisted, thereby interrupting its blood supply and leading to necrosis of the section of bowel involved.

In turn, infarction leads to failure of the gut to canalize and failure of a segment to develop during fetal growth.

Anorectal anomalies

Numerous anorectal anomalies exist, the commonest of which are imperforate anus and anorectal agenesis.

Imperforate anus

This common anomaly affects 1 per 5000 live births, males more so than females. The anus is in the normal position but a thin layer of tissue separates the anal canal from the exterior. The membrane is thin enough to bulge on straining and appears blue from the presence of meconium above it.

Its cause is the failure of the anal membrane to perforate at the end of the eighth week.

Anorectal agenesis

The rectum ends superior to the puborectalis muscle, accounting for about two-thirds of anorectal defects. There are two types:
- With fistula (most common): in males—rectovesical fistula (to bladder) or rectourethral fistula (to urethra). Meconium may be observed in the urine. In females—rectovaginal fistula (to vagina) or rectovestibular fistula (to vestibule of vagina). Meconium may be present in the vestibule of the vagina.
- Without fistula (rectal agenesis): anal canal and rectum are present but they are separated.

Infections and enterocolitis
Diarrhoea and dysentery
Definitions

'Diarrhoea' means frequent bowel evacuation or the passage of abnormally soft or liquid faeces. Dysentery is an inflammatory disorder of the intestinal tract causing severe diarrhoea with blood and mucus.

Classification

Diarrhoea can be classified as:

- Secretory: diarrhoea caused by a combined effect of excessive intestinal secretions and decreased absorption. Stool volumes may be very high, and diarrhoea persists even when there is total fasting.
- Osmotic: diarrhoea caused by the presence of unabsorbed solute in the colon which prevents the absorption of fluid. Ceases on fasting long enough to empty the small bowel.
- Exudative: diarrhoea due to inflammatory exudate consisting of extracellular fluid and pus mixed with blood.
- Deranged motility: diarrhoea as a result of either increased or decreased motility of the small intestine.
- Malabsorption: diarrhoea occurring as a result of malabsorption (see below).

The classification and causes of diarrhoea are described in Fig. 9.28.

Infectious enterocolitis

Enterocolitis (inflammation of the colon and small intestine) is common and is often a result of infection.

Viral gastroenteritis

Viruses are the commonest cause of gastroenteritis in infants and young children, and account for 10% of all food poisoning outbreaks in the UK. Transmission is typically by a faecal–oral route. Symptoms are cramps, vomiting, fever, but no blood in stools.

In children:

- Rotavirus: causes 50% of infantile diarrhoea and accounts for some adult cases.
- Adenovirus (especially types 40, 41): second to rotavirus as cause of acute diarrhoea in young children.
- Astrovirus: most infections occur in childhood and are mild.

Classification and causes of diarrhoea	
Type	**Causes**
secretory	infections: bacteria producing enterotoxins, viral diarrhoea, *Giardia* irritants: laxatives, bile acids, hydroxy fatty acids hormonal: VIP, glucagon, medullary carcinoma of the thyroid, Addison's disease mucosal infiltration: villous adenoma, lymphoma, collagen diseases congenital: chloridorrhoea
osmotic	osmotic laxatives, e.g. lactulose, magnesium sulphate disaccharidase deficiency malabsorption syndromes congenital, e.g. chloridorrhoea (secretory and osmotic), hexose malabsorption
exudative	inflammatory diseases, e.g. ulcerative colitis, Crohn's disease infections: bacteria causing invasion of the mucosa, i.e. enteroinvasive bacteria such as *Shigella*, *Campylobacter*, enterohaemorrhagic *Escherichia coli*; and *Entamoeba histolytica*
deranged motility	decreased motility: • systemic sclerosis and other collagen disorders • intestinal pseudo-obstruction • diabetic autonomic neuropathy increased motility: • carcinoid syndrome • postvagotomy state • thyrotoxicosis • unabsorbed bile salts entering colon
malabsorption	may be a mixture of secretory, osmotic and exudative diarrhoea (see Fig. 9.33)

Fig. 9.28 Classification and causes of diarrhoea.

In adults, the Norwalk virus accounts for 30% of cases of gastroenteritis, and is responsible for the 'winter vomiting disease'.

Bacterial enterocolitis

The types of pathogenic mechanisms are as follows:

- Preformed toxin: ingestion of food contaminated with bacterial toxins, e.g. from *S. aureus*, *Bacillus cereus*, *Clostridium botulinum*. Incubation period is very short (1–7 hours).
- Toxigenic organism: ingestion of bacteria that produce toxins in the gut, e.g. *Vibrio cholerae*, enterotoxigenic *E. coli* (ETEC) and *C. perfringens*.
- Enteroinvasive organism: ingestion of bacteria that invade the intestinal mucosa and may cause dysentery as a result of severe inflammation, e.g. *Salmonella typhi*, *Campylobacter jejuni*, *Shigella*, enterohaemorrhagic *E. coli* (EHEC).
- Antibiotic-associated diarrhoea: occurs as a result of overgrowth of one type of bacteria due to disruption of normal gut flora following antibiotic treatment. Main culprit is *C. difficile*, which causes a condition known as pseudomembranous colitis

(forms a false membrane in the colon). Other pathogens are *C. perfringens* and *S. aureus*.

- Necrotizing enterocolitis: rare condition arising through a combination of ischaemia and infection. Ischaemia progresses to intestinal infarction and necrosis of the intestines. Infection of infarcted tissue results in gas gangrene (see Chapter 3), sepsis and shock with paralytic ileus. Most cases are seen in neonates. Adult cases are related to *C. perfringens* infection.

See Fig. 9.29 for a summary of common bacterial GI infections.

Pseudomembranous colitis

Caused by overgrowth with *C. difficile*, this is almost invariably associated with antibiotic therapy.

Clostridial toxin produced by bacteria causes necrosis of colonic mucosa. Patients develop fever, abdominal pain and diarrhoea.

Other diseases of the colon which allow clostridial overgrowth (gastrointestinal surgery, ischaemia, shock and burns) also predispose to its development.

Summary of common bacterial GI infections							
Mechanism	Bacterium	Incubation period	Duration (days)	V	C	F	B
preformed toxin	*Staphylococcus aureus*	2–7 hours	1	+	+	±	–
	B. cereus	1–6 hours	1	+	+	–	–
toxigenic organisms	*Vibrio cholerae*	2–3 days	up to 7	+	–	–	–
	Escherichia coli (ETEC)	12 hours–3 days	2–4	+	–	–	–
	Clostridium perfringens	8 hours–1 day	0.5–1	–	+	–	–
enteroinvasive bacteria	non-typhoidal *Salmonella*	8–48 hours	4–7	+	±	+	±
	Campylobacter jejuni	2–11 days	3–21	–	+	+	+
	Shigella	1–4 days	2–3	–	+	+	+
	E. coli (EHEC)	1–5 days	1–4	+	+	+	+
antibiotic-associated bacteria	*C. difficile*	–	–	–	+	+	±

Fig. 9.29 Summary of common bacterial GI infections. (V, vomiting; C, abdominal cramps; F, fever; B, blood in the stools; ETEC, enterotoxigenic *Escherichia coli*; EHEC, enterohaemorrhagic *E. coli*..)

Protozoa and other parasites

Chagas' disease

Infection by *Trypanosoma cruzi* results in the destruction of the myenteric plexus over a period of years with resulting dilatation of various parts of the alimentary canal, especially the colon and oesophagus. Common in South America.

Amoebic dysentery

This infection by *Entamoeba histolytica* is common throughout the tropics and occasionally seen in Britain. Cysts are ingested in water or uncooked food. The condition follows a chronic course with abdominal pains and two or more unformed stools a day. Periods of diarrhoea alternating with constipation are common.

Inflammatory disorders of the bowel
The idiopathic inflammatory bowel diseases

This group of disorders are characterized by primary inflammation of the intestinal wall.

Crohn's disease

A granulomatous inflammation of unknown cause that affects the full thickness of the bowel wall anywhere in the GI tract from mouth to anus, this disease is characterized by a relapsing and remitting course. Its prevalence is about 30–50 per 100 000 in the UK.

It usually presents in early adult life, with 90% of patients between 10 and 40 years, although a secondary peak occurs in the elderly. Females are affected more than males. There is a higher incidence in northern Europe and the US than elsewhere.

Cause and pathogenesis are unknown but several hypotheses have been suggested:

- Infectious, e.g. mycobacteria, *Chlamydia* and viruses, but no direct evidence.
- Immune: abnormal immune response to gut antigens.
- Dietary: increased carbohydrate, decreased fibre.
- Genetic: often associated with family history.
- Vascular: focal small vessel narrowing claimed to precede development of inflammation.
- Smoking: increased incidence in smokers. (Note: this is different from ulcerative colitis.)
- Miscellaneous: food antigens, psychosomatic and other factors have been proposed.

Macroscopic appearance

Site—Most commonly affects the terminal ileum but may affect any part of the GI tract from the mouth to the anus in a discontinuous pattern. Two-thirds of cases affect only the terminal ileum, one-sixth affect only the colon, and one-sixth are in the terminal ileum and colon.

Pattern:

- 'Skip' lesions: disease is characterized by a discontinuous distribution with normal bowel areas present between diseased segments.
- Oedema of submucosa and mucosa.
- Haemorrhagic ulcers: initially small and discrete, progress to form deep, linear, fissured ulcers ('rose thorn' ulcers).
- Cobblestone pattern: of bowel mucosa due to submucosal oedema and interconnecting deep fissured ulcers.
- Thickened bowel wall due to oedema and fibrosis.
- Fibrous strictures may cause partial obstruction.
- Dilatation of normal bowel proximal to diseased segment due to partial obstruction.
- Enlargement of mesenteric lymph nodes.

Microscopic appearance

- Transmural inflammation: all layers of bowel wall may be affected. Forms basis of fissures, adhesions, fistulae and sinuses.
- Lymphoid aggregates develop deep in bowel wall.
- Submucosal oedema.
- Ulceration.
- Non-caseating granulomas present in inflamed bowel wall and in mesenteric lymph nodes in about 60% of cases.

Clinical features are symptoms of abdominal pain, diarrhoea and weight loss, with signs of anaemia, clubbing, fever, mouth ulcers, and abdominal mass (inflamed bowel loops, abscesses).

Complications—The natural history of Crohn's disease is one of remissions and relapses of inflammation punctuated by complications.

Local complications are:

- Fistulae and sinuses: inflammation of serosal layer leads to formation adhesions to other bowel loops, to parietal peritoneum of anterior abdominal wall or to bladder.
- Stricture formations lead to intestinal obstruction.
- Fibrous adhesions lead to intestinal obstruction.
- Perforation of bowel by deep fissured ulcers leads to intra-abdominal abscesses.

- Carcinoma of bowel: increased incidence after many years.
- Haemorrhage: significant bleeding from areas of ulceration (rare).

Systemic complications, which develop in a minority of patients with Crohn's, are:

- Malabsorption due to diseased bowel or surgical resections.
- Skin disease: pyoderma gangrenosum, erythema nodosum.
- Eye disease: uveitis.
- Joint disease: polyarthropathy, sacroiliitis, ankylosing spondylitis.

- Chronic liver disease: pericholangitis, gallstones.
- Finger clubbing.
- Systemic amyloidosis: rare.

Ulcerative colitis

This diffuse superficial inflammation of the colorectum is of unknown cause, and characterized by relapses and remissions. It affects about 80 per 100 000 in the UK, with much lower rates in underdeveloped countries with warmer climates. (Ulcerative colitis has a similar age distribution to Crohn's, but the sex incidence is equal.)

Aetiopathogenesis—Unknown, but same hypotheses as for Crohn's have been proposed with the exception of smoking, which is associated with a decreased risk for ulcerative colitis.

Macroscopic appearance—The site and pattern are important to note as described below.

Site—Ulcerative colitis usually begins distally as proctitis and then spreads proximally to affect the whole of the large bowel, and may affect the terminal ileum ('backwash' ileitis).

The pattern is one of shallow ulceration (which may become confluent), with 'pseudopolyps', hyperaemia, and haemorrhage.

Microscopically, inflammation is diffuse and is limited to mucosa, with infiltration at both acute and chronic inflammatory cells. Other features are crypt

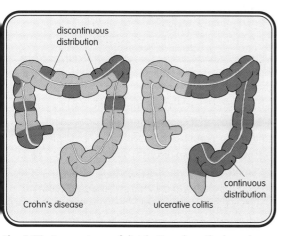

Fig. 9.30 Comparisons of distribution along the bowel.

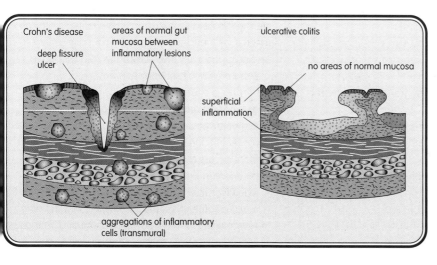

Fig. 9.31 Depth and distribution of lesions in the bowel wall.

Comparison of the basic features of Crohn's disease and ulcerative colitis		
	Crohn's disease	**Ulcerative colitis**
prevalence in UK	~30–50 per 100 000 in UK	~80 per 100 000
site	any part of GI system but typically terminal ileum	colon and rectum only
macroscopic:		
• disease continuity	discontinuous	continuous
• bowel wall	thickened with strictures and adhesions	not thickened
• ulcers	deep fissures form basis of fistulae	flat based; do not extend to submucosa
microscopic:		
• pattern of inflammation	transmural focal granulomas (in 60% of cases)	mucosal and submucosal diffuse no granulomas
• crypt pattern	little distortion	distorted in long-standing disease; crypt abscesses
anal lesions	present in 75%; anal fistulae; ulceration or chronic fissure	present in <25%
frequency of fistula	10–20% of cases	uncommon
risk of developing cancer	slightly increased	significantly increased

Fig. 9.32 Comparison of the basic features of Crohn's disease and ulcerative colitis.

abscesses with ulceration, crypt atrophy, and Paneth's cell metaplasia.

Clinical features are symptoms of bloody diarrhoea, mucus, cramping discomfort, and weight loss, and signs of fever, tachycardia, pallor, and abdominal tenderness.

Acute local complications include perforation, dilatation, haemorrhage, and dehydration (blood and fluid loss from extensive ulceration).

Chronic local complications include strictures, dysplasia, and carcinoma.

Systemic complications are:
• Anaemia.
• Malabsorption due to diseased bowel or surgical resections.
• Skin disease: pyoderma gangrenosum, erythema nodosum.
• Eye disease: uveitis, hypopyon.
• Joint disease: polyarthropathy, sacroiliitis, ankylosing spondylitis.
• Chronic liver disease: primary sclerosing cholangitis.
• Finger clubbing.
• Systemic amyloidosis (rare).

A comparison of Crohn's and ulcerative colitis

Both Crohn's and ulcerative colitis are examples of inflammatory bowel disease, and have many features in common. However, in the majority of cases (about 90%), it is possible to distinguish between these two conditions (Figs 9.30–9.32).

Diagnosis is by colonoscopy, barium and small bowel enema. With colonoscopy, biopsy specimens can be taken for histological examination (see Fig. 9.32 for differences in microscopical appearance). This investigation is also important in the surveillance of patients with long-standing colitis as it allows severe dysplasia and early invasive cancer to be detected.

Barium and small bowel enema:
• Crohn's is characterized by a discontinuous distribution, often with rectal sparing. Diseased segments have a 'cobblestone' appearance caused by deep longitudinal and transverse ulcers. 'Rose thorn' ulcers may be present, which sometimes perforate to produce fistulous tracks.
• Mild ulcerative colitis is characterized by a disturbed mucosal pattern with small ulcers. Long-standing severe disease may show loss of haustral markings with a featureless, shortened hosepipe colon.

Management can be medical or surgical.

Medical:

- Corticosteroids: effective in inducing remission (Local—topical steroid enemas used for exacerbations of distal proctocolitis; systemic—oral prednisolone).
- Sulphasalazine: can be used to maintain remission once remission has been induced by corticosteroids.
- Azathioprine: helpful in patients with chronic disease for whom surgery is inappropriate.

Surgical:

- Minimal resections for strictures, fistulae or perforations.
- Colectomy: indicated in cases of chronic disease, side effects from long-term high dosages of steroids, premalignant change on colonoscopic surveillance and in patients at high risk of developing chronic cancer (early onset disease, extensive colonic involvement and continuous rather than episodic symptoms).
- Colectomy and pouch formation: younger patients with ulcerative colitis can have a sphincter preserving operation in which a pouch is constructed from a duplicated (J pouch) or triplicated (Park's pouch) loop of ileum. Pouch is anastomosed to dentate line following excision of the rectum. Crohn's patients are not suitable for pouch formation as recurrent disease may affect the ileum used in constructing the pouch.

Miscellaneous intestinal inflammatory disorders

GI manifestations of HIV disease

AIDS is associated with fulminant bowel infection which often causes severe diarrhoea.

Malabsorptive or colitic syndromes

These are described below.

Diarrhoea in bone marrow transplantation graft versus host disease

Bone marrow transplants contain competent T lymphocytes which can react against HLA antigens of the recipient, causing skin rash, liver toxicity and diarrhoea, which may be torrential in severe forms.

Malabsorption syndromes

General aspects of malabsorption syndromes

Malabsorption may be caused by disorders of:

- Intraluminal digestion: pancreas secretes digestive enzymes into the gut lumen (these are necessary for breakdown of macromolecules).
- Intraluminal solubilization: liver secretes bile acids required for solubilization and absorption of fats.
- Terminal digestion: mucosa is the site of a set of enzymes located on the brush border which hydrolyse large molecules for absorption, especially complex sugars (e.g. sucrose and lactose).
- Transepithelial transport: mucosa is specialized for absorption—transverse mucosal folds and finger-like villi provide a vast surface area.

Systemic effects of the malabsorption syndromes:

- Weight loss.
- Abdominal distension.
- Diarrhoea (loose, bulky stools).
- Steatorrhoea: malabsorption of fat producing pale, foul-smelling stools which characteristically float in water.
- Anaemia.

Classification of malabsorption syndromes

This is described in Fig. 9.33.

Specific malabsorption syndromes

Coeliac disease

There is atrophy of small intestinal villi due to an abnormal sensitivity to gluten, which is a protein in wheat flour. It affects about 1 per 2000 in most populations in western Europe (but 1 per 300 in western Ireland).

It can present at any age but is an important cause of failure to thrive in infants and children.

Caused by an immune response to the protein gliadin, a component of gluten. Anti-gliadin antibodies are present in the majority of cases. There is an increased incidence of disease in first-degree relatives of those affected, and linkage with certain HLA-B8 groups has been shown. It often occurs concurrently with dermatitis herpetiformis (itchy, blistering skin disease).

Macroscopically, the lumenal surface becomes flattened developing a mosaic-like pattern of crypt

Causes of malabsorption	
defective intraluminal digestion or solubilization	pancreatic insufficiency: • chronic pancreatitis • cystic fibrosis • carcinoma of the pancreas liver disease: failure of bile secretion into gut
primary mucosal cell abnormalities	lactase deficiency
reduced surface area of small intestine	conditions that cause villous atrophy: • coeliac disease • tropical sprue • Crohn's disease • malnutrition iatrogenic: • extensive small intestine resection • jejunal ileal bypass procedures • postradiotherapy
infection	parasitic infestation of gut bacterial overgrowth in blind loops of diverticulae postinfective malabsorption giardiasis Whipple's disease
lymphatic obstruction	primary lymphangiectasia lymphoma
drug-induced	cytotoxic drugs drugs that bind bile salts, e.g. cholestyramine and some antibiotics such as neomycin (which cause steatorrhoea)
miscellaneous	thyrotoxicosis → increased gastric emptying and motility Zollinger–Ellison syndrome diabetes mellitus → bacterial overgrowth hypogammaglobulinaemia → infection

Fig. 9.33 Causes of malabsorption.

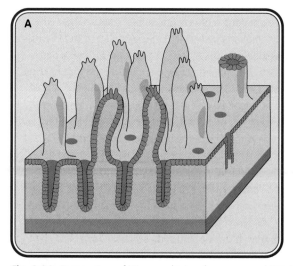
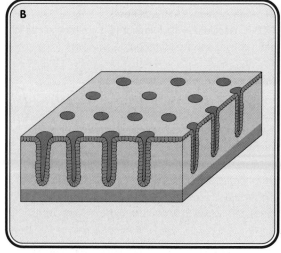

Fig. 9.34 Comparison of (A) normal jejunal mucosa and (B) jejunal mucosa in coeliac disease with total villous atrophy.

openings (Fig. 9.34).

Microscopically there is:

- Mucosal inflammation with lymphocytic infiltration.
- Loss of villous architecture ranging from blunting (partial villous atrophy) to complete flattening (total villous atrophy).
- Increase in depth of crypts with epithelial cell hyperplasia to compensate for those lost through damage.

Long-term complications are:

- Chronic ulceration of the small intestine: may lead to strictures.
- Development of primary T cell lymphoma of the small intestine.
- Development of adenocarcinoma (rare).

Diagnosis is by biopsy of the small bowel mucosa; and by the gluten-challenge, in which gluten is withdrawn from the diet. Improvement should result, followed by relapse of the disease on the subsequent reintroduction of gluten.

Management is by the complete withdrawal of gliadin from the diet (i.e. a gluten-free diet), which leads to gradual recovery of the villous structure which may be partial or complete.

Causes of small intestinal bacterial overgrowth	
Cause	**Example**
excessive entry of bacteria	achlorrhydria infected bile ducts gastrocolic fistula gastric surgery resection of ileocaecal valve
defective immune mechanisms	immune deficiencies malnutrition old age
stagnant region	blind loops enterocolic fistulae jejunal diverticula strictures or other obstruction continent ileostomy
disturbed motility	systemic sclerosis intestinal pseudo-obstruction diabetes autonomic neuropathy

Fig. 9.35 Causes of small intestinal bacterial overgrowth.

Tropical sprue

This persistent malabsorption syndrome without a definable cause is seen in patients who live or have lived in the tropics, and in the absence of other intestinal disease or parasites. The disease occurs mainly in the West Indies including Sri Lanka, southern India, Malaysia and Indonesia.

Aetiology is unclear; however the condition is thought to be infective, probably toxigenic *E. coli.*

Clinical features and histological appearances resemble those of coeliac disease.

Whipple's disease

This rare condition is characterized by tissue infiltration with foamy macrophages staining with periodic acid–Schiff (PAS) stain. PAS-staining material has been shown to be derived from an unknown bacterium.

Bacterial overgrowth syndrome

Here, there is malabsorption secondary to excessive bacteria in the small intestine, usually the jejunum. (It is also known as contaminated bowel syndrome, blind loop syndrome and small intestine stasis syndrome.)

Causes of small intestinal bacterial overgrowth are outlined in Fig. 9.35.

Malabsorption is as a result of:

- Deconjugation of bile salts by the bacteria, hence steatorrhoea.
- Damage to the small intestinal mucosa, probably by bacterial products.
- Binding of vitamin B_{12} by bacteria, hence vitamin B_{12} deficiency.

Diarrhoea is both secretory (due to bacterial products affecting mucosa) and osmotic (due to unabsorbed products and deficiency of disaccharidases because of mucosal damage).

Clinical features are weight loss, diarrhoea and anaemia (due to vitamin B_{12} deficiency).

Diagnosis is by the reversal of symptoms by broad spectrum antibiotics and by demonstration of the causative lesion.

Management is by antibiotic therapy and surgical resection for a localized abnormality, e.g. stricture, fistula.

Giardiasis

This disease is caused by the parasitic protozoan,

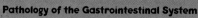
Giardia lamblia, in the small intestine. Infection occurs by eating food or water contaminated with parasitic cysts. Symptoms include diarrhoea, nausea, abdominal pain and flatulence, as well as the passage of pale fatty stools. The disease occurs worldwide and is particularly common in children.

Disaccharidase deficiency (alactasia)

This is the absence or deficiency of the enzyme lactase which is essential for the digestion of milk sugar (lactose). All babies have lactase in their intestines but the enzyme disappears during childhood in about 10% of northern Europeans, 40% of Greeks and Italians, and 80% of Africans and Asians. The presence of undigested lactose in the small intestine (following consumption of raw milk) causes diarrhoea and abdominal pain.

Abetalipoproteinaemia

This rare condition is characterized by the absence of plasma β-lipoproteins resulting in:

- Abnormally shaped red blood cells with spikes on the surface (acanthocytosis).
- Retinitis pigmentosa leading to blindness.
- Progressive ataxia.
- Fatty infiltration of enterocytes.
- Steatorrhoea.

β-Lipoproteins are thought to be necessary for the transport of lipids from enterocyte into lacteals, and for the transport of nutrients into the CNS and red blood cells. Plasma vitamin E levels are very low since vitamin E is carried primarily on the β-lipoproteins.

Early intensive and continued repletion with vitamin E prevents neurological deterioration. Steatorrhoea is managed by a low fat diet and nutritional supplements.

Obstruction of the bowel

Major causes of bowel obstruction

Classification of obstruction and pseudo-obstruction

Simple mechanical obstruction

The bowel above the obstructing lesion becomes distended with fluid and gas, stimulating excessive peristalsis, producing colic. Impairment of mucosal function causes net loss of water and electrolytes into the lumen (with ECF depletion).

Strangulation obstruction

Here, there is occlusion of the venous system by constricting agents, e.g. tight neck of a hernial sac or twist of a volvulus, results in ischaemia and infarction of bowel and ultimately causes obstruction.

Paralytic ileus

This may arise as a consequence of peritonitis, pancreatitis or retroperitoneal bleeding, but can also complicate mechanical obstruction. The abdomen is distended, bowel sounds are absent but colic is not a feature of ileus.

Pseudo-obstruction

This is a rare syndrome in which gaseous abdominal distension and obstructive bowel sounds suggest a mechanical intestinal obstruction when none is present. The disorder is caused by abnormal gut motility rather than by an organic obstructive lesion. There are two types of cause:

- Primary (rare): abnormalities of smooth muscle or nerve plexuses in gut.
- Secondary (common): connective tissue diseases, particularly scleroderma, diabetic neuropathy and amyloidosis of gut.

Examples of simple mechanical obstruction, strangulation obstruction, and paralytic ileus types of obstructions are listed in Fig. 9.36.

Hernias

Definition

This is the protrusion of the whole or part of a viscus from its normal position through a defect in the cavity wall in which it is contained. About 1 per 100 people have a hernia at some time. Hernias can be congenital or acquired.

Acquired:
- Secondary to increased intra-abdominal pressure: cough, straining at the stool, cysts, carcinoma, pregnancy.
- Iatrogenic: incisional hernias.

Classification:

- Reducible: contents of sac can be completely returned to abdominal cavity.
- Irreducible/incarcerated: content of sac cannot be completely returned to the abdominal cavity.

Common sites of abdominal hernias are inguinal (70%), femoral (20%), and umbilical (10%). Others are supraumbilical or linea alba, incisional hernias, and hiatus hernia (see pp. 136–137).

Complications:

- Obstruction: constriction at neck of hernial sac causes obstruction of bowel loops within it.
- Strangulation: constriction at neck of sac prevents venous return leading to venous congestion, arterial occlusion and gangrene. May result in perforation leading to peritonitis/groin abscess.

Note that strangulation can occur without obstruction if only one wall of viscus pouches into sac (Richter's hernia).

Hernias must be repaired because of the potential complications. The principles of surgical repair are identification of sac and contents, mobilization of sac, reduction of contents, ligation of sac, and repairing the fascial defect.

Inguinal hernia

The commonest type of hernia, this is much more prevalent in men than in women. There are two types: indirect inguinal (85%) and direct inguinal (15%).

Indirect inguinal hernia

The hernial sac enters the inguinal canal through the deep ring (lateral to the inferior epigastric artery) and then traverses through the canal to the superficial ring, where it may eventually reach the scrotum or labium major.

Its origin is congenital (due to patency of processus vaginalis) and is most common in children and young adults. Males are more affected than females by 20:1!

Strangulation is a common complication due to the narrow neck of the hernial sac.

Direct inguinal hernia

The hernial sac protrudes through a weakness in fascia transversalis (medial to inferior epigastric artery) and does not normally descend into the scrotum.

It originates as a result of weakened abdominal muscles. It is most common in the elderly and affects males more than females. The neck of the sac is wide and so strangulation is rare.

Major causes of bowel obstruction	
Cause	Example
simple mechanical obstruction	intraluminal: • foreign bodies • gallstone ileus • fecaliths • meconium in cystic fibrosis bowel wall: • adhesions • carcinoma • strictures • atresia • imperforate anus
strangulation obstruction	intussusception infarction volvulus internal/external hernias bands
adynamic obstruction (paralytic ileus)	abdominal causes: postoperative, peritonitis, vascular occlusion systemic causes: electrolyte disorders, uraemia, hypothyroidism drugs: anticholinergics, opiates

Fig. 9.36 Major causes of bowel obstruction.

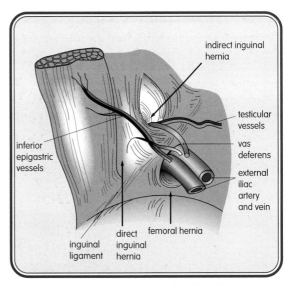

Fig. 9.37 Sites of direct inguinal, indirect inguinal and femoral herniations. (Adapted with permission from *Principles and Practice of Surgery*, 3rd edn, by APM Forrest, PC Carter and IB Macleod, Churchill Livingstone, 1995.)

177

Clinically, it is difficult (often impossible) to distinguish between direct and indirect inguinal hernias. Often, differentiation can only be made at operation from the position of the neck of the hernial sac relative to the inferior epigastric artery.

Femoral hernia

The hernial sac protrudes through the femoral canal inferior to the inguinal ligament (Fig. 9.37). There is an increasing incidence with age, and females are affected more than males by 2:1 (but inguinal hernia is still more common in both males and females). The most common complication is strangulation.

Adhesions

Adhesions are by far the commonest cause of mechanical obstruction in the small bowel and are defined as areas of fibrosis between adjacent membranes or organs resulting in their fusion. The causes can be congenital (e.g. bands in small children) or acquired.

Acquired causes are as follows:

- Inflammation, e.g. Crohn's disease, sclerosing peritonitis.
- Infection, e.g. appendicitis, diverticulitis, tuberculosis, peritonitis.
- Trauma, e.g. stab wounds.
- Iatrogenic: post-surgery introduction of foreign bodies (starch granules, talc, non-absorbable sutures), irradiation.
- Vascular: infarction/gangrene.
- Malignancies.

Intussusception

This is invagination of one part of the bowel into the adjoining segment (Fig. 9.38). The ileocaecal valve is the most common site with the ileum invaginating into the caecum. It typically affects children under the age of four.

Adult cases are extremely rare, and are almost invariably precipitated by structural abnormalities of the small intestinal wall, e.g. benign tumours (leiomyoma or lipoma) or Meckel's diverticulum.

As the contents of the intestine are pushed onwards by muscular contraction, more and more intestine is dragged into the adjoining bowel. The net effect is venous congestion of the invaginated portion causing bleeding from the mucosa as well as intestinal obstruction.

Symptoms are intermittent colic or pain, vomiting, and the passing of 'redcurrant jelly' with the stools.

Complications—If the bowel remains invaginated, infarction and shock from gangrene may result.

Management is by barium reduction in children or

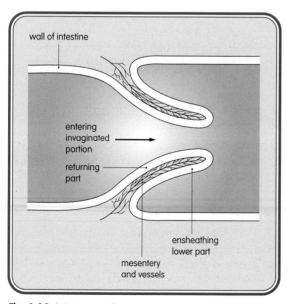

Fig. 9.38 Intussusception.

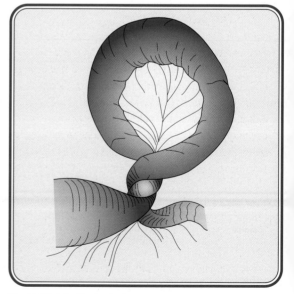

Fig. 9.39 Intestinal volvulus.

by resection in adults because of the high incidence of organic causes.

Volvulus

This is a twisting of part of the GI tract, usually leading to partial, or complete obstruction (Fig. 9.39). Sites:

- Gastric volvulus: twisting of the stomach, usually in a hiatus hernia.
- Small intestinal volvulus: twisting of part of the bowel around an adhesion.
- Sigmoid volvulus: twist of the sigmoid colon, usually when this loop is particularly long.

The most common complication is strangulation (reduction of blood supply causing infarction and possibly gangrene).

Management—May untwist spontaneously but surgical manipulation is usually performed.

Colonic diverticulosis

Definitions

'Diverticulum' means a sac or pouch formed at weak points in the wall of the alimentary tract, and 'diverticulosis' means a condition in which diverticula exist in a segment of the intestine without evidence of inflammation. Diverticulitis is inflammation of a diverticulum, most commonly of one or more colonic diverticula.

Aetiopathogenesis of diverticula

Congenital diverticula are true diverticula containing all three coats of the bowel wall, e.g. Meckel's diverticulum (see p. 166).

Acquired diverticula may contain some (false diverticula) or all (true diverticula) coats of the bowel wall.

Pathogenesis of acquired diverticula—Typically develop during adult life as a result of:

- Pulsion from increased intraluminal pressure causing protrusion at points of focal weakness (e.g. at the sites of penetration of blood vessels).
- Traction due to extrinsic disease.

Colonic diverticulosis

This acquired diverticulosis of the colon is caused by chronic lack of dietary fibre. It is also known as colonic diverticular disease.

Though rare before 35 years, by 65 years at least one-third of the population of developed countries are affected—but it is rare in countries with high fibre diets.

Diverticula are most common in sigmoid colon emerging between mesenteric and antimesenteric taeniae.

Pathogenesis—Increased intraluminal pressure (e.g. as a result of straining at the stool) causes herniation of intestinal mucosa through the circular muscle at points of weakness, notably sites of penetration of blood vessels.

The clinical course may be either asymptomatic or symptomatic, with left-sided colicky abdominal pain and alteration of bowel habit (usually constipation) or rectal bleeding.

Complications are:

- Inflammation (peridiverticulitis): may cause pain and tenderness in left iliac fossa, alteration of bowel habit, fever, leukocytosis and may produce a palpable mass.
- Perforation: results in peritonitis.
- Obstruction: due to oedema or fibrosis in the inflamed segment of colon or to adherence of small bowel loops.
- Stricture formation: long-standing diverticular disease may cause stricture formation and subacute intestinal obstruction.
- Fistula: commonest cause of colovesical fistula.
- Bleeding: common complication.

Diagnosis is by barium enema and colonoscopy.

Treatment:

- Conservative: high fibre diet results in improvement in most patients.
- Surgery: sigmoid colectomy with end-to-end anastomosis if there are persistent symptoms or when carcinoma cannot be excluded by radiology or colonoscopy.

Vascular disorders of the bowel

Ischaemic bowel disease

Ischaemic bowel disease may affect the small or large bowel and is most commonly seen in elderly patients with severe atherosclerosis.

Causes of bowel ischaemia

Vessel disease

These are:

- Vascular occlusion: emboli lodge in superior mesenteric artery which supplies entire small intestine except for first part of duodenum. Extent of bowel infarction depends on whether occlusion is in proximal or distal branch. Emboli are derived from mural thrombus from myocardial infarct, thrombotic vegetations on mitral or aortic valves, left atrial thrombosis.

- Vascular stenosis (less common): thrombosis in severely atherosclerotic mesenteric artery typically located in its proximal part shortly after its origin from aorta. Resultant small bowel infarction is extensive and usually fatal.
- Vasculitic syndromes (pp. 97–99), e.g. polyarteritis nodosa, Henoch–Schönlein purpura, SLE.

Strangulation
Thin-walled veins which drain blood from the small bowel become occluded by extrinsic pressure, e.g. from:
- Loop of bowel in a narrow hernial sac.
- Intussusception.
- Volvulus.
- Adhesions.

Venous occlusion causes congestion and oedema of the bowel wall. Increased pressure prevents entry of oxygenated arterial blood leading to ischaemic necrosis.

Hypoperfusion
In severe hypotension, blood is shunted preferentially away from the superficial mucosa, which is the layer of the wall most susceptible to injury due to its high metabolic requirements.

In infants, poor perfusion of the mucosa followed by infection produces a rapidly fatal condition known as neonatal necrotizing enterocolitis. The bowel wall is thickened from congestion and there is extensive superficial mucosal ulceration. Predisposing factors are prematurity, ARDS, Hirschsprung's disease and cystic fibrosis with meconium ileus.

Classification of severity
Ischaemic infarcts are classified according to the depth of involvement, either mucosal infarction, mural infarction or transmural infarction.

Mucosal infarction
This transient or reversible infarction may be followed by complete regeneration. However, increased permeability to toxic substances can bring about further cardiovascular deterioration and gradual progression to a transmural infarct.

Mural infarction
Here, there is infarction of mucosa and submucosa up to muscularis propria. Mucosa is ulcerated, oedematous and haemorrhagic. Healing occurs by granulation tissue formation and may lead to development of fibrous strictures.

Transmural infarction
Necrosis extends through muscularis propria and is synonymous with gangrene. The bowel is flaccid, dilated and liable to perforation. Surgical resection is an option, but many patients already have peritonitis, endotoxaemia and severe circulatory problems at the time of diagnosis so that prognosis is poor.

Watersheds of ischaemic bowel disease
Progression of mural infarction to stricture formation occurs in about 50% of patients with ischaemic bowel disease. The splenic flexure and left colon are the common sites affected. Most patients ultimately require resection but a minority improve spontaneously.

Angiodysplasia
In this condition, abnormal venous dilatations develop in submucosa of the large intestine (typically the right side) often causing occult or massive intestinal

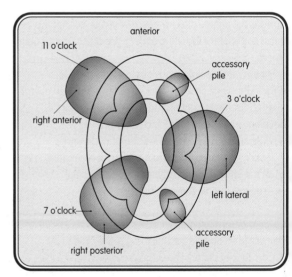

Fig. 9.40 Diagram to illustrate the 3, 7, 11 distribution of haemorrhoids around the anus. (Adapted with permission from *Surgery of the Anus, Rectum and Colon*, 5th edn, by J. Goligher, Baillière Tindall, 1984.)

bleeding. It occurs in the elderly and is associated with hypertension and left-sided valvular heart disease.

It is thought to be a degenerative process resulting in increasing obstruction of mucosal veins. Obstruction results in repeated episodes of transient elevated pressure causing dilatation and tortuosity of the submucosal veins and subsequently of the venules and capillaries of the mucosal units draining into the veins.

Haemorrhoids (piles)

These are dilated varicose veins forming in the anal canal. The commonest of all anal conditions, they affect as much as 40% of the population at some time.

Aetiology:
- Increased intra-abdominal pressure: constipation and straining at the stool, pregnancy.
- Portal hypertension (rare).

Classification:
- Internal haemorrhoids: proximal to superior haemorrhoidal plexus, above anorectal margin.
- External haemorrhoids: below the anorectal margin.

Internal haemorrhoids

These are caused by the enlargement of the normal, spongy, blood-filled cushions in the wall of the anus, most commonly occurring at three main points equidistant around the circumference of the anus (Fig. 9.40). There are four types of internal haemorrhoids:
- First degree: present in the lumen but do not prolapse.
- Second degree: prolapse on defecation but return spontaneously.
- Third degree: remain prolapsed but can be digitally replaced.
- Fourth degree: long-standing prolapsed haemorrhoids which cannot be replaced in the anal canal.

Types of intestinal tumours		
	Small intestine	**Large bowel**
non-neoplastic polyps	hamartomas juvenile polyps adenomatous polyps (in familial adenomatous polyposis and Gardner's syndrome) inflammatory fibroid polyps	hyperplastic polyps: small, flat, pale lesions typically 5 mm in size, which occur most commonly in the rectum and sigmoid colon hamartomatous polyps: typically occur in childhood and in adolescence: • Peutz–Jeghers syndrome • juvenile polyps (autosomal dominant) • sporadic inflammatory 'pseudopolyps' (of ulcerative colitis)

neoplastic epithelial lesions	adenocarcinomas	pre-malignant:
		• adenomas (dysplastic):
		    tubular adenoma
		    villous adenoma
		    tubulovillous adenoma
		• familial adenomatous polyposis
		malignant:
		• colorectal carcinoma

mesenchymal lesions	benign: lipoma, neurogenic tumours, leiomyoma and haemangioma malignant: some smooth muscle tumours (leiomyosarcomas)	rare; usually incidental findings or at post mortem; seldom responsible for symptoms; lipomas, leiomyomas, haemangiomas, neurofibromas
lymphoma	common site for primary lymphoma of the GI tract; coeliac disease is a major predisposing factor	very uncommon in large bowel
carcinoid tumours (neuroendocrine tumours)	commonest site for carcinoid tumours (especially appendix); lesions typically scattered singly throughout GI tract; may secrete gut hormones, e.g. somatostatin, cholecystokinin, pancreatic polypeptide and vasoactive intestinal polypeptide (VIP)	rare; do not usually produce functioning hormones

Fig. 9.41 Types of intestinal tumours.

Diagnosis is by proctoscopy (to visualize the haemorrhoids) or by sigmoidoscopy (to exclude coexisting rectal pathology).

Treatment:

- Sclerotherapy: injection with 5% phenol in almond oil induces submucosal fibrosis.
- Rubber-band ligation: haemorrhoid is pulled down through proctoscope and a rubber band is applied around the mucosa-covered part.
- Infrared photocoagulation: causes coagulation within haemorrhoid with reduction in size.
- Haemorrhoidectomy.

External haemorrhoids

There are two types: prolapsed internal haemorrhoids, and perianal haematomas or residual skin tags remaining after a perianal haematoma has healed.

Complications—Both internal and external haemorrhoids have the following complications:

- Prolapse.
- Bleeding.
- Ulceration.
- Thrombosis.
- Strangulation.

Neoplastic disease of the intestine

Primary tumours of the small intestine are rare. Those that do arise are outlined in Fig. 9.41. In contrast, tumours of the large bowel are extremely common. The colon and rectum are frequently affected by both benign and malignant tumours.

Classification of intestinal tumours
Intestinal tumours can be classified according to Fig. 9.41.

Neoplastic epithelial lesions
Adenomas
These premalignant tumours are derived from the glandular epithelium of the large bowel. Common in older subjects, they are present in up to 50% of persons aged over 60, males more than females by 2:1.

Aetiology is probably multifactorial. Both genetic and environmental (dietary) factors have been implied.

There are three types:

- Tubular: rounded lesions (0.5–2 cm in size). Often pendunculated (i.e. have a stalk of normal mucosa). Microscopically composed of tube-shaped glands.
- Villous: frond-like lesions about 0.6 cm thick, which occupy a broad area of mucosa (about 1–5 cm in diameter). Microscopically composed of finger-like epithelial projections.
- Tubulovillous: raised lesions (1–4 cm in size). Pendunculated but composed of both tube-shaped glands and finger-like epithelial projections.

Epithelia of all three types show dysplastic features which can be subjectively graded as mild, moderate or severe.

Progression from adenoma to carcinoma
Most carcinomas of the colon develop from previous adenomata. Progression from adenoma to carcinoma is the well-established basis of the polyp–cancer sequence for development of carcinoma of the colon.

Risk of malignant change is greatest where adenomas show the following features:

- Large: less than 1 cm (1% malignant), 1–2 cm (12% malignant), more than 2 cm (30% malignant).
- Villous: villous adenomas are more likely to undergo malignant transformation.
- Severe dysplasia.

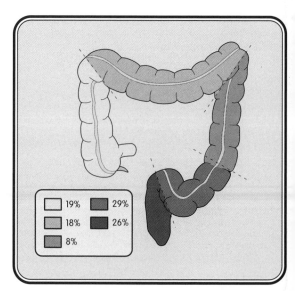

Fig. 9.42 Site and incidence of carcinomas of the large intestine.

Familial adenomatous polyposis

This autosomal dominant condition is due to a mutation in a tumour suppressor gene, and characterized by the presence of innumerable adenomata of the large bowel from about the age of 25, with a 100% risk of developing a carcinoma of the colon by the age of 45.

Colorectal carcinoma

This adenocarcinoma is derived from the glandular epithelium of the large bowel mucosa.

It is the second most common cause of death from neoplasia, with a peak incidence between 60 and 70 years; it is rare under the age of 40.

It is rare in Africa but there is a high incidence in developed countries. It is related to environmental factors (probably diet) rather than genetic.

Risk factors are:
- Presence of multiple sporadic adenomatous polyps.
- Ulcerative colitis.
- Familial adenomatous polyposis.

Macroscopically, the commonest sites for colorectal carcinomas are illustrated in Fig. 9.42.

Types of colorectal carcinomas are:
- Polypoid: cauliflower-like growth.
- Annular: small, circumferential carcinomas which may cause stenosis.
- Ulcerated: tumours that present mainly with bleeding.
- Diffusely infiltrative: rare, but virtually identical to that seen in stomach. Often associated with carcinoma that develops in association with inflammatory bowel disease.

Right-sided carcinomas (ascending colon):
- Type of growth: polypoid.
- Pathogenesis: faecal material is soft in ascending colon, and so lesions grow to large size before causing obstruction.
- Presentation: later than for left-sided carcinomas.

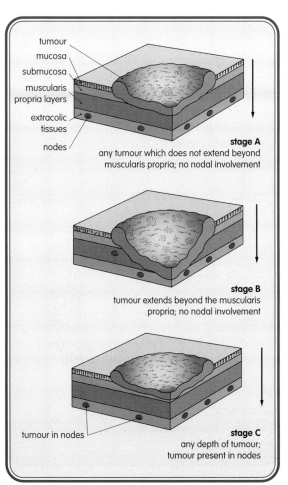

Fig. 9.43 Staging of carcinoma of the colon.

- Describe the features of a Meckel's diverticulum.
- Name the types of pathogenic mechanisms of bacterial enterocolitis and give examples of the micro-organisms responsible.
- Compare and contrast the features of Crohn's disease with those of ulcerative colitis.
- Describe the pathology of coeliac disease.
- State the major causes of bowel obstruction.
- Outline the complications of colonic diverticulosis.
- What are the causes of ischaemic bowel disease?
- Summarize the features colorectal carcinomas.

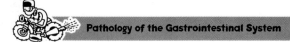

Left-sided carcinomas (descending colon):
- Type of growth: annular, ulcerating.
- Pathogenesis: lesions develop where faecal material is more solid.
- Presentation: earlier due to mechanical obstruction to passage of faeces.

Microscopical features—The majority of colorectal carcinomas are moderately or well-differentiated adenocarcinomas forming recognizable glandular structures. Poorly differentiated carcinomas have a poorer prognosis.
 Spread:
- Local: into adjacent bowel wall and adherent structures (e.g. bladder).
- Lymphatic: to draining nodes.
- Blood: to liver and then elsewhere.
- Transcoelomic: along peritoneal cavity.

Prognosis of carcinoma of the colon is related to the stage of the disease which is assessed using a modification of a staging system originally proposed for carcinoma of the rectum by Dukes (Fig. 9.43).

DISORDERS OF THE PERITONEUM

Inflammation—peritonitis
Peritoneal infection
This can be a primary or secondary infection. Primary infection (less common) is seen in patients with nephrotic syndrome (peritoneal dialysis), cirrhosis with ascites, or abdominal trauma.
 Secondary infection (most common) is typically an extension of inflammatory processes from abdominal cavity, e.g.:
- Appendicitis.
- Ruptured ulcers: peptic, ulcerative colitis, typhoid ulcers, ulcerated neoplasms.
- Cholecystitis, pancreatitis, salpingitis.
- Diverticulitis.
- Strangulated bowel.

Organisms involved are typically a mixture of normal gut commensals with anaerobic bacteria and coliforms predominating.
 Irritation of the peritoneum by leaking bile, gastric juice, pancreatic enzymes or urine produces an exudate which is initially sterile but which usually becomes infected within 6–12 hours.

As peritonitis develops, inflammation of visceral and parietal peritoneum produces a purulent exudate, the intestine becomes flaccid, dilated and covered with fibrinous plaques which form adhesions between bowel loops.
 Clinical features are:
- Tenderness, guarding and rebound tenderness.
- Board-like abdominal rigidity.
- Absent bowel sounds (paralytic ileus).
- Increased pulse and temperature.

Complications are:
- Hypovolaemic shock.
- Severe toxaemia from absorbed bacterial products.
- Ileus: paralysis of gut motility as a result of inflammation of the serosa of the small bowel.
- Fibrous adhesions as a result of organization of fibrinous adhesion by granulation tissue.
- Abscesses, particularly in the paracolic gutters and beneath the diaphragm (subphrenic recesses).
- Portal pyophlebitis: spread via the portal vein to the liver.

Diagnosis is by clinical examination and erect abdominal X-ray, which may show air under the diaphragm from perforated viscus.
 Management is by:
- Treatment of shock.
- Antibiotic therapy.
- Surgery: removal of contaminating source, e.g. appendicitis or perforated bowel.
- Peritoneal toilet and lavage.

See Fig. 9.44 for a summary of peritoneal infection.

Sclerosis retroperitonitis
This dense progressive fibrosis of peritoneum particularly affects the visceral peritoneum of the small intestine. It is thought to be a side effect of practolol (β-blocker), now withdrawn from use. It is also seen in patients undergoing long-term continuous ambulatory peritoneal dialysis.

Mesenteric cysts
Sequestered lymphatic channels (cystic lymphangiomas)
These cystic developmental abnormalities of lymphoid type are typically asymptomatic and discovered incidentally at laparotomy or autopsy.

Punched-off enteric diverticula (enterogenous cysts)
These common lesions are found either incorporated in the bowel wall or in mesentery detached and separated from the tract. They are usually surrounded by smooth muscle and have a mucosal lining of alimentary type epithelium.

Urogenital ridge derivations
These developmental cysts are of urogenital origin.

'Walled-off' infections
This localized peritonitis is due to the capacity of omentum to wall off infection.

Neoplasms
Primary mesothelioma
A rare condition, this is associated with exposure to asbestos. It corresponds to the much more common pleural mesothelioma.

The peritoneal cavity is a common site of metastases; malignancy of any organ within the peritoneal cavity may lead to peritonitis.

Secondary
The most common tumours to metastasize to the peritoneal cavity are of the stomach, ovary, pancreas and colon.

Metastases result in the effusion of protein-rich fluid into the cavity (i.e. an exudate) containing neoplastic cells which also grow as tiny white nodules on the mesothelial surface of the cavity. Nodules eventually coalesce to form tumour sheets over the surface of the viscera.

	Summary of peritoneal infection
aetiology	primary infection (less common): nephrotic syndrome, peritoneal dialysis, cirrhosis with ascites, abdominal trauma; secondary infection (most common): typically an extension of inflammatory processes from abdominal cavity, e.g. appendicitis, ruptured ulcers (peptic, ulcerative colitis, typhoid ulcers, ulcerated neoplasms), cholecystitis, pancreatitis, salpingitis, diverticulitis, strangulated bowel
organisms involved	normal gut commensals with anaerobic bacteria and coliforms predominating
pathogenesis	leaking bile, gastric juice, pancreatic enzymes or urine cause irritation and inflammation of peritoneum producing an exudate that typically becomes infected; intestine becomes flaccid, dilated and covered with fibrinous plaques forming adhesions between bowel loops
clinical features	guarding and rebound tenderness; board-like abdominal rigidity; absent bowel sounds (paralytic ileus); increased pulse and temperature
complications	local: ileus, fibrinous adhesions, abscesses, portal pyophlebitis; systemic: hypovolaemic shock, severe toxaemia

Fig. 9.44 Summary of peritoneal infection.

- State the causes of peritoneal infection.
- What are the complications of peritonitis?
- Name the tumours that may metastasize to the peritoneum.

10. Pathology of the Kidney and Urinary Tract

ABNORMALITIES OF KIDNEY STRUCTURE

Congenital abnormalities of the kidney
Congenital anomalies of kidneys are common, affecting 3–4% of newborn infants.

Agenesis of the kidney
Unilateral
This occurs in 1 in 1000 births, is asymptomatic, and affects males more than females by 2:1; the left kidney is usually the absent one.

Bilateral
Occurrence is in 1 in 3000 births, as part of Potter's syndrome. Affected infants have abnormal facies and often have abnormalities of the lower urinary tract, lungs and nervous system.

Characteristically, there is oligohydramnios in pregnancy as kidneys are not present to contribute to amniotic fluid. The disorder is not compatible with postnatal life.

Hypoplasia
Kidneys fail to reach the normal adult size either as a result of a congenital maldevelopment or due to shrinkage, which may have occurred as a result of chronic infection in early life.

Ectopic kidneys
One or both kidneys may be in an abnormal position, most commonly the pelvis, but some lie in the inferior part of the abdomen.

Pancake kidney
Here, there is fusion of the pelvic kidneys to form a round discoid mass.

Unilateral fused kidney
Kidneys fuse together in the pelvis, then, as one kidney ascends to the 'normal' position, the other is carried with it so that both kidneys end up on the same side.

Horseshoe kidney
Poles of the kidneys are fused, usually inferiorly, to form a large U-shaped (horseshoe) kidney. This affects about 1 in 500 people, but is typically asymptomatic as its collecting system develops normally. However, Wilms' tumours are 2 to 8 times more frequent in children with horseshoe kidneys than in the general population (p. 208).

Cystic diseases of the kidney
Overview of cystic kidney disease
This heterogeneous group of diseases comprises of:
- Hereditary disorders.
- Developmental (but not hereditary) disorders.
- Acquired disorders.

Each disease is distinguished by a characteristic distribution of cysts, illustrated in Fig. 10.1. Fig. 10.2 provides a summary of cystic diseases of the kidney.

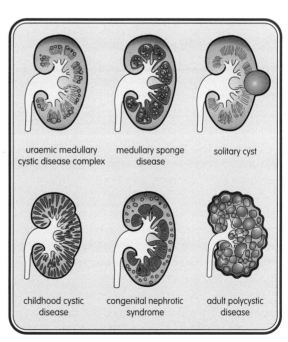

Fig. 10.1 Macroscopic features of cystic diseases of the kidney.

Accurate diagnosis of cystic diseases is important for two reasons:
- **Appropriate patient management to delay onset of renal failure.**
- **Appropriate genetic counselling to patients/relatives in the case of hereditary cystic diseases.**

Cystic diseases

Cystic renal dysplasia

Here, the failure of differentiation of metanephric tissues affects the whole or just one segment of a kidney, either unilaterally or bilaterally. Affected areas are replaced by solid or cystic masses in which cartilage is usually prominent.

The condition often presents in childhood as an abdominal mass and requires surgical excision to exclude a malignant tumour (e.g. nephroblastoma). Prognosis is good for unilateral lesions.

Adult polycystic kidney disease (APKD)

In this hereditary disease, both kidneys are progressively replaced by cysts, which develop and enlarge over a period of years.

Incidence is 1 per 1250 live births, accounting for 10% of all end-stage renal disease, with the sexes equally affected.

It is inherited as an autosomal dominant disorder (but about 50% are new mutations). The affected gene sequence and function are unknown.

Associations are berry aneurysms of the cerebral arteries, and cysts of the liver, pancreas and lung.

The condition is asymptomatic at first, but eventually replacement and compression of the functioning renal parenchyma by the enlarging cysts lead to slowly progressive impairment of renal function.

Macroscopically, in fully developed APKD, the kidneys are asymmetrically enlarged and are composed of a mass of large cysts (which may be up to 5 cm in diameter). Haemorrhage into cysts is common, leading to bloodstained contents.

Microscopically, cysts are lined by flattened cuboidal epithelium and communicate both with calyces and

with each other. Surrounding parenchyma often shows extensive fibrosis and arteriosclerosis.

Clinical features—This presents in adult life (typically fourth decade or later) usually with a large lobulated abdominal mass, pain or haematuria. There is progressive renal insufficiency and hypertension.

Complications are as follows:
- Uraemia.
- Hypertension: often preceding development of cardiac failure.
- Intracranial haemorrhage (10% of cases): combination of berry aneurysms and hypertension predisposes to cerebral haemorrhage.

Diagnosis is by:
- Intravenous urography: reveals irregular renal enlargement with calyceal distortion.
- Ultrasound: shows multiple cysts of variable sizes.

Management is by:
- Control of blood pressure: uncontrolled hypertension accelerates development of renal failure.
- Treatment of urinary infections.
- Relief of cardiac failure.
- Eventual dialysis or transplantation.

Infantile (childhood) polycystic disease

A less common autosomal recessive disorder in which there is cystic replacement of both kidneys present at birth. Cysts are composed of dilated tubules and collecting ducts.

This is a rare condition (at 1 per 10 000 live births), with associations of cysts of the liver, pancreas and lungs.

It presents in stillborn or neonates with enlarged kidneys (12–16 times normal size) containing a radiating cystic pattern in the medulla and cortex ('sunburst' pattern; Fig. 10.1). Rarely, it may present in childhood with renal insufficiency.

Prognosis—Affected infants usually die within the first 2 months of life.

Cystic diseases of the renal medulla

Medullary sponge kidney (tubular ectasia)

In this condition, multiple cysts develop in renal papillae, with an incidence of 1 in 20 000. Renal function is not impaired and the main clinical problem is development of renal stones which predispose to renal colic and infection.

Nephronophthisis complex (uraemic medullary cystic disease complex)

This complex describes two hereditary diseases both of which are characterized by development of cysts at the corticomedullary junction of the kidney and associated with interstitial fibrosis:

- Juvenile nephronophthisis: autosomal recessive disease presenting at about 11 years of age.
- Medullary cystic disease: autosomal dominant trait presenting at about 20 years of age.

Clinically, conditions are characterized by thirst and polyuria (due to nephrogenic diabetes insipidus; see Chapter 11) and eventually result in early-onset chronic renal failure. Together, conditions account for about 20–25% of cases of end-stage renal failure in the first three decades.

Acquired dialysis-associated cystic disease

This is seen in kidneys left *in situ* while patients are treated by dialysis or transplantation for chronic renal failure.

Simple cysts

These common lesions occur as solitary or occasionally multiple cystic spaces in otherwise normal kidneys, and are extremely common, incidence increasing with age.

Abnormality is widely held to be acquired but the cause is unknown.

Macroscopically, cysts are of variable size (generally being no larger than 5–6 cm) and contain clear watery fluid.

Microscopically, they are lined by flattened cuboidal epithelium and surrounded by a thin fibrous capsule.

Clinically, cysts may cause renal enlargement, but have no effect on renal function. However, they require clinical differentiation from tumours and other cystic disorders.

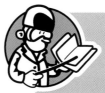

- Name four common congenital abnormalities of the kidney.
- List the types of cystic diseases of the kidney.
- Describe the pathology of adult polycystic kidney disease. Compare with infantile polycystic disease.
- Which of the cystic diseases affect the renal medulla?

Summary of cystic diseases of the kidney	
Type of cystic disease	**Clinical features**
hereditary:	
• adult polycystic disease (autosomal dominant) • infantile polycystic disease (autosomal recessive)	chronic renal failure and hypertension
• medullary cystic disease (autosomal dominant) • juvenile nephronophthisis (autosomal recessive)	early-onset chronic renal failure
• medullary sponge kidney (occasionally familial)	renal stones predispose to renal colic and infection
developmental:	
• cystic renal dysplasia	typically asymptomatic
acquired:	
• simple renal cysts • dialysis-associated cystic disease	typically asymptomatic

Fig. 10.2 Summary of cystic diseases of the kidney.

DISEASES OF THE GLOMERULUS

Overview of glomerular disease

Glomerular diseases are typically caused by disturbances of structure. There are four significant components of the glomerulus which may be damaged:

- Endothelial cells lining the capillary.
- Glomerular basement membrane.
- Mesangium: supporting mesentery to the capillary comprised of mesangial cells (phagocytic support cells) and associated extracellular material (mesangial matrix).
- Epithelial cells or podocytes, which form an outer coating to the capillary. These cells are in contact with the outer surface of the basement membrane via a series of foot processes.

Patterns of glomerular disease

Although a small number of diseases affect all glomeruli in a uniform manner, most glomerular diseases affect

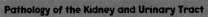
different glomeruli to varying degrees. A nomenclature has been agreed for the various patterns of disease:

- Global: affecting the whole glomerulus uniformly.
- Segmental: affecting one glomerular segment while sparing the others within that glomerulus.
- Diffuse: affecting all glomeruli in both kidneys.
- Focal: affecting a proportion of glomeruli, sparing others.

Thus a glomerular disease may be described as one of 'diffuse global', 'diffuse segmental', 'focal global' or 'focal segmental'. The vast majority are either 'diffuse global' or 'focal segmental'.

This explains how some glomerular diseases cause sudden acute renal failure (diffuse global diseases) whereas others cause a selective partial renal failure (focal segmental diseases).

Aetiology of glomerular diseases

Glomerular diseases may be classified as (Fig. 10.3):

- Primary (majority): disease process appears

to start within the glomerulus. These are further classified into four main histological types—proliferative (majority), membranous, glomerulosclerotic, and minimal change lesions.

- Secondary: disease process is secondary to systemic disease, either immune complex-mediated, metabolic or vascular conditions. These are covered on pp. 197–198.
- Hereditary: Alport's syndrome, Fabry's disease and congenital nephrotic syndrome.

Steps in diagnoses of glomerular lesions

Clinical presentation

This is to identify the type of urinary abnormality (see below).

Histological identification

This is to identifiy the pattern of glomerular response to injury. Percutaneous needle biopsy of the kidney allows

Aetiology of glomerular disorders		
Type	**Aetiology**	**Example**
primary	Antiglomerular basement membrane disease: • proliferative	Goodpasture's syndrome
	Immune complex-mediated lesions: • proliferative	diffuse proliferative glomerulonephritis focal proliferative glomerulonephritis membranoproliferative glomerulonephritis crescentic glomerulonephritis
	• membranous	membranous glomerulopathy
	• glomerulosclerosis	focal glomerulosclerosis
	• minimal change	minimal change disease
secondary	Immune complex-mediated conditions	systemic lupus erythematosus Henoch–Schönlein purpura infective endocarditis
	Metabolic conditions	diabetes mellitus renal amyloidosis multiple myeloma
	Vascular conditions	polyarteritis nodosa Wegener's granulomatosis haemolytic uraemic syndrome idiopathic thrombocytopenic purpura disseminated intravascular coagulation
hereditary		Alport's and Fabry's syndromes

Fig. 10.3 Aetiology of glomerular disorders.

histological examination of glomeruli and tubules to identify structural abnormalities and to characterize patterns of damage.

Immunological investigation
This is for the detection of immune complex deposition and serological changes (see below).

Clinical manifestations of glomerular disease
Patients with glomerular disease usually present with one of five possible syndromes (described below).

Asymptomatic haematuria
A haematuria without significant proteinaemia, this may be continuous or intermittent, and varies in severity from macro- to microscopic. The condition does not cause renal failure.

Asymptomatic proteinuria
This proteinuria (>0.3 g every 24 hours) without haematuria may be continuous, orthostatic (postural) or transient. It is typically detected at a routine medical examination.

Acute nephritic syndrome
This presents with a sudden onset of haematuria, proteinuria (often with urinary casts) and hypertension. Loin pain and headache may be present and the patient will often feel unwell. In children there is often generalized oedema, especially around the eyes.

Nephrotic syndrome
Here, there is proteinuria (usually >3.5 g every 24 hours) with hypoproteinaemia and oedema. There is also hypercholesterolaemia.

Chronic renal failure
This is an irreversible deterioration in renal function caused by the destruction of more and more individual nephrons over a long period of time. Impairment of excretory, metabolic and endocrine functions of the kidney leads to the clinical syndrome of uraemia.

Fig. 10.4 gives the symptoms and signs of renal failure.

Management—Excretory function of the kidney can be partially replaced by dialysis. However, replacement of the endocrine and metabolic functions can only be achieved by successful renal transplantation.

Unless some form of supportive therapy, such as dialysis or transplantation, is available, chronic renal failure is eventually fatal.

Summary
Many of the diseases causing the above clinical syndromes are listed in Fig. 10.5.

However, there is considerable overlap—several diseases may give rise to the same clinical picture, and conversely many conditions fall into more than one clinical group.

The mechanism of glomerular injury
Many glomerular diseases are caused by immune-mediated damage with five main mechanisms (listed below). Different patterns of immune-mediated damage point to different diagnoses, thus it is important to identify the site, type, and pattern of immune complexes and complement within the glomerulus by immunohistochemistry and electron microscopy.

Circulating immune complex nephritis
This is the most common pattern of immunological disease.

Mechanism
Antigen–antibody complexes circulating in the blood are trapped at the basement membrane, the mesangium or both. Complexes activate the complement cascade via the classical pathway (see Fig. 3.6). Activated components

Symptoms and signs of renal failure	
Symptoms	**Signs**
general malaise	uraemia
breathlessness on exertion	anaemia
nausea and vomiting	metabolic bone disease (renal osteodystrophy)
disordered GI motility	hypertension
headaches	acidosis
pruritus	neuropathy
pigmentation	generalized myopathy endocrine abnormalities

Fig. 10.4 Symptoms and signs of renal failure.

191

Clinical manifestations of glomerular disease and the conditions that cause them	
Clinical manifestations	**Causative renal disease**
asymptomatic haematuria	exercise haematuria IgA nephropathy Henoch–Schönlein purpura bacterial endocarditis systemic lupus erythematosus (SLE) polyarteritis nodosa (PAN)
asymptomatic proteinuria	primary: • focal segmental glomerulosclerosis • membranoproliferative glomerulonephritis secondary: • Henoch–Schönlein purpura • SLE • PAN • bacterial endocarditis
acute nephritic syndrome	primary: • poststreptococcal glomerulonephritis • rapidly progressive glomerulonephritis • Goodpasture's syndrome secondary: • SLE • PAN • Wegener's granulomatosis • Henoch–Schönlein purpura • essential cryoglobulinaemia

nephrotic syndrome	primary:
	• minimal change disease
	• membranous glomerulopathy
	• membranoproliferative glomerulonephritis
	• focal proliferative glomerulonephritis
	• focal glomerulosclerosis
	secondary:
	• immune complex-mediated conditions
	  SLE
	  Henoch–Schönlein purpura
	  infective endocarditis
	• metabolic conditions
	  diabetes mellitus
	  renal amyloidosis
	• vascular conditions
	  PAN
	  Wegener's granulomatosis
	  haemolytic uraemic syndrome
	• infections
	  malaria, syphilis, hepatitis B

chronic renal failure	all of above except minimal change disease

Fig. 10.5 Clinical manifestations of glomerular disease and the conditions that cause them.

of complement bring about the characteristic acute inflammation of glomerulonephritis by attracting neutrophil polylmorphs, increasing vascular permeability, and causing membrane damage (Fig. 3.7). Damage to the basement membrane results in alteration of its properties leading to some of the urinary abnormalities observed clinically.

Example
Poststreptococcal glomerulonephritis.

In-situ immune complex formation
Mechanism
Circulating antigens become trapped in the glomerulus, where they are targeted by circulating antibodies such that immune complexes are formed within the glomerulus. This in-situ formation explains why, in contrast to circulating immune complex nephritis described above, there is little complement and no inflammatory or proliferative responses.

Example
This is believed to occur in certain cases of SLE when free DNA in the blood is trapped in the glomerular basement membrane, subsequently binding to anti-DNA antibodies.

Cytotoxic antibodies
Mechanism
Autoantibodies are directed to a component of the glomerular basement membrane (anti-GBM antibodies). This is an uncommon form of immune-mediated damage.

Example
This is the basis of Goodpasture's syndrome in which autoantibodies cause direct damage to the glomerular basement membrane. The Goodpasture antigen (which is the target of the anti-GBM antibodies) has been identified as a domain on the α_3 type IV collagen chain.

Activation of the alternate complement pathway
Mechanism
The alternate complement pathway is normally activated by the presence of bacterial cell walls and is independent of immune complex formation (Fig. 3.6). However, in certain disease conditions, the alternate pathway can be activated by different mechanisms.

Example
In type II membranoproliferative glomerulonephritis, a circulating autoantibody (termed 'C3 nephritic factor') activates complement via the alternate pathway by

stabilizing the enzyme, C3-convertase. This enzyme normally activates C3 but has a very short half life. Thus, stabilization of C3-convertase prolongs the activation of C3.

Cell-mediated immunity

Cell-mediated immunological mechanisms are uncommon in the initiation of acute glomerular diseases, but are thought to play a role in the progression of acute glomerulonephritis to a chronic phase.

Proliferative glomerulonephritis

This group of disorders are characterized histologically by varying degrees of proliferation of mesangial and epithelial (and sometimes endothelial) cells within the glomerulus.

The majority of cases of glomerulonephritis (over 70%) belong to this group.

Proliferative glomerulonephritis can be divided according to certain histological appearances into:

- Diffuse proliferative.
- Rapidly progressive.
- Focal proliferative.
- Membranoproliferative.

However, it must be emphasized that these subdivisions are not diagnoses, but rather describe a pattern of reaction caused by glomerular insult.

Diffuse proliferative glomerulonephritis

Diffuse, global, acute inflammation of glomeruli is caused by the deposition of immune complexes in glomeruli, stimulated by a preceding infection.

This affects all ages, but children are more commonly affected. There is a much higher incidence in poorer countries, e.g. India, but a falling incidence in the UK.

Aetiology is as follows:

- Poststreptococcal (most common): onset is 1–2 weeks after a primary pharyngeal infection with β-haemolytic streptococci of Lancefield group A.
- Non-streptococcal (less common): a range of bacterial, viral and protozoal infections can also stimulate this pattern of disease.

Those antibodies produced to combat initial infection cross-react with cellular antigens producing immune complexes. These complexes circulate in the blood, and are filtered out in the glomerulus producing four main histological changes:

- Immune complex deposition: in lumps on the epithelial side of glomerular basement membrane.
- Neutrophil infiltration: activation of complement attracts neutrophils into glomerulus.
- Endothelial cell proliferation: degranulation of neutrophils damages endothelial cells, stimulating their proliferation.
- Mild mesangial cell proliferation: mediated by factors derived from complement and platelets.

Rapidly progressive glomerulonephritis (RPGN; crescentic glomerulonephritis)

RPGN is a manifestation of severe glomerular injury characterized by the formation of cellular crescent-shaped masses within the Bowman's space. It occurs in a small percentage of patients with poststreptococcal glomerulonephritis (see above), but can also be associated with many other forms of glomerular damage.

If damage to the glomerular capillaries is severe, fibrin and blood leak into Bowman's space stimulating epithelial cell proliferation, and infiltration of macrophages and neutrophils. Crescent-shaped cellular masses composed of epithelial cells and macrophages are formed within the Bowman's space. These crescents are associated with glomerular ischaemia and ultimately result in permanent glomerular damage.

Focal proliferative glomerulonephritis

Here, there is an acute inflammation with cellular proliferation occurring in only a proportion of all glomeruli (focal) and usually affecting only one segment of the glomerular tufts (segmental). Thus, the condition is more accurately described as focal segmental proliferative glomerulonephritis.

Several diseases can cause this pattern of response. These can be classified into two groups:

- Primary: mainly mesangial IgA disease and Goodpasture's syndrome.
- Secondary: associated with other systemic diseases including infective endocarditis, vasculitis and connective tissue diseases.

Immunohistochemistry and electron microscopy are required to distinguish them.

Mesangial IgA disease (IgA nephropathy; Berger's disease)

This is the most common cause of glomerulonephritis in adults, and also affects children and young adults. There is a geographical variation with high incidences in France, Australia and Singapore.

Its aetiology is unknown.

Pathogenesis—Serum IgA levels are raised and IgA is deposited in the mesangium and at the junction between the mesangium and basement membrane (paramesangial). Activation of complement results in a mild mesangial proliferation, followed by mesangial matrix deposition and eventual sclerosis of the damaged segment.

Goodpasture's syndrome

This is a very rare cause of primary proliferative glomerulonephritis occurring predominantly in young men.

Aetiology—Autoimmune, but the mechanism of sensitization is unknown.

Pathogenesis—Autoantibodies (usually IgG type) bind to the glomerular basement membrane (anti-GBM antibodies). Resultant activation of complement causes severe basement membrane damage. The Goodpasture antigen (which is the target of the anti-GBM antibodies) has been identified as a domain on type IV collagen of the basement membrane.

The clinical presentation is:
- Episodic haematuria with mild proteinuria or very occasionally nephritic syndrome.
- Hypertension.
- Haemoptysis: autoantibody also reacts with alveolar basement membrane causing pulmonary alveolar haemorrhage.

In advanced disease, there may be diffuse involvement of glomeruli with signs of rapidly progressive renal failure (usually due to progression to 'rapidly progressive glomerulonephritis').

Prognosis is poor without treatment, but the outlook improves with plasmaphoresis.

Membranoproliferative glomerulonephritis (MPGN)

This is a diffuse, global pattern of glomerulonephritis with features of both proliferation and membrane thickening (hence the name). It is also known as mesangiocapillary glomerulonephritis.

Diseases causing MPGN can be classified into two groups:
- Primary (majority): idiopathic. Subdivided according to clinical and pathological features into type I (90% of cases) and type II (10% of cases).
- Secondary: a few are secondary to systemic disorders such as SLE, infective endocarditis, malaria and infected ventricular CSF shunts.

Type I MPGN (subendothelial type)

The aetiology is unclear but it is thought to be an immune complex disease associated with an abnormality of complement.

Pathogenesis—Subendothelial deposition of immune complexes and C3 causes a reactive inflammation.

Capillaries are greatly thickened in appearance as a result of:
- Large subendothelial immune complex deposits.
- Proliferation of mesangial cells: also causes characteristic exaggerated lobularity of glomeruli.
- Thickening of glomerular basement membrane: due to extension of mesangial cytoplasm into basement membrane.

Type II MPGN (dense deposit disease)

Aetiology—Autoimmune-mediated abnormality of complement.

Pathogenesis—Described on p. 192.

Morphological features—Capillaries are greatly thickened in appearance as a result of the following:
- Dense continuous deposits of C3 in the basement membrane.
- Mild mesangial proliferation (not as prominent as in type I).
- Extension of mesangial cytoplasm into basement membrane.

Clinical features of type I and type II MPGN

The two types have many clinical similarities: they are both mostly seen in adolescents and young adults, and they both have a slight female preponderance.

They may cause asymptomatic haematuria, nephrotic syndrome or mixed nephritic/nephrotic syndrome.

Hypocomplementaemia is caused by activation of the classical pathway in type I MPGN and of the alternate pathway in type II.

Typically, there is progressive deterioration in renal function over a period of about 10 years, resulting in chronic renal failure. Type II MPGN tends to recur in transplants.

Membranous nephropathy

Here, there is a pattern of reaction in which the glomerular capillary basement membrane is uniformly thickened. Unlike the proliferative types of glomerulonephritis, there is no associated inflammation or endothelial/epithelial proliferation, although the mesangial cell population may be slightly increased.

It affects all age groups, but the highest incidence is between fifth and seventh decades. Males are affected more than females.

Aetiology is as follows:
- Primary: 80–90% of cases have no apparent reason for development of immune complexes, and are classed as primary or idiopathic membranous nephropathy.
- Secondary: membranous nephropathy is found in association with a number of conditions which are listed in Fig. 10.6.

There are four pathological stages:
- In-situ formation of immune complexes on the epithelial side of the basement membrane (diffuse, global pattern).
- Mild mesangial increase.
- New basement membrane is deposited around immune complex deposits.
- Immune complex deposits disappear, leaving thickened 'lacy' basement membrane.

Over many years, the abnormal glomeruli develop increased mesangial matrix produced by the mesangial cells. This, together with membrane thickening, causes gradual hyalinization of the glomeruli (glomerulosclerosis) and death of individual nephrons.

Abnormality of the basement membrane renders it unusually permeable resulting in heavy proteinuria and the nephrotic syndrome. Indeed, membranous nephropathy is one of the most important causes of the nephrotic syndrome.

Prognosis is variable and related to cause, but in crude figures 25% of patients undergo remission and 25% develop stable persisting proteinuria; 50% develop chronic renal failure over a period of about 10 years.

Minimal change disease (lipoid nephrosis)

The characteristic feature in this neuropathy (and the reason for the name) is that no significant abnormalities can be detected by light microscopy.

It mainly affects children under the age of 6 years and is less common in adults, but still accounts for 10–25% of cases of nephrotic syndrome. Males are affected more than females.

Aetiology is unknown.

Pathogenesis is postulated to be immunologically related because of the universal satisfactory response to corticosteroid therapy. Ultimately, polyanionic charges of the glomerular basement membrane are depleted, leading to failure of protein retention.

Morphological features—With electron microscopy, there is a diagnostic loss of epithelial foot processes. Tubules may show accumulation of lipid in lining cells, giving rise to the alternative name of 'lipoid nephrosis'.

Prognosis in children is good, with no permanent renal damage. In adults, the outlook is variable.

Focal segmental glomerulosclerosis

The glomerulus is partially replaced by hyaline material which, in most cases, is excess mesangial matrix.

Aetiology is variable and related to age:
- Primary (most common): idiopathic disease affecting children and young adults.
- Secondary: in later adult life condition is usually

Conditions associated with membranous nephropathy	
Type	**Example**
infections	malaria syphilis hepatitis B
malignancy	carcinoma (lung, breast, GI) lymphoma
drugs	gold, mercury, penicillamine, captopril
systemic disease	SLE (10% of renal involvement is of the membranous pattern)

Fig. 10.6 Conditions associated with membranous nephropathy.

secondary to other disorders, especially previous focal proliferative glomerulonephritis.

Pathogenesis is unknown but is probably immune mediated.

Focal glomerulosclerosis initially affects the juxtamedullary glomeruli, causing an increase in mesangial matrix, which gradually expands to destroy the surrounding lobule, until global sclerosis occurs. In time similar lesions appear in glomeruli throughout the cortex.

The patient presents with nephrotic syndrome. Later, haematuria, hypertension and renal failure are common.

Prognosis is poor with progression of disease over many years leading to chronic renal failure.

It is useful to remember that the clinical syndromes of glomerulonephritis broadly relate to histological findings:

○ Asymptomatic proteinuria and nephrotic syndrome are associated with basement membrane thickening as a result of either structural change or deposition of excessive mesangial matrix, e.g. membranous nephropathy, glomerulosclerosis.

○ Asymptomatic haematuria and nephritic syndrome are associated with proliferation of the endothelial or mesangial cells, e.g. diffuse, global glomerulonephritis.

○ Mixed nephritic/nephrotic syndrome is associated with combined damage to the basement membrane and cell proliferation, e.g. membranoproliferative glomerulonephritis.

Hereditary glomerulonephritis
Alport's syndrome

Syndrome characterized by the clinical triad of deafness, glomerulonephritis and ocular lesions. Inheritance is complex but is basically autosomal dominant with incomplete penetrance.

The clinical features are:

- Glomerulonephritis: usually presents as microscopic haematuria and proteinuria in childhood. There is subsequent development of nephrotic syndrome with progression to renal failure, occurring by the second decade in males, but often not until the fifth decade in females.
- Ocular disease: occurs in only severely affected patients.
- Deafness: only for high-pitched sounds and may be difficult to demonstrate.

Fabry's syndrome

A rare, X-linked recessive syndrome of glycosphingolipid metabolism resulting in painful extremities, red hyperkeratotic papules on skin, proteinuria and renal failure.

Congenital nephrotic syndrome

A rare disorder characterized by nephrotic syndrome occurring at or shortly after birth, often associated with bulky placenta, congenital heart disease and raised α-fetoprotein level in maternal amniotic fluid. Aetiology is an autosomal recessive pattern of inheritance.

There are two types:

- Finnish type: shows slight glomerular mesangial proliferation and progressive glomerulosclerosis.
- Non-Finnish type: shows focal and segmental glomerulosclerosis.

Both types ultimately progress to renal failure.

Chronic glomerulonephritis

Chronic renal failure associated with small, contracted kidneys in which all the glomeruli are hyalinized (end-stage kidneys).

This may be caused by many diseases, particularly proliferative types of acute glomerulonephritis.

In patients who present for the first time with chronic glomerulonephritis, it is often not possible to ascertain the cause due to diffuse global glomerular destruction.

However, it is likely that many patients presenting for the first time have had IgA mesangial disease.

Macroscopically, affected kidneys are small and there is granularity of external surface, reflecting fine scarring due to nephron hyalinization. However, the pelvicalyceal system is normal, an important distinction from cases of end-stage kidney due to chronic pyelonephritis.

Microscopically, there is hyalinization of glomeruli, tubular atrophy and interstitial fibrosis.

It is helpful to remember that the patterns of glomerular damage that occur secondary to systemic disease mimic the various patterns of primary glomerulonephritis.

- List the distribution patterns of glomerular disease.
- Explain the differences between nephritic and nephrotic syndrome.
- State the mechanisms of immune-mediated glomerulonephritic injury.
- Name the types of proliferative glomerulonephritis.
- Describe the two types of membranoproliferative glomerulonephritis.
- What is minimal change nephropathy?
- Name the hereditary glomerulonephritic syndromes.

GLOMERULAR LESIONS IN SYSTEMIC DISEASE

Systemic lupus erythematosus (SLE)

Glomerular lesions are the main abnormalities of renal involvement in SLE. These vary in severity from minor abnormalities such as asymptomatic proteinuria to severe glomerular disease leading to renal failure.

The basis of glomerular damage is immune complex deposition in the basement membrane (leading to basement membrane thickening), or in the mesangium (leading to mesangial expansion).

Patterns of glomerular damage that may occur include:
- Diffuse MPGN: associated with a mixed nephritic/nephrotic syndrome and rapid progression to renal failure.
- Focal segmental proliferative glomerulonephritis: associated with haematuria, proteinuria and slow progression.
- Diffuse membranous nephropathy: associated with nephrotic syndrome and slow progression to chronic renal failure.

SLE immune complexes

The immune complexes are characterized by the presence of IgG, IgA, IgM, C3 and C1q (known as a 'full-house' of deposits). The detection of this pattern of immunoglobulins and complement factors, together with the particular location of the immune complexes in relation to the glomerular basement membrane, is an important factor in distinguishing lupus glomerulonephritis from non-lupus patterns.

Note that although glomerular lesions are the main abnormalities of renal involvement in SLE, there may also be extraglomerular vascular abnormalities and tubular damage, particularly interstitial nephritis.

Henoch–Schönlein purpura

This immune complex-mediated systemic vasculitis affects small arteries in the skin, joints, intestine and kidneys (see Chapters 7 and 14).

Significant renal damage occurs in over one-third of cases, ranging from proteinuria, possibly with nephrotic syndrome, to RPGN.

Bacterial endocarditis

Renal lesions in infective endocarditis are caused by two mechanisms:

- Immune complex deposition—immune complexes (formed with antigens of infecting organisms) are deposited in the glomerulus causing a focal segmental proliferative glomerulonephritis or a diffuse proliferative glomerulonephritis.
- Embolism-mediated infarction—embolic vegetations from heart valves cause multiple renal infarcts.

Renal lesions typically subside when the bacterial source of the antigen is removed by intensive antibiotic therapy.

Diabetic glomerulosclerosis

Diabetic glomerular damage causes an increase in the permeability of the glomerular capillary basement membrane, leading to proteinuria and occasionally the nephrotic syndrome.

Pathogenesis of the basement membrane changes is not known, but histologically there are three types of glomerular lesions that occur, representing a continuous spectrum of increasing severity:

- Capillary wall thickening: mild proteinuria.
- Diffuse glomerulosclerosis: excess mesangial matrix formation in an even pattern throughout the glomerulus combined with capillary thickening eventually encroaches on the capillaries.
- Nodular glomerulosclerosis (Kimmelstiel–Wilson nodules): nodular expansion of the mesangium at the tips of the glomerular lobules is very characteristic of diabetes.

Diabetic sclerosis causes progressive hyalinization of glomeruli with obliteration of capillary loops and death of individual nephrons. Over a period of years this leads to chronic renal failure.

Prognosis—Approximately 10% of all diabetics die in renal failure. This rises to 50% if patients developing diabetes in childhood are considered separately.

Amyloidosis

This is a condition in which amyloid, an extracellular fibrillar protein, is deposited in a variety of tissues (see Chapter 14). Amyloidosis is an important cause of the nephrotic syndrome in adults.

Amyloid is deposited as fibrils in the glomerular basement membrane and in the mesangium of the kidney, resulting in membrane thickening and increased mesangial matrix formation. The net result is the development of:

- Proteinuria: membrane thickening leads to an

increase in membrane permeability so that the first manifestation of amyloidosis is often proteinuria.
- Nephrotic syndrome: increased deposition of amyloid causes increased protein loss until the patient develops features of the nephrotic syndrome.
- Chronic renal failure: combined effect of amyloid deposition and increased mesangial matrix formation eventually leads to expansion of the mesangium causing compression of the glomerular capillary system and transition into chronic renal failure.

Amyloid is also deposited in the walls of intrarenal vessels, particularly afferent arterioles.

Polyarteritis nodosa

Systemic disease characterized by inflammatory necrosis of the walls of small and medium-sized arteries (see Chapter 7). Necrosis of medium-sized arteries causes small infarcts in the kidney, and necrosis of arterioles and the glomerular tuft produces infarction of entire glomeruli or segments, visible as fibrinoid necrosis.

Wegener's granulomatosis

This immune complex-mediated systemic necrotizing vasculitis primarily affects the nose, upper respiratory tract and kidneys. Renal involvement is of variable severity causing one of the following:

- Focal segmental glomerulonephritis (asymptomatic haematuria or nephritic syndrome).
- Rapidly progressive glomerulonephritis (rapidly progressive acute renal failure).

This condition usually responds to immunosuppressive therapy.

- Describe the patterns of glomerulonephritis that may occur in SLE.
- Name the vasculitic diseases that cause glomerulonephritis.
- Describe the glomerular lesions that occur in diabetic glomerulosclerosis.
- What are the clinical effects of amyloid deposition in the kidney?

DISEASES OF THE TUBULES AND INTERSTITIUM

Acute tubular necrosis (ATN)

This acute, but usually reversible, renal failure is caused by necrosis of renal tubular epithelial cells resulting from metabolic or toxic disturbances. The causes of ATN are shown in Fig. 10.7.

The aetiology is:
- Ischaemic (most common): caused by failure of renal perfusion, typically the result of hypotension and hypovolaemia in shock.
- Toxic: uncommon.

There are three phases to ATN (oliguric, polyuric and recovery) as follows.

Oliguric phase

A damaging stimulus causes necrosis of renal tubular epithelial cells. Necrotic cells cause tubule blockage, accompanied by a secondary reduction in glomerular blood flow (caused by arteriolar constriction) reducing glomerular filtration. Patients develop acute renal failure and oliguria.

Polyuric phase

Regeneration of tubular epithelium takes place over 1–3 weeks. Necrotic material is partially removed by phagocytic cells and partially excreted in the form of casts in urine. As tubules slowly open up, the glomerular blood flow is increased. However, the regenerated tubular cells are undifferentiated and have not yet developed the necessary specializations for resorption, thus there is development of polyuria.

Recovery phase

Tubular cells differentiate and there is restoration of renal function.

The morphological features are:
- Ischaemic ATN: kidneys are pale and swollen. Histology reveals flattened, vacuolated epithelial cells along the entire length of the tubules.
- Necrotic ATN: kidneys are red and swollen. Histology reveals flattened, vacuolated epithelial cells restricted to proximal tubular cells, those of the distal tubule being spared.

Clinical features are oliguria (50–500 mL daily) with features of renal failure (Fig. 10.4), and polyuria.

A knowledge of the aetiology (ischaemic versus toxic) and an understanding of the pathogenesis (oliguric and polyuric phases) of ATN make the morphological and clinical features easy to remember.

Treatment:
- Oliguric phase: supportive measures to prevent hyperkalaemia and fluid overload.
- Polyuric phase: replacement of fluid and electrolytes to compensate for excessive loss from urine.

The prognosis depends on the speed and efficiency with which corrective measures are put into operation, on the prompt recognition and effective treatment of complications, and on the nature and severity of causal disorder.

Tubulointerstitial nephritis
Urinary tract infection and pyelonephritis
Acute pyelonephritis

Inflammation of the tubules and interstitium is caused by bacterial infection. There are three age peaks—

Causes of acute tubular necrosis	
Type of ATN	**Causes**
ischaemic	major surgery extensive acute blood loss severe burns haemorrhage
toxic	endogenous products: haemoglobinuria and myoglobinuria heavy metals: lead, mercury organic solvents: chloroform, carbon tetrachloride drugs: antibiotics, NSAIDs, cyclosporin others: paraquat, phenol, ethylene glycol, poisonous fungi

Fig. 10.7 Causes of acute tubular necrosis.

childhood, pregnancy and in the elderly.
Gender differences are as follows:
- Infancy: males more than females due to anatomical abnormalities.
- Puberty to middle age: females more than males; related to urethral trauma and pregnancy.
- Post-40 years: males more than females due to obstructive aetiology of prostatic disease.

Most cases of infection are caused by enterobacteria from the patient's faecal flora (e.g. *E. coli*, *Proteus* and *Klebsiella*) or by staphylococci from skin (perineal) flora. The organism may enter the kidney by one of two routes:
- Ascending infection (most common): from lower urinary tract. Risk factors include pregnancy, diabetes mellitus, stasis of urine, structural defects of urinary tract, urethral trauma (e.g. caused by sexual intercourse in women or instrumentation of urinary tract) and reflux of urine from bladder into ureter (vesicoureteric reflux).
- Bloodstream spread: in bacteraemic or septicaemic states (rare). More likely in elderly patients who develop pyrexia of unknown origin, often with rigors and acute renal failure.

Macroscopically, the condition is characterized by numerous abscesses throughout the kidney:
- Cortical abscesses: small, yellowish-white abscesses, usually spherical, under 2 mm in diameter and sometimes surrounded by zone of hyperaemia. Most prominent on subcapsular surface.
- Medullary abscesses: yellowish-white linear streaks which converge on the papilla. Pelvicalyceal mucosa is hyperaemic or covered with a fibrinopurulent exudate.

Microscopically, there is focal inflammation with infiltration of tubules by neutrophils and interstitial oedema.
Clinical features are fever, rigors and pain in the back.
This condition is often associated with dysuria and urgency of micturition, signs of a lower urinary tract infection.
Complications and sequelae:
- Resolution: occurs in the absence of frank suppuration; however, some scarring usually occurs.
- Healing: with scarring.
- Chronicity: development of chronic pyelonephritis.
- Pyonephrosis: obstruction of urinary tract near the kidney causes stagnation and suppuration of fluid in the pelvis and calyceal system. Eventually the kidney becomes grossly distended with pus.
- Renal papillary necrosis: associated with severe infections, particularly in diabetics, and caused by compromised medullary blood supply due to inflammatory thrombosis of vasa recta supplying the papillae.
- Perinephric abscess: infection breaches the renal capsule and extends into the perirenal tissues.
- Death (in uraemia).

Diagnosis is by examination of midstream urine, especially cultured to demonstrate responsible organisms:
- Significant bacteriuria is defined as $>10^5$ culture-forming units per mL (to eliminate cases of extraneous bacterial contamination).
- Significant pyuria is defined as >10 neutrophil polymorphs per high power field.

Treatment is by oral antibiotic therapy (e.g. trimethoprim, ampicillin or amoxycillin: active against *E. coli*). Intravenous antibiotic therapy is used for more severe or septicaemic cases.
Untreated, infection may spread to cause Gram-negative septicaemia with shock.

Chronic pyelonephritis
Chronic inflammation of the tubules and interstitium is associated with nephron destruction and coarse scarring of the kidneys. There are two forms (obstructive and reflux-associated) as described below.

Obstructive chronic pyelonephritis
Obstruction of pelvicalyceal drainage causes recurrent episodes of infection (discussed in more detail on p. 207).

Reflux-associated chronic pyelonephritis
Reflux of urine from the bladder into the ureter predisposes to recurrent bouts of inflammation. It is most common in childhood and early adult life, with males more affected than females.

Normally, the ureter enters the bladder obliquely so that contraction of the bladder wall during micturition closes the ureteric orifice. In patients with vesicourethral reflux, the terminal portion of the ureter is short and orientated at approximately 90° to the mucosal surface. Contraction of the bladder tends to hold the ureteric orifice open thus facilitating reflux of urine, enabling organisms to gain access to the kidney from the bladder.

Macroscopically, kidneys have irregular areas of scarring seen as depressed areas, 1–2 cm in size, most commonly sited in the renal calyces at the poles of the kidney, but often associated with fibrous scarring of the renal papilla. Involvement may be either bilateral or unilateral.

Microscopically, kidneys have irregular areas of interstitial fibrosis with chronic inflammatory cell infiltration. Tubules are atrophic or may be dilated and contain proteinaceous casts. Glomeruli show periglomerular fibrosis and many demonstrate complete hyalinization.

Clinical features are symptoms of urinary tract infection (p. 209) and of uraemia.

Diagnosis is by:
- Intravenous urography: reveals reduction in kidney size and localized contraction of renal substance associated with clubbing of the adjacent calyces.
- Urine culture: for identification of infecting organism.

Treatment is by antibiotic therapy, control of hypertension, and removal of the source of obstruction.

Prognosis—The course is usually long and punctuated by acute exacerbations.

Toxin- and drug-induced tubulointerstitial nephritis

This group of disorders is characterized by inflammation of the renal interstitium and tubules. There are a wide range of causes, the main one of which is exposure to drugs, particularly certain analgesics and antibiotics. Less commonly, physical agents such as irradiation cause a similar pattern of tubulointerstitial damage.

There are two types of this nephritis: acute interstitial and chronic interstitial.

Acute interstitial nephritis
Morphological features are oedema of the interstitium associated with lymphocytic and eosinophilic inflammatory infiltration. Tubules may show epithelial degeneration or necrosis.

Clinical features present 2–3 weeks after exposure to a causative agent, and include fever, haematuria, proteinuria and elevated blood urea. In some cases acute renal failure develops.

Prognosis—Recovery usually takes place on withdrawal of the causative agent.

Chronic interstitial nephritis
Morphological features are interstitial fibrosis, chronic inflammation and atrophy of tubules. The condition typically presents with chronic renal failure. Establishing a cause is often very difficult.

Prognosis—Chronic renal failure is irreversible.

Urate (gouty) nephropathy
This affects a small proportion of patients with hyperuricaemia (see Chapter 13). Precipitation of urate crystals in the renal collecting ducts causes tubular damage, inflammation and later scarring.

Hypercalcaemia and nephrocalcinosis
Persistent hypercalcaemia causes calcification of the renal parenchyma particularly the tubular basement membrane with tubular damage and later fibrosis (nephrocalcinosis). There is eventual failure of tubular function, with development of polyuria.

Multiple myeloma
In some types of myeloma, the proliferating plasma cells produce monoclonal free light chains which are small enough to enter the urine, where they are called Bence Jones proteins. During passage through the tubules, these proteins precipitate as casts causing physical obstruction of tubules and damage to the tubular epithelial cells.

Furthermore, light chains which pass through capillaries may be incorporated into amyloid (AL type) within glomeruli, and if the myeloma is associated with hypercalcaemia from bone destruction there may be superimposed nephrocalcinosis.

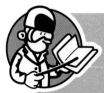

- State the causes of acute tubular necrosis.
- Describe the pathogenesis of acute tubular necrosis.
- List the complications of acute pyelonephritis.
- Name the two types of pathogenesis for chronic pyelonephritis.
- What is nephrocalcinosis?
- How does multiple myeloma cause tubular interstitial nephritis?

DISEASES OF THE RENAL BLOOD VESSELS

Benign nephrosclerosis

This is hyaline arteriosclerosis of the kidney is associated with benign hypertension.

The condition is an important complication of long-standing benign hypertension (pp. 77–78), chronic renal failure being one of its major sequelae.

This is the most common form of nephropathy, found in approximately 75% of autopsies over the age of 60 years.

(The causes of hypertension are listed in Fig. 7.11.)

In long-standing benign hypertension, there is reduced flow of blood to the glomeruli caused by vascular changes which affect:

- Branches of the renal artery: thickening of arterial walls due to fibroelastic intimal proliferation, elastic lamina reduplication, and muscular hypertrophy of the media. Results in focal areas of ischaemia with scarring.
- Afferent arterioles: undergo hyalinization (arteriolosclerosis), their muscular walls being replaced by a rigid and inelastic amorphous material.

A progressive reduction in blood flow to nephrons leads to chronic ischaemia with slow conversion of individual glomeruli into a mass of hyaline tissue devoid of capillary lumina (Fig. 10.8).

Blood supply to the tubules is also derived from glomerular blood flow, thus there is eventual ischaemic destruction of the associated tubule.

The process gradually destroys individual nephrons over a period of many years.

Clinical features—Initially, there are no clinical symptoms, although a gradual increase in blood levels of urea and a reduction in creatinine clearance occur.

Eventually, sufficient numbers of nephrons become non-functioning for the patient to develop manifestations of chronic renal failure.

Prognosis—Less than 5% of patients with well-developed benign nephrosclerosis die from renal failure. Death in the great majority of cases of benign hypertension occurs from congestive heart failure, coronary insufficiency and cerebral vascular accidents.

Malignant nephrosclerosis

Renal disease is associated with malignant, accelerated hypertension.

(The causes of malignant hypertension are listed in Fig. 7.11.)

Pathogenesis—In accelerated hypertension, the rise in blood pressure is very rapid, causing a pattern of renal damage which differs from that seen in benign hypertension:

- Larger muscular vessels undergo fibroelastic proliferation of the intima, but no muscular hypertrophy.
- Afferent arterioles frequently undergo necrosis, often with fibrin in their damaged walls (fibrinoid necrosis) following exposure to the sudden high pressures.
- Glomerular capillary network: segmental fibrinoid necrosis of glomerular tuft.

The patient develops acute renal failure when sufficient nephrons are rendered non-functional because of damage to glomerular tufts and afferent arterioles.

The renal changes seen in benign and accelerated hypertensive nephrosclerosis are summarized in Fig. 10.8.

Untreated accelerated hypertension causes death from renal failure in 90% of cases, usually with marked rapidity. However, if hypertension is

Pathology of the Kidney and Urinary Tract

treated adequately, before there is evidence of impairment of renal function by a raised blood urea, then prognosis is good and subsequent renal failure unusual.

Renal artery stenosis

This is a narrowing of renal arteries, typically caused by generalized atherosclerosis, but may rarely be caused by arterial fibromuscular dysplasia.

Atherosclerotic occlusion of the renal artery is usually most severe at its origin from the aorta. Renal artery stenosis at this point can lead to two main pathological processes:

- Chronic ischaemia of the affected kidney: reduction in function of all nephrons on that side produces an end-stage shrunken kidney. However, contralateral kidney undergoes compensatory hypertrophy, so that renal function is largely unaffected.
- Renovascular hypertension: inadequate perfusion of the kidney caused by renal artery stenosis may lead to hyperreninism, and so to abnormal activation of the renin–angiotensin system. This condition is important in that it is one of the recognized causes of hypertension that is amenable to surgical correction.

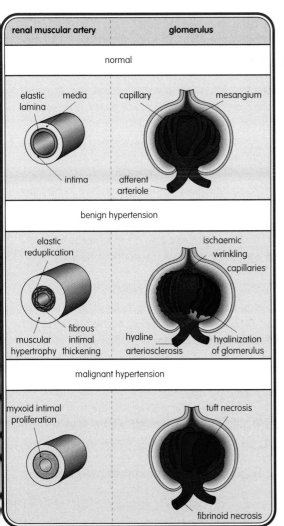

Fig. 10.8 Vascular changes associated with hypertensive renal disease.

A useful diagnostic pointer for renal artery stenosis is to look for associated features of:
○ **Vascular disease elsewhere.**
○ **Severe or drug-resistant hypertension.**
○ **Abdominal bruits.**

Thrombotic microangiopathies
Haemolytic uraemic syndrome (HUS)

This complex syndrome of disordered platelet function is characterized by the triad of thrombocytopenia, haemolysis and acute renal failure.

Classification

There are three subtypes of HUS—childhood, adult and secondary.

Childhood HUS

This usually affects children under 4 years of age. The aetiology is unknown, but the prognosis is better than for the other two types.

Adult HUS

This is more frequently fatal than childhood HUS and is associated with the following conditions:
- Pregnancy: occurring postpartum even several months after delivery.
- Oestrogen therapy: contraceptive pills or oestrogen

therapy for men with prostatic carcinoma.
- Infections, e.g. typhoid, viruses and shigellosis.

Secondary HUS
This occurs as a complication of:
- Malignant hypertension.
- Progressive systemic sclerosis.
- SLE.
- Transplant rejection.

Pathogenesis—Platelets adhere to the endothelium of small vessels, including the glomerular capillaries, where they undergo aggregation and trigger fibrin deposition. Fibrin strands form a tight mesh which deforms the erythrocytes as they are forced through (microangiopathic haemolysis).
   Morphological features are:
- Endocapillary proliferation: in response to fibrin and platelet deposition in glomerular tufts.
- Luminal narrowing: arterioles and small arteries show fibrin and erythrocytes in the walls, often with thrombosis which, when extensive, can result in cortical necrosis.

Clinical features are:
- Sudden onset of oliguria with haematuria and occasionally melaena.
- Jaundice.
- Anaemia with schistocytes (fragmented erythrocytes) and thrombocytopenia.
- Hypertension in 50% of cases.

In childhood HUS, symptoms are often preceded by a prodromal episode of diarrhoea or flu-like illness lasting for 5–15 days.
   Prognosis depends on the severity of attack but mortality may be as high as 40%.

Thrombotic thrombocytopaenic purpura (TTP)
TTP and HUS are thought to represent the same disease process but with a different distribution of thrombotic lesions. In TTP, occlusive plugs lead to widespread ischaemic organ damage, especially of the brain and kidney, resulting in neurological abnormalities and progressive renal impairment.

Renal infarcts
There are two mechanisms of renal infarction: embolic infarction and diffuse cortical necrosis.

Embolic renal disease
Renal infarcts are usually due to the passage of emboli down renal arterial branches. The most common causes are:
- Embolization of atheromatous material.
- Thrombotic material arising from left side of heart.
- Bacterial vegetation from infective endocarditis.

Resultant infarcts may be clinically silent or may result in haematuria and loin pain. Macroscopically, infarcts are pale or white and have a characteristic wedge shape with the apex directed towards the hilum (see Fig. 3.15).

Diffuse cortical necrosis
This rare pattern of renal infarction is associated with conditions resulting in severe hypotension, the most common of which are hypovolaemic shock, severe sepsis, and eclampsia of pregnancy.
   The pathogenesis is uncertain but diffuse spasm of renal blood vessels is thought to play a major part in precipitating ischaemic damage.
   Macroscopically, necrosis is confined to the outer part of the renal cortex, which in the acute stages is pale and focally haemorrhagic.
   This condition results in acute renal failure, and prognosis depends on the extent of the damage.

Sickle cell disease nephropathy
Vascular occlusion of vasae rectae in sickle cell disease (pp. 312–313) causes papillary necrosis, leading to the development of haematuria and polyuria.

- **Compare the features of benign and malignant hypertension.**
- **Describe the effects of renal artery stenosis.**
- **What is HUS? Describe the clinical features.**
- **Describe the mechanisms of renal infarctions.**

NEOPLASTIC DISEASE OF THE KIDNEY

Benign tumours of the kidney
These are common incidental findings at post mortem examination in about 20% of all patients; however, they rarely cause clinical problems.

Cortical adenoma
These are benign epithelial tumours derived from renal tubular epithelium.

Macroscopically, they are discrete nodules usually less than 20 mm in diameter, situated in the cortex of the kidney.

Microscopically, appearances are similar to those of renal cell carcinomas, both being composed of well-differentiated large clear cells with small nuclei.

Difficulty in differentiating between these tumours has prompted the adoption of an arbitrary cut-off of 3 cm in size to distinguish between the smaller adenomas and the typically larger carcinomas. However, the distinction is unreliable since some small lesions suspected of being adenomas may in fact be carcinomas going on to metastasize.

Renal fibroma or hamartoma (renomedullary interstitial cell tumour)
This is the commonest benign tumour of the kidney and is composed of spindle cells.

Macroscopically, there are firm white nodules situated in the medulla, typically 3–10 mm in size.

Microscopically, it is composed of spindle cells which surround the adjacent tubules.

They are of no functional or clinical significance.

Angiomyolipoma
This hamartoma is composed of a mixture of smooth muscle, blood vessels and fat, and situated either in the cortex or in the medulla. It is mainly seen in association with tuberose sclerosis (see Chapter 6).

Oncocytoma
This benign epithelial tumour is composed of large cells with granular, eosinophilic cytoplasm filled with mitochondria. It is a variant of the renal adenomas, and can attain a considerable size and may be confused with renal cell carcinoma.

Malignant tumours of the kidney
Renal cell carcinoma (renal adenocarcinoma; hypernephroma)
An adenocarcinoma derived from the renal tubular epithelium in adults, this tumour accounts for about 3% of all carcinomas, and about 90% of primary malignant renal tumours. It is usually seen after the age of 50 years. Males are more often affected than female by 3:1.

There is an increased incidence in those who smoke tobacco and also in patients with von Hippel–Lindau syndrome, a rare hereditary condition (suggesting a genetic predisposition).

Associations—Paraneoplastic syndromes of hypercalcaemia, hypertension, polycythaemia or Cushing's syndrome caused by ectopic or inappropriate hormone secretion.

Macroscopically, tumours occur most commonly at the upper pole of a kidney. They are usually rounded masses, with a yellowish cut surface marked with areas of haemorrhage and necrosis.

Microscopically, they are composed of either clear or granular cell types. The most common is the 'clear cell pattern' in which tumour cells have clear cytoplasm due to the high content of glycogen and lipid. Granular cell types are derived from tubular and papillary carcinomas.

Route of spread is:
- Local: eroding through renal capsule into perinephric fat.
- Lymphatic: to para-aortic and other nodes.
- Blood-borne metastasis: involving lungs, bone, brain and other sites as a result of tumour invasion of the renal vein. A characteristic feature is that large tumours may grow as a solid core along the main renal vein even entering the inferior vena cava.

Clinical features are:
- Common presenting symptoms: haematuria, loin pain, loin mass.
- Occasional presenting symptoms: bone metastasis, brain metastasis or polycythaemia.

Prognosis depends on the stage at presentation. If the tumour is confined within a renal capsule there is a 70% chance of 10 years' survival. However, prognosis is very poor if metastases are present at diagnosis.

Differential diagnosis of unilateral enlargement of the kidney is:
- Hydronephrosis.
- Tumour.
- Renal vein thrombosis.
- Postcontralateral nephrectomy.
- Contralateral kidney failure.

Prognosis is related to the spread of the tumour at diagnosis. Treatment is by a combination of radiotherapy and intensive chemotherapy, achieving a high cure rate.

- Name the common benign tumours of the kidney.
- What is the differential diagnosis of a unilaterally enlarged kidney?
- Describe the pathology of renal cell carcinoma.
- Define 'Wilms' tumour' and describe its presenting features.

Urothelial carcinoma of the renal pelvis

This malignant tumour of the renal pelvis derived from the transitional cells of the urothelium is mainly caused by environmental agents. It is associated with analgesic abuse and exposure to aniline dyes used in the dye, rubber, and plastics industries. Some cases have also been reported to develop many years after the use of 'Thorotrast', an α-particle-emitting contrast agent used in retrograde pyelography.

Tumours generally present early with haematuria or obstruction.

Histologically, tumours are similar in nature to those seen in the bladder (p. 206).

Wilms' tumour (nephroblastoma)

This malignant embryonal tumour is derived from the primitive metanephros. A common malignant tumour of childhood, its peak incidence is between the ages of 1 and 4 years. Males and females are equally affected.

Macroscopically, large amounts of kidney are replaced by rounded masses of solid, fleshy, white lesions with frequent areas of necrosis. The tumour is aggressive and rapidly growing; extension beyond the capsule into perinephric fat and even into the root of mesentery is frequent. Spread to lungs is identified in a high proportion of cases at time of diagnosis.

Microscopically, it is composed of up to four elements:
- Primitive, small-cell, blastematous tissue: resembles developing metanephric blastema.
- Immature-looking, glomerular structures.
- Epithelial tubules.
- Stroma composed of spindle cells and striated muscle.

Clinical presentation—Abdominal mass or haematuria.

DISORDERS OF THE URINARY TRACT

Congenital abnormalities of the urinary tract

Ureteric abnormalities

Double and bifid ureters

The commonest ureteric abnormality, these often occur in association with duplication of renal pelvis. They may be associated with vesicoureteric reflux, and predispose to recurrent infections.

Ureteropelvic junction obstruction

This is most commonly caused by a stricture which may be either intrinsic (within the wall of the ureter) or extrinsic (associated with external factors such as an aberrant vessel). The condition causes an increase in the relative amount of fibrous tissue at the site of the stricture. This appears to provide a barrier to the conduction of a wave of contraction of the ureter.

Diverticulum

This is a rare outpouching of the ureter.

Megaloureter

In this common congenital anomaly, retention of urine within the enlarged ureter results in hydroureter. The condition predisposes to reflux and recurrent infections.

Bladder abnormalities
Diverticula
Congenital diverticula are rare and are more often acquired as a result of bladder outlet obstruction. Symptoms are due to stasis and the resultant infection.

Urethral abnormalities
Hypospadias
The urethra opens on to the underside of the penis, either on the glans (glandular hypospadias), at the junction of the glans with the shaft (coronal hypospadias) or on the shaft itself (penile hypospadias).

Epispadias
The urethra opens on to the dorsal (upper) surface of the penis.

All varieties can be corrected surgically.

Urinary tract obstruction and urolithiasis
Urinary tract obstruction
This is obstruction of urine drainage from the kidney occurring at any level within the urinary tract. Obstruction may be caused by either a structural lesion (majority) or congenital neuromuscular defects which prevent contraction waves and thus the flow of urine.

Structural lesions can be classified into:
- Intrinsic lesions: within ureteric wall or lumen, e.g. urinary calculus (most common), caseous or necrotic debris, fibrosis following trauma or infection, tumour.
- Extrinsic lesions: cause pressure from without, e.g. tumours of the rectum, prostate and the bladder, aberrant renal arteries, retroperitoneal fibrosis, pregnancy.

Causes vary according to site of obstruction (Fig. 10.9) where * indicates the most common sites of obstruction:
- Renal pelvis: calculi, tumours.
- Pelviureteric junction*: stricture, calculi, extrinsic compression.
- Ureter: calculi, extrinsic compression (pregnancy, tumour, fibrosis).
- Bladder neck*: tumour, calculi.
- Urethra*: prostatic hyperplasia or carcinoma, urethral valves, urethral stricture.

Pathogenesis—Obstruction at any point in the urinary tract causes increased pressure superior to blockage, with dilatation of the renal pelvis and calyces (hydronephrosis):
- Obstruction at the pelviureteric junction → hydronephrosis.
- Obstruction of the ureter → hydroureter with subsequent development of hydronephrosis.
- Obstruction of the bladder neck or urethra → bladder distension with hypertrophy of its muscle (seen on cystoscopic examination as trabeculation). Subsequently leads to hydroureter and hydronephrosis.

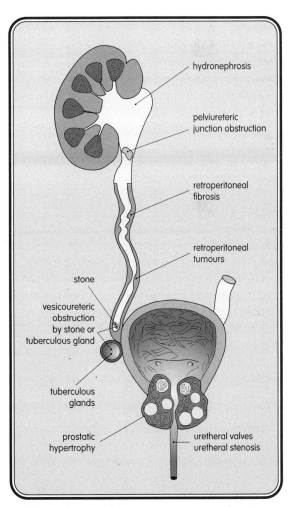

Fig. 10.9 Urinary tract showing common sites of obstruction.

Hydronephrosis may be:
- Unilateral: caused by obstruction at the level of the ureter, pelviureteric junction or renal pelvis. Obstruction is typically detected late, because renal function is maintained by the non-obstructed kidney. Renal parenchyma becomes severely atrophic and renal function is permanently impaired (end-stage hydronephrosis).
- Bilateral: caused by obstruction at the level of the bladder or urethra. Obstruction is typically detected at an earlier stage, as renal failure develops before severe atrophy of both kidneys.

In both forms, urinary tract obstruction predisposes to infection of the bladder (cystitis) and kidney (pyelonephritis or pyonephrosis) as well as stone formation.

Effects of hydronephrosis

The net result of hydronephrosis is that fluid entering the collecting ducts cannot empty into renal pelvis, and intrarenal resorption of fluid occurs.

If obstruction is removed at this stage, then renal function returns to normal. However, persistence of obstruction leads to atrophy of renal tubules with glomerular hyalinization and fibrosis.

Clinical features depend on the cause and site of the lesion.

Obstruction above the bladder will cause either an acute onset of renal colic or a gradual onset of aching pain in the loins, sometimes aggravated by drinking.

The clinical feature of obstruction below the bladder is difficulty in micturition, occasionally with distension of the bladder; it may progress to a bilateral ache in the loins.

Superimposed infection causes malaise, fever, dysuria and sometimes septicaemia.

Management is by removal of the obstruction and treatment of the infection.

Urolithiasis (urinary calculi)

This is the formation of stones in the urinary tract. It affects 1–5% of the population in the UK and onset is typically after 30 years of age, with males affected more than females.

Stones can form anywhere in the urinary tract but the commonest site is within the renal pelvis.

Composition of stones:
- Calcium oxalate (75–80%).
- Triple phosphates (15%): magnesium ammonium

phosphate stones.
- Uric acid (5%).
- Calculi in cystinuria and oxalosis.

Aetiology is:
- Acquired: as a result of urinary tract obstruction, persistent urinary tract infection, reduced urine volume (low fluid intake or excessive sweating).
- Inherited: primary metabolic disturbances, e.g. cystinuria, xanthinuria, etc.

The mechanism of stone formation is not well understood, but is thought to involve an excess of solute in urine (due to either primary increase in metabolite, or stasis) or reduced solubility of solute in urine (due to persistently abnormal urinary pH).

Calculi vary greatly in size, from sand-like particles to large round stones. 'Staghorn calculi' fill the whole renal pelvis and branch into calyces. Deposits of calcium may be present throughout renal parenchyma giving rise to nephrocalcinosis (p. 201).

The condition may present with:
- Renal colic often with nausea and vomiting: caused by the passage of small stones along the ureter.
- Dull ache in the loins: due to the presence of stones in the kidney.
- Strangury (the desire to pass something that will not pass): caused by stones in the bladder.
- Recurrent and intractable urinary tract infection, haematuria or renal failure.

Occasionally, the condition is asymptomatic, discovered only during radiological examination for another disease.

Management is by bed rest, application of warmth to the site of pain and administration of analgesia.

Small stones (<0.5 cm) in diameter are usually passed naturally. Larger stones may require surgical intervention.

Inflammation of the urinary tract
Cystitis

This is inflammation of the bladder and is extremely common—most women will have one or more episodes of cystitis. Females are affected more often than males because they have a short urethra (i.e. less travelling distance for bacteria).

Aetiology

The condition is most commonly due to infection, but is occasionally caused by physical agents, e.g. radiation or mechanical irritants.

Infective causes:

- Bacterial infection (most common): usually Gram-negative coliform bacilli, e.g. *E. coli* and *Proteus*, but *Streptococcus faecalis*, *Pseudomonas aeruginosa* and staphylococci are also common.
- Viral infection: adenovirus may cause haemorrhagic cystitis in children.
- Parasites: *Schistosoma haematobium*, which is common in Africa.
- Fungi: *Candida*.

Risk factors are:

- Urinary retention: due to obstruction, bladder paralysis, diverticula, calculi, foreign bodies, tumours, uterine prolapse.
- Infection of adjacent structures, e.g. prostatitis, urethritis, and diverticular disease of the colon.
- Diabetes mellitus.
- Pregnancy.
- Trauma, e.g. catheterization.

Routes of infection are:

- Ascending infection (most common): from urethral infection, or introduction of bacteria directly into the bladder via the urethra, e.g. on catheterization.
- Descending infection: from the kidney, e.g. renal tuberculosis.
- Direct spread: from adjacent organs, e.g. diverticulitis.
- Haematogenous: rare.
- Lymphatic: extremely rare.

Macroscopically, there is acute inflammation with oedema, erythema and later ulceration of bladder mucosa.

Microscopically, there is infiltration of mucosa with acute inflammatory cells.

Clinical features—Urinary tract infections may present with any of the following features:

- Disorders of micturition: increases in frequency, urgency, dysuria, haematuria, and incontinence.
- Pain in the right iliac fossa, loin, and suprapubic area.
- Pyrexia.

Investigations—Examination of midstream urine (see p. 200 for definitions of significant bacteruria and pyuria).

Treatment is by:

- Increased fluid intake to flush out organisms.
- Antibiotic therapy, e.g. trimethoprim.
- Treatment of any underlying causes, e.g. obstruction.

Sequelae:

- resolution (which is common)
- chronicity if the underlying cause is untreatable.
- development of pyelonephritis and associated complications, see pp. 199–201.

Interstitial cystitis (Hunner's ulcer)

This is a condition of unknown aetiology in which the bladder is inflamed, fibrotic and of small capacity, but the urine is sterile. It is characterized clinically by suprapubic pain and increased frequency.

Macroscopically, there is linear ulceration and erythema.

Microscopically, there is fibrosis and lymphocytic infiltration through the full thickness of the bladder wall.

Malakoplakia

A rare variant of cystitis, the bladder mucosa develops yellow plaques composed of a mixture of chronic inflammatory cells including characteristic granule-containing macrophages. Granules (known as Michaelis–Gutmann bodies) are composed of calcified bacterial debris and are thought to reflect defective macrophage functions.

Plaques may subsequently undergo ulceration thus mimicking a bladder tumour.

Ureteritis

This inflammation of the ureter is usually due to an ascending urinary tract infection.

Causative organisms are the same as for cystitis.

Pathogenesis—In most cases, lower urinary tract infection remains localized to the urethra and bladder. Occasionally, organisms may ascend the ureter and enter the pelvicalyceal system, particularly when there is an obstructive lesion. Thus, an acute bacterial cystitis may lead to an ascending ureteritis and pyelitis (inflammation of the renal pelvis and calyces).

Complications—Organisms may gain access to renal parenchyma to produce acute pyelonephritis, with the formation of abscesses in the renal medulla and cortex.

Ureteritis follicularis
This ureteritis presents with large aggregates of lymphoid cells.

Ureteritis cystica
This is a complication of chronic ureteritis in which epithelial nests become trapped by fibrosis and subsequently develop into thin-walled cysts.

Neoplastic disease of the urinary tract
Tumours of the ureter
Tumours of the ureter are extremely rare and are almost always epithelial.

Fibroepithelial polyps
These are benign papillary tumours.

Malignant urothelial tumours
These tumours arise from the transitional cell epithelium of the ureter. They are mainly caused by environmental agents (see below), and are identical to those seen in the bladder.

Tumours of the bladder
Metaplasia
Glandular metaplasia (cystitis glandularis)
These small, rounded collections of urothelial cells are found just below the urothelial surface (Brunn's nests), which develop a central lumen surrounded by cuboidal or columnar cells. These are quite common and often seen in the normal bladder.

Occasionally, there is metaplasia to an intestinal variant of cystitis glandularis, lined by colonic, mucin-secreting epithelium.

Adenomatous metaplasia (nephrogenic adenoma)
This benign condition is characterized by metaplasia of the urothelium to cuboidal epithelium. Metaplastic areas resemble collecting tubules of the kidney. It is associated with chronic infections, e.g. tuberculosis.

Squamous metaplasia
There are two types:
- Keratinizing squamous metaplasia (leukoplakia): the bladder mucosa develops white plaques which are often secondary to chronic irritation, e.g. calculi. Occurs in both males and females, and a significant proportion progress to squamous carcinoma of the bladder.
- Non-keratinizing squamous metaplasia (vaginal metaplasia): white plaques are seen on trigone. This only occurs in women and has no pathological significance.

Transitional cell carcinoma
These are tumours of the urothelium, affecting 1 in 5000 in the UK and accounting for 3% of all cancer deaths. They are found in those aged 60–70 years, with males more often affected than females by 3:1.

Aetiology is as follows:
- Chemicals: exposure to environmental agents excreted in high concentrations in the urine. Known carcinogens are associated with cigarette smoking, aniline dyes and the rubber industry.
- Schistosomiasis: bladder cancer is extremely common in endemic areas.
- Leukoplakia (see above): associated with bladder stones.
- Bladder diverticula: about 3% are complicated with tumour.

Most tumours are at the base of trigone and around the ureteric orifices.

Morphological types:
- Papillary (most common): warty masses projecting into the lumen with little or no invasion of the bladder wall. Only a small percentage evolve into invasive carcinoma.
- Solid: tumours grow directly into the bladder wall and are often ulcerated or encrusted. Most are invasive from the outset.
- Mixed papillary and solid.
- Flat in-situ carcinoma: reddened mucosal surface due to underlying telangectatic blood vessels. May become invasive.

The majority of urothelial cancers are caused by exposure to environmental agents. Thus, bladder tumours are usually multiple and are often found in conjunction with urothelial tumours at other sites of the lower urinary tract, e.g. renal pelvis, ureters or urethra.

Grading and staging of bladder carcinomas

The degree of differentiation (grade) and extent of spread (stage) are important indicators for prognosis.

Grading

The grading is as follows:
- Grade I (well differentiated): vast majority are papillary growths with no evidence of invasion.
- Grade II (moderately well differentiated): usually papillary, but many are either invasive at presentation or become so. Cells show significant atypicality and an increase in mitotic figures.
- Grade III (poorly differentiated): mainly solid lesions which are extensively invasive. Cells are pleomorphic with numerous mitoses.

TNM (tumour–node–metastasis) staging

The TNM staging is as follows:
- T1: tumour confined to mucosa or submucosa.
- T2: superficial muscle involved.
- T3: deep muscle involved.
- T4: invasion beyond the bladder.

Spread is as follows:
- Local: to pelvic structures.
- Lymphatic: to iliac and para-aortic lymph nodes.
- Haematogenous: to liver and lung.

Clinically, the disease commonly presents with painless (or painful) haematuria or recurrent urinary tract infections. Rarely, it may present with hydronephrosis (from ureteric obstruction), pneumaturia from vesicocolic fistula, or incontinence from vesicovaginal fistula.

Treatment depends on the stage at diagnosis:
- Diathermy via cystoscope: for T1 and T2 (± chemo- or radiotherapy).
- Radical radiotherapy, cystectomy or a combination of the two for T3.
- Palliative radiotherapy for T4.

Prognosis depends on the histological type of tumour and extent of spread. Papillary, non-invasive tumours have an excellent prognosis, whereas solid, invasive, urothelial tumours only have an overall 35% 5 year survival rate.

- What are the common congenital abnormalities of the ureter, bladder and urethra?
- List the causes of urinary tract obstruction.
- What are the effects of hydronephrosis?
- Name the different types of kidney stones according to their composition.
- State the risk factors for development of cystitis.
- Name the metaplastic tumours of the bladder.
- What are the chemical causes of urothelial tumours?

DISORDERS OF THE PITUITARY

The pituitary (hypophysis) is a small gland lying in the sella turcica in the base of the skull. It is composed of two parts:

- Anterior lobe (adenohypophysis): synthesizes and secretes a number of hormones (Fig. 11.1), most of which act on other endocrine glands.
- Posterior lobe (neurohypophysis): stores and secretes two hormones synthesized in the hypothalamus, namely antidiuretic hormone and oxytocin. This lobe is in direct continuity with the hypothalamus.

Secretion of the pituitary hormones is regulated by neural and chemical stimuli from the hypothalamus, diseases of which cause secondary abnormalities in pituitary function.

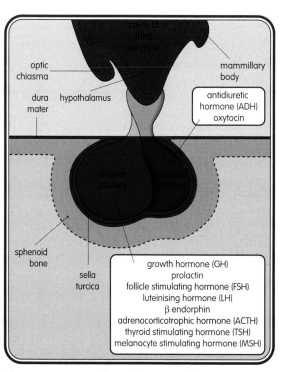

Fig. 11.1 Pituitary and hypothalamus and their hormones.

The anterior pituitary: hyperpituitarism

Hyperpituitarism is defined as excessive secretion of one or more of the pituitary hormones. Its commonest causes are functioning (hormone-secreting) adenomas of the anterior lobe.

Anterior lobe adenomas

Anterior lobe adenomas comprise about 15% of all intracranial tumours (posterior lobe adenomas do not occur). These tumours do not usually metastasize but are often life threatening due to their position and ability to secrete excess hormone.

Effects of pituitary adenomas

Pituitary adenomas cause problems due to a combination of endocrine effects (excessive secretion of a particular hormone) and compressive effects, caused by local compression of:

- Remainder of the pituitary → hypopituitarism.
- Optic chiasm → visual field defects, notably bitemporal hemianopia.
- Brain (large tumours) → distortion of the midbrain with internal hydrocephalus.
- Dura → headaches.
- Cavernous sinus → III, IV or VI nerve palsies.

The endocrine effects depend on which hormone is being excessively secreted (see below).
  Investigations:
- Imaging: plain X-ray (can detect enlargement of sella turcica and erosion of the clinoid processes), CT scans, MRI, cisternography.
- Hormone assays (e.g. growth hormone, prolactin).
- Functional testing of the pituitary–adrenal axis.
- Visual field assessment.

Types of functioning adenomas

Functioning adenomas may produce any of the adenophyseal (anterior lobe) hormones, but the majority produce either prolactin (produced by prolactinomas—lactotroph adenomas), growth hormone (produced by somatotroph adenomas) or ACTH (produced by corticotroph adenomas).

Prolactinomas

Abnormally increased prolactin secretion is associated in women with menstrual irregularity and infertility, and in men with ejaculatory failure or impotence.

Galactorrhoea is present in about 30% of affected women, but is rare in men since oestrogen priming is required for lactation.

Somatotroph adenoma

This results in hypersecretion of growth hormone, the effects of which depend on the developmental stage of the affected individual:

- Pre-epiphyseal union (prepubertal) leads to gigantism (syn. giantism), i.e. excessive growth in a regular and initially well-proportioned manner. Most giants also show some features of acromegaly with disproportionate enlargement, e.g. of the hands and jaw.
- Postepiphyseal union (adults) leads to

acromegaly, which is characterized by enlargement of the hands, feet and head, but may also present with secondary diabetes (growth hormone is an insulin antagonist) or cardiovascular effects (Fig. 11.2).

There are three types of treatment:
- Surgery: hypophysectomy (transfrontal or transphenoidal), especially where there are signs of compression of adjacent structures.
- Radiotherapy: less complications than surgery, but less successful.
- Drug therapy: bromocriptine lowers growth hormone levels in uncomplicated acromegaly.

Corticotroph adenoma

Overproduction of ACTH by the pituitary gland (Cushing's disease) causes adrenal hyperplasia, resulting in the excessive secretion of glucocorticoids causing Cushing's syndrome, the effects of which are described in 'Disorders of the Adrenal Gland' (pp. 227–229).

Other functioning adenomas

Other endocrine secreting adenomas, e.g. of TSH, LH and FSH, are extremely rare.

The anterior pituitary—hypopituitarism

Hypopituitarism is defined as insufficient secretion of the pituitary hormones. The clinical features are dependent on the patient's age, and the type and severity of the hormone deficiencies (Fig. 11.3).

Hypopituitarism can be caused by either hypothalamic lesions or pituitary lesions.

Hypothalamic lesions are:
- Idiopathic deficiency of one or more of the releasing factors, e.g. GnRH (Kallmann's syndrome), GHRH, or more rarely TRH or CRF.
- Infarction.
- Inflammation.
- Suprasellar tumours, e.g. craniopharyngioma, or more rarely pinealoma, teratoma or secondary from other sites.

Pituitary lesions are:
- Idiopathic deficiency of one or more of the pituitary hormones.

skull
- enlarged head circumference

brain
- mental disturbances
- insomnia

face
- large lower jaw
- spaces between lower teeth due to jaw growth
- large nose
- large tongue

heart
- enlarged

liver and kidneys
- enlarged organs

hands
- large, square and spade like

blood pressure
- hypertension

blood
- hypercalcaemia

bones
- predisposes to osteoarthritis

skin
- increased greasy sweating
- temperature intolerance

feet
- large and wide

Fig. 11.2 Features of acromegaly.

- Non-functioning chromophobe pituitary adenomas: adenomas of the anterior pituitary (usually derived from non-hormone-secreting chromophobe cells) may cause hypopituitarism by compression or obliteration of normal pituitary tissue.
- Sheehan's syndrome: ischaemic necrosis of the adenohypophysis due to hypotensive shock occurring as a result of intrapartum or postpartum haemorrhage.
- Empty sella syndrome: occupation of the sella by a CSF-containing arachnoid space. This may be a primary anatomical variant or it may follow spontaneous infarction, surgery or radiotherapy of a tumour.
- Trauma, including surgery and radiotherapy.
- Granulomatous lesions: sarcoidosis, tuberculosis, histiocytosis.

Management

Management is by substitution therapy according to the deficiencies demonstrated, e.g. cortisol replacement for ACTH deficiency, thyroid hormone replacement for TSH deficiency.

The posterior pituitary

Diseases of the posterior pituitary are much less common than those of the anterior pituitary, and are usually the result of damage to the hypothalamus due to tumour invasion or infarction. Posterior pituitary diseases typically cause disorders of abnormal ADH secretion. There are no known effects of abnormal oxytocin secretion.

Diabetes insipidus (DI)

This rare condition is characterized by the persistent excretion of excessive quantities of dilute urine and by constant thirst.

The aetiology and features of diabetes insipidus are common topics in MCQs.

Clinical features associated with specific forms of hypopituitarism		
Hormone deficiency	Clinical features	Tests to exclude hypofunction of anterior pituitary
gonadotrophin deficiency	prepubertal: • failure to enter puberty • undescended testes • obesity • eunuchoidism postpubertal: • infertility • amenorrhoea • oligospermia • progressive loss of secondary sex characteristics (hypogonadism) • osteoporotic collapse of spine → loss of stature	LH reserves adequate if: • males have a normal testosterone • females are ovulating FSH reserves adequate if: • males have normal spermatogenesis • females are ovulating
GH deficiency	children: failure of longitudinal growth adults: tendency to hypoglycaemia	GH reserves adequate if: • random plasma level >20 mU/l • stress or otherwise elevated GH peak >20 mU/l
TSH deficiency	fetus or newborn: cretinism adults: hypothyroidism	TSH reserves adequate if serum thyroxine within normal range
ACTH deficiency	features of primary hypoadrenalism but with decreased pigmentation (rather than an increase)	ACTH reserves adequate if: • random plasma cortisol >550 nmol/l • stress-induced cortisol rise >550 nmol/l

Fig. 11.3 Clinical features associated with specific forms of hypopituitarism.

There are two types:
- Cranial DI: caused by the failure of ADH (vasopressin) production.
- Nephrogenic DI: distal tubules are refractory to the water reabsorptive action of ADH (Fig. 11.4).

Clinical features—Irrespective of aetiology, reabsorption of water from the glomerular filtrate in the renal collecting ducts does not occur, resulting in the excretion of large quantities of dilute urine (polyuria) with a high risk of body water depletion. DI is potentially lethal without appropriate therapy.

Investigations—Water deprivation test for 8 hours or until 3% of the body weight is lost. Demonstration of continued polyuria and increased haemoconcentration indicates DI. This test serves to differentiate DI from psychogenic polydipsia. The test is then followed by ADH administration to demonstrate whether the kidneys can (cranial DI) or cannot (nephrogenic DI) respond.

Treatment of mild DI—The effects of dehydration can be counteracted by greatly increasing water intake (polydipsia).

Treatment of moderate to severe DI:
- Cranial DI: treatment with desmopressin (vasopressin analogue but without vasoactive effects).

- Nephrogenic DI: treatment with thiazide diuretics, producing a decrease in urine volume by approximately 50%.

Syndrome of inappropriate ADH secretion

Increased secretion of ADH occurs as a complication of other diseases. (Primary hypersecretion of ADH is not recognized.) The condition is characterized by water retention with haemodilution, and in severe cases cerebral oedema supervenes with impaired consciousness.

The causes are:
- Idiopathic.
- Tumours: ectopic secretion of ADH, especially by oat cell carcinomas of the lung and some neuroendocrine tumours.
- Trauma: skull fracture, head injury or surgery may produce transiently increased ADH.
- Intracranial inflammation: meningitis, tuberculosis, syphilis.
- Thoracic diseases, e.g. pneumonia, pulmonary embolus, etc., probably due to involvement of intrathoracic baroreceptors.

Fig. 11.5 shows a comparison table of features of DI with those of inappropriate ADH secretion.

Causes of cranial and nephrogenic diabetes insipidus (DI)		
	Cause	**Features**
cranial DI	hypothalamic or pituitary stalk damage	surgical damage, usually in the course of tumour removal head injury, usually transient hypothalamic tumour (either primary or secondary) hypothalamic inflammatory lesions, e.g. sarcoidosis, encephalitis, meningitis
	genetic defects	dominant recessive: DIDMOAD syndrome—association of DI with diabetes mellitus (DM), optic atrophy (OA) and deafness (D)
	idiopathic	about 30% of cases have no known cause
nephrogenic DI	hereditary	abnormality of ADH receptors
	metabolic abnormalities	hypokalaemia hypercalcaemia
	drug therapy	lithium demethylchlortetracycline
	poisoning	heavy metals

Fig. 11.4 Causes of cranial and nephrogenic diabetes insipidus (DI).

Disorders of the pineal gland
Pinealomas
These common tumours of young adults and children are often called germinomas. They are thought to originate from primitive germ cells, and histologically resemble testicular seminomas and/or teratomas:

- Pressure on the midbrain may produce Parinaud's syndrome (paralysis of the conjugate upward gaze without paralysis of convergence).
- Pressure on the hypothalamus can produce symptoms of DI, emaciation or precocious puberty.

- **Describe the effects of local compression caused by pituitary tumours.**
- **What are the commonest adenomas of the anterior lobe? Describe their effects.**
- **State the causes of hypopituitarism.**
- **Describe the individual forms of hypopituitarism.**
- **What are the causes of diabetes insipidus?**

THYROID DISORDERS

Thyrotoxicosis (hyperthyroidism)
This syndrome is caused by the excessive secretion of thyroid hormones (typically both thyroxine, T_4 and tri-iodothyronine, T_3) in the bloodstream, characterized by tachycardia, sweating, tremor, anxiety, increased appetite, loss of weight and intolerance of heat.

Hyperthyroidism can be classified on the basis of aetiology into:

- Primary hyperthyroidism ($\uparrow$ thyroid hormones, $\downarrow$ TSH): hypersecretion of thyroid hormones, which is not secondary to increased levels of TSH.
- Secondary hyperthyroidism ($\uparrow$ thyroid hormones, $\uparrow$ TSH): overstimulation of the thyroid gland caused by excess TSH produced by a tumour in the pituitary or elsewhere (rare).

The causes of primary hyperthyroidism:

- Graves' disease (exophthalmic goitre): commonest cause of thyrotoxicosis, characterized by a diffusely enlarged thyroid gland, which is stimulated to produce excess hormone by an IgG autoantibody (see p. 221).
- Toxic multinodular goitre (Plummer's disease): second commonest cause of hyperthyroidism (see p. 222).
- Toxic adenoma: solitary thyroid nodule producing excess hormone with remainder of the thyroid gland being suppressed.
- Ingestion of large doses of thyroid hormone (thyrotoxicosis factitia).

Effects of thyrotoxicosis
Signs and symptoms of thyrotoxicosis are a consequence of an increase in the body's metabolism, which occurs as a direct result of increased concentrations of thyroid hormones. The most important symptoms diagnostically are:

Comparison of features of diabetes insipidus with those of inappropriate ADH secretion			
Condition	**Imbalance**	**Urinary and plasma osmolality**	**Symptoms**
diabetes insipidus	$\downarrow$ ADH	low urinary osmolality high plasma osmolality	polyuria (5–20 l/day) thirst polydipsia (may lead to severe dehydration, exhaustion, coma)
syndrome of inappropriate ADH secretion	$\uparrow$ ADH	high urinary osmolality low plasma osmolality (dilutional hyponatraemia)	oliguria water intoxication (may lead to confusion, neurological disturbances, coma)

Fig. 11.5 Comparison of features of diabetes insipidus with those of inappropriate ADH secretion.

- Heat intolerance and excessive sweating.
- Nervousness and irritability.
- Weight loss with normal or increased appetite.
- Usually a goitre of some sort.

Other symptoms are summarized in Fig. 11.6.

Investigations—Hyperthyroidism is confirmed by raised serum thyroxine and/or lowered serum TSH.

Management is by:

- Surgery: reduces the amount of functioning thyroid tissue.
- Radioactive iodine to destroy part of the gland.
- Drugs (such as carbimazole or propylthiouracil) that interfere with the production of thyroid hormones.

Hypothyroidism

Decreased activity of the thyroid gland results in decreased production of thyroid hormones. There are two forms:

- Hypothyroidism present at birth → cretinism or congenital hypothyroidism.
- Hypothyroidism in adults → myxoedema.

Cretinism (congenital hypothyroidism)

This condition occurs as a result of extreme hypothyroidism during fetal life, infancy or childhood. It has the following types and aetiology:

- Endemic cretinism, which occurs in iodine-deficient countries where goitre is common. The mother almost always has a goitre and the thyroid of the affected infant is usually enlarged and nodular.
- Sporadic cretinism, which is caused by congenital hypoplasia or absence of the thyroid gland and often associated with deaf mutism.
- Dyshormonogenesis, which is a congenital familial recessive enzyme defect leading to inability to complete the formation of thyroid hormones. TSH is increased, and the thyroid gland is enlarged and shows epithelial hyperplasia.

The clinical features of cretinism are:

- Mental retardation.
- Retarded growth: skeletal growth is inhibited more than soft tissue growth, hence the cretinism appearance of the obese, stocky, short child.
- Coarse, dry skin.
- Lack of hair and teeth.
- Pot belly (often with umbilical hernia).
- Protruding tongue.

Management is by early detection and treatment with thyroxine, which can prevent an irreversible mental defect and cerebellar damage. Many countries now have screening programmes measuring serum TSH and/or thyroxine levels on heel-prick blood samples taken on the fourth or fifth day of life.

Hypothyroidism in adults (myxoedema)

This common clinical condition is associated with decreased function of the thyroid gland and a decrease in the circulating level of thyroid hormones. It affects 8 per 10 000 people in the UK, with females more than males by 4 to 1, and can present at any age but most commonly between 30 and 50 years.

Note that, strictly speaking, myxoedema describes a non-pitting, oedematous reaction characteristic of hypothyroidism caused by the deposition of a mucoid substance ('myxo–' is a prefix denoting mucus) in the

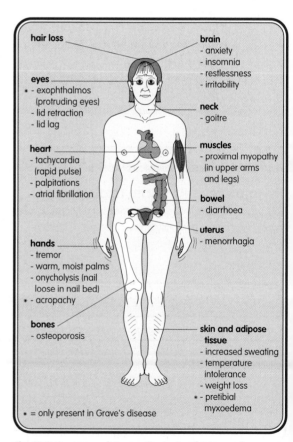

Fig. 11.6 Summary diagram illustrating features of thyrotoxicosis. (* = additional features seen only in Graves' disease.)

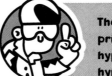

skin and elsewhere in the body. However, the terms 'myxoedema' and 'hypothyroidism of adults' are now frequently used interchangeably.

Hypothyroidism can be classified according to aetiology:

- Primary (↓ thyroid hormones, ↑ TSH): failure of the thyroid gland itself. (This is much more common than secondary hypothyroidism.)
- Secondary (↓ thyroid hormones, ↓ TSH): failure of TSH production due to pituitary disease.

The causes of primary hypothyroidism are:

- Autoimmune thyroiditis: atrophic form, e.g. primary atrophic thyroiditis, and goitrous form (such as Hashimoto's thyroiditis).
- Graves' disease: approximately 5% of patients with thyrotoxicosis develop hypothyroidism in later years, unrelated to treatment. Probably caused by a spectrum of antithyroid antibodies, some of which stimulate TSH receptor and some of which are destructive.
- Treatment of hyperthyroidism: surgical ablation, radioiodine or drug treatment.
- Severe iodine deficiency (rare in the UK): iodine must be virtually absent from the diet before myxoedema develops.

The effects of hypothyroidism are shown in Fig.11.7.

Signs and symptoms of hypothyroidism are a consequence of widespread effects (which decrease the body's metabolism due to reduced concentrations of thyroid hormones) and of localized effects (myxoedema due to the accumulation of mucoproteins). The most important symptoms diagnostically are:

- Mental and physical slowness.
- Tiredness.
- Cold intolerance.
- Dryness of skin and hair.

Investigations are:

- Serum thyroxine concentration (decreased in hypothyroidism).
- Serum TSH concentration (reduced in secondary hypothyroidism but increased in primary hypothyroidism).

The treatment is oral thyroxine daily for life.

The differences between primary and secondary hyperthyroidism and hypothyroidism:

- **Primary hyperthyroidism:** ↑ **thyroid hormones, ↓ TSH.**
- **Secondary hyperthyroidism:** ↑ **thyroid hormones, ↑ TSH (excess TSH production due to pituitary tumour).**
- **Primary hypothyroidism:** ↓ **thyroid hormones, ↑ TSH.**
- **Secondary hypothyroidism:** ↓ **thyroid hormones, ↓ TSH (failure of TSH production due to pituitary disease).**

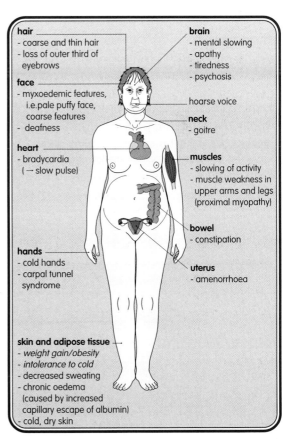

Fig. 11.7 Summary diagram illustrating features of hypothyroidism in the adult (myxoedema).

Congenital disorders of the thyroid
Development of the thyroid
The thyroid gland develops from an endodermal thickening in the floor of the primitive pharynx at a point later indicated by the foramen caecum of tongue (Fig. 11.8). As the embryo grows, the thyroid descends into the neck, passing anterior to the hyoid and laryngeal cartilages. During migration, the gland remains connected to the tongue by a narrow canal, the thyroglossal duct, which later becomes solid and finally disappears.

Thyroglossal cysts
Cystic remnants of parts of the thyroglossal duct are known as thyroglossal cysts (Fig. 11.8). These cysts may form anywhere along the course of descent but are always located near or in the midline of the neck, most commonly just inferior to the hyoid bone. Cysts usually develop as painless, progressively enlarging, and movable masses. Infection of cysts may result in the formation of sinuses that open through the skin.

Thyroiditis
This is inflammation of the thyroid gland, which may have a viral or autoimmune aetiology.

Hashimoto's thyroiditis (commonest cause of hypothyroidism)
This organ-specific autoimmune disease results in destructive thyroiditis. It can occur at any age but typically affects the middle-aged, and females more than males by 12:1.

The most common autoantibodies are antimicrosomal antibody and antithyroglobulin. The disease is associated with the HLA-DR5 and -B8 haplotypes, and patients with Hashimoto's disease (and Graves' disease) show a high incidence of other autoimmune diseases.

Macroscopically, the thyroid gland is usually:
- Diffusely enlarged (typically 2–5 × normal size).
- Firm in consistency.
- White or grey on a cut surface as a result of the disappearance of brown (iodine-rich) colloid, and its replacement by lymphocytes.

Microscopically, the thyroid gland shows:
- Small thyroid follicles infiltrated by lymphocytes and plasma cells.
- Lymphoid follicle formation and increased fibrous tissue stroma.
- Acini lined with abnormal, highly eosinophilic epithelial cells termed Askanazy cells, Hürthle cells, or oncocytes.
- Reduced colloid content of disrupted acini.

The condition may present with a goitre or with hypothyroidism. However, damage to thyroid follicles may lead to the release of thyroglobulin into the circulation causing a transient phase of thyrotoxicosis. Some cases proceed to primary atrophic thyroiditis.

Treatment is by oral thyroxine, which overcomes hypothyroidism and reduces the size of the goitre.

De Quervain's thyroiditis
A rare, viral thyroiditis seen in young and middle-aged women as a slight diffuse tender swelling of the thyroid, this is also known as subacute, giant cell or granulomatous thyroiditis. The condition usually occurs in association with a transient febrile illness, often during various viral epidemics.

Characteristic features are:
- Painful enlargement of thyroid (about twice normal size).
- History of usually short duration.
- Preceded by general malaise, pyrexia or upper respiratory infection.

Histological examination shows:
- Inflammation with a giant cell granulomatous reaction engulfing leaked colloid (hence the synonyms giant cell or granulomatous thyroiditis).

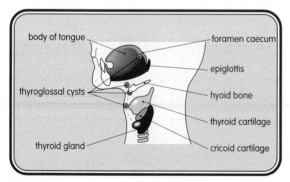

Fig. 11.8 Path of descent of thyroid gland (broken line) and localization of thyroglossal cysts.

- Degeneration of follicles with inflammatory cell infiltration (neutrophils, plasma cells, lymphocytes and histiocytes).
- Fibrous scarring.

The illness is usually self limiting and settles in a few weeks. Transient hyperthyroidism can result from the release of thyroglobulin and excessive amounts of thyroid hormone.

Severe thyroiditis may be fatal in the elderly and debilitated.

Subacute lymphocytic thyroiditis

This form of autoimmune thyroiditis is characterized by focal lymphocytic infiltration of the thyroid (also known as focal lymphocytic thyroiditis).

Histological changes are similar to those in Hashimoto's thyroiditis but are focal rather than diffuse. The disease is less severe than Hashimoto's thyroiditis, and is often asymptomatic (Fig. 11.9).

Note that some degree of progressive lymphocytic infiltration of the thyroid is noted in 5–10% of thyroid autopsies, and these are thought to be a normal ageing change. However, in subacute lymphocytic thyroiditis, lymphocytic infiltration is in excess of what would be expected for the age of the patients.

GRAVES' DISEASE

This organ-specific autoimmune disorder results in thyrotoxicosis due to overstimulation of the thyroid gland by autoantibodies. It is the commonest form of thyrotoxicosis, females being affected more than males by 8:1, and is usually associated with a diffuse enlargement of the thyroid.

Pathogenesis—IgG-type immunoglobulins bind to TSH membrane receptors and cause prolonged stimulation of the thyroid, lasting for as long as 12 hours (cf. 1 hour for TSH). The autoantibody binds at a site different to the hormone-binding locus, and is termed long-acting thyroid stimulator (LATS) or thyroid-stimulating immunoglobulin (TSI).

Histologically, the gland shows hyperplasia of acinar epithelium, reduction of stored colloid, and local accumulations of lymphocytes with lymphoid follicle formation.

The clinical features of Graves' disease are similar to those of general thyrotoxicosis but with some additional features, namely:
- Exophthalmos (protrusion of the eyeballs in their sockets) due to the infiltration of orbital tissues by fat, mucopolysaccharides and lymphocytes. May cause compression of the optic nerve, hence blindness. However, only about 5% of Graves' patients show signs of exophthalmos.
- Thyroid acropachy: enlargement of fingernails.
- Pretibial myxoedema: accumulation of mucoproteins in the deep dermis of the skin.
- Clubbing of the fingers.

Treatment is as for thyrotoxicosis (p. 218).

Thyroid goitres
Definitions

A goitre is any enlargement of part or whole of the thyroid gland. There are two types:
- Toxic goitre, i.e. goitre associated with thyrotoxicosis.

Summary of features of thyroiditis			
	Hashimoto's thyroiditis	De Quervain's thyroiditis	Subacute lymphocytic thyroiditis
aetiology	autoimmune	viral	autoimmune
histological features	diffuse lymphocytic infiltration of thyroid	giant cell granulomatous inflammatory reaction	focal lymphocytic infiltration of thyroid
hypothyroidism	common	rare	rare

Fig. 11.9 Summary of features of thyroiditis.

- Non-toxic goitre, i.e. goitre associated with normal or reduced levels of thyroid hormones.

Toxic goitre
Graves' disease
This is the commonest cause of toxic goitre (described above).

Toxic multinodular goitre
This results from the development of hyperthyroidism in a multinodular goitre (see below).

Non-toxic goitres
Diffuse non-toxic goitre (simple goitre)
This diffuse enlargement of the thyroid gland is classified into:
- Endemic goitre: due to iodine deficiency. Rare in the UK but still common in geographical areas remote from the sea.
- Sporadic goitre: caused by goitrogenic agents (substances that induce goitre formation) or may be familial in origin. Examples of goitrogenic agents include certain cabbage species because of their thiourea content, and specific drugs or chemicals, such as iodide, paraminosalicylic acid and drugs used in the treatment of thyrotoxicosis. Familial cases show inherited autosomal recessive traits, which interfere with hormone synthesis at differing enzyme pathways (these are dyshormonogenic goitres).
- Physiological goitre: enlargement of the thyroid gland in females during puberty or pregnancy; the reason is unclear.

Multinodular goitre
This is the commonest cause of thyroid enlargement, and seen particularly in the elderly. The aetiology is uncertain but may represent an uneven responsiveness of various parts of the thyroid to fluctuating TSH levels over a period of many years.

Morphological features are:
- Irregular hyperplastic enlargement of the entire thyroid gland due to the development of well-circumscribed nodules of varying size.
- Larger nodules filled with brown, gelatinous colloid, thus laoften termed multinodular colloid goitres.

Most patients have normal thyroid function and generally seek treatment for cosmetic reasons (an unsightly swelling in the neck) or compression symptoms, e.g.

pressure on the trachea producing stridor, or pressure on the recurrent laryngeal nerve producing hoarseness.

However, toxic changes occasionally occur in a multinodular goitre resulting in hyperthyroidism, and the goitre is then termed a toxic multinodular goitre.

Neoplasms of the thyroid
Tumours of the thyroid are generally benign. Carcinomas are rare, and lymphomas are rarer still.

Benign tumours
Thyroid adenomas
These are solitary or multiple, encapsulated solid nodules. Compression of the adjacent gland is a common feature, and the centre may show areas of haemorrhage and cystic changes. The commonest type is follicular adenoma, which consists of colloid-containing microfollicles and columns of larger cells of alveolar arrangement.

Rarely, follicular adenomas may synthesize excess thyroid hormones, causing thyrotoxicosis.

Malignant tumours
These rare tumours account for less than 1% of total cancer deaths in the UK, with females affected more than males by 3:1. Types of malignant thyroid tumours and their basic features are outlined in Fig. 11.10.

Papillary adenocarcinoma
This is a well-differentiated tumour most commonly found in younger patients. It presents as a non-encapsulated infiltrative mass, but is a slow growing tumour with an excellent prognosis.

Histologically, it consists of epithelial papillary projections between which calcified spherules may be present. Epithelial cell nuclei are characteristically large with optically clear areas centrally ('Orphan Annie nuclei').

Follicular adenocarcinoma
This well-differentiated, single, encapsulated lesion is histologically similar to follicular adenoma but can be differentiated by its invasion of the capsule and/or blood vessels. Spread is usually to bones and the lungs via the blood stream.

Many of these tumours retain the ability to take up radioactive iodine, which may be used as a highly effective targeted form of radiotherapy. The prognosis is therefore good.

Anaplastic carcinoma

This highly malignant, poorly differentiated adenocarcinoma usually presents in the elderly as a diffusely infiltrative mass.

Histologically, the dominant features are those of a spindle cell tumour with or without giant cell areas, or a small cell pattern.

The prognosis is very poor due to the rapid local invasion of structures such as the trachea, producing respiratory obstruction.

Medullary carcinoma

This rare tumour arises from parafollicular C cells, which commonly synthesize and secrete calcitonin but may also secrete serotonin, various peptides of the tachykinin family, ACTH and prostaglandins. As a consequence, carcinoid syndrome and Cushing's syndrome have been described in association with medullary carcinoma.

High levels of serum calcitonin are useful diagnostically but produce no clinical effects.

Although medullary carcinoma is most common in the elderly, it also occurs in younger individuals where it is commonly associated with other endocrine tumours—MEN syndromes IIa and IIb (p. 226).

Lymphomas

Non-Hodgkin's B-cell lymphomas occasionally arise in long-standing, autoimmune thyroiditis, especially Hashimoto's disease.

- State the causes of hyperthyroidism.
- Describe the effects of thyrotoxicosis.
- State the causes of hypothyroidism.
- Compare the clinical features of untreated hypothyroidism in the neonate and in the adult.
- Name three types of thyroiditis, and outline their basic features.
- Describe the pathogenesis of Graves' disease and its clinical features.
- What are the types and features of malignant thyroid tumours?

PARATHYROID DISORDERS

Parathyroid hormone (PTH)

PTH is a polypeptide secreted by chief cells of the parathyroid glands (four glands, two in each of the superior and inferior lobes of the thyroid).

The main action of PTH is to increase serum calcium

	Tumour type	Origin of tumour	Frequency (%)	Typical age range (years)	Spread	Prognosis (% for 10-year survival)
differentiated carcinoma	papillary	follicular cells	70	20–40	lymph nodes	90
	follicular	follicular cells	10	40–60	blood stream	60
undifferentiated carcinoma	anaplastic	follicular cells	5	>60	aggressive local invasion; blood stream	1
medullary carcinoma	–	parafollicular C cells	5–10	>40	local, lymphatic and blood	50 (but very variable)
lymphoma	–	lymphocytes	5–10	>60	lymphatic	10

Types and features of malignant thyroid tumours

Fig. 11.10 Types and features of malignant thyroid tumours.

Understanding the physiological functions of PTH is essential towards an understanding of the clinical effects produced by its hypo- or hypersecretion.

and decrease serum phosphate. Its actions are mediated by the bones and kidneys as described below.

In bone, PTH stimulates osteoclastic bone resorption and inhibits osteoblastic bone deposition. The net effect is the release of calcium from bone.

In the kidney, PTH has the following effects:
- Increases calcium reabsorption.
- Decreases phosphate reabsorption.
- Increases 1-hydroxylation of 25-hydroxyvitamin D (i.e. activates vitamin D).

Hyperparathyroidism

Hyperparathyroidism is defined as an elevated secretion of PTH, of which there are three main types:
- Primary: hypersecretion of PTH by adenoma or hyperplasia of gland.
- Secondary: physiological increase in PTH secretions in response to hypocalcaemia of any cause.
- Tertiary: supervention of an autonomous hypersecreting adenoma in long-standing secondary hyperparathyroidism.

Primary hyperparathyroidism

This is the commonest of the parathyroid disorders with a prevalence of about 1 per 800 in the UK. More than 90% of patients are over 50 years of age, and the condition affects females more than males by about 2:1. The aetiology of primary hyperparathyroidism is outlined in Fig. 11.11.

Effects of hyperparathyroidism

The clinical effects are the result of hypercalcaemia and bone resorption (as described below).

Hypercalcaemia:
- Renal stones due to hypercalcuria.
- Excessive calcification of blood vessels.
- Corneal calcification.
- General muscle weakness.
- Tiredness.

- Thirst and polyuria.
- Anorexia and constipation.
- Peptic ulceration (rare) due to enhanced gastrin secretion.

Bone resorption:
- Osteitis fibrosa: increased bone resorption with fibrous replacement in the lacunae.
- 'Brown tumours': haemorrhagic and cystic tumour-like areas in the bone containing large masses of giant osteoclastic cells.
- Osteitis fibrosa cystica (von Recklinghausen's disease of bone): multiple brown tumours combined with osteitis fibrosa.
- Changes may present clinically as bone pain, fracture or deformity.

However, about 50% of patients with biochemical evidence of primary hyperparathyroidism are asymptomatic.
Investigations are:
- Biochemical: increased PTH and Ca^{2+}, and decreased Po_4^{3-}.
- Radiological: 90% normal; 10% show evidence of bone resorption, particularly phalangeal erosions.

Management is by the surgical removal of abnormal parathyroid and by conservative treatment with oral phosphate to reduce plasma calcium.

Secondary hyperparathyroidism

This is compensatory hyperplasia of the parathyroid glands, occurring in response to diseases of low serum calcium or increased serum phosphate.
Its causes are:
- Chronic renal failure and some renal tubular disorders.
- Steatorrhoea and other malabsorption syndromes.
- Osteomalacia and rickets.
- Pregnancy and lactation.

Morphological changes of the parathyroid glands are:
- Enlargement of all parathyroid glands, but to a lesser degree than in primary hyperplasia.
- Increase in 'water clear' cells and chief cells of the parathyroid glands, with loss of stromal fat cells.

Clinical manifestations—Symptoms of bone resorption are dominant.

Renal osteodystrophy

Skeletal abnormalities, arising as a result of raised PTH secondary to chronic renal disease, are known as renal osteodystrophy.

The pathogenesis of renal osteodystrophy is shown in Fig. 11.12.

Abnormalities vary widely according to the nature of the renal lesion, its duration and the age of the patient, but include:

- Osteitis fibrosa (see above).
- Rickets or osteomalacia due to reduced activation of vitamin D.
- Osteosclerosis: increased radiodensity of certain bones, particularly the parts of vertebrae adjacent to the intervertebral discs—'rugger jersey spine'.

Note that the symptoms of hypercalcaemia are not a feature of secondary hyperparathyroidism as calcium levels are usually normal or reduced (PTH is secreted as a compensatory response to reduced calcium levels).

The investigations are both biochemical (raised PTH and normal or lowered Ca^{2+}) and radiological (higher incidence of bone resorption than in primary hyperparathyroidism).

Management is by treatment of the underlying disease, and oral calcium supplements to correct hypocalcaemia.

Tertiary hyperparathyroidism

This condition resulting from chronic overstimulation of the parathyroid glands in renal failure causes one or more of the glands to become an autonomous hypersecreting adenoma with resultant hypercalcaemia.

Fig. 11.13 gives a comparison of primary, secondary and tertiary hyperparathyroidism.

Aetiology of primary hyperparathyroidism		
Type	**Frequency**	**Features**
adenoma	75%	orange–brown, well-encapsulated tumour of variable size but seldom >1 cm diameter tumours are usually solitary, affecting only one of the parathyroids, the others often showing atrophy; they are deep seated and rarely palpable
primary hyperplasia	20%	diffuse enlargement of all the parathyroid glands
parathyroid carcinoma	5%	usually resembles adenoma but is poorly encapsulated and invasive locally

Fig. 11.11 Aetiology of primary hyperparathyroidism.

$$\text{renal disease} \rightarrow \begin{array}{c} \downarrow \text{vit. D activation} \\ + \\ \downarrow Ca^{2+} \text{ reabsorption} \end{array} \rightarrow \downarrow \text{serum } Ca^{2+} \rightarrow \quad \uparrow \text{PTH} \rightarrow \quad \uparrow \text{bone resorption}$$

Fig. 11.12 Pathogenesis of renal osteodystrophy.

Comparison of primary, secondary and tertiary hyperparathyroidism			
	Primary	**Secondary**	**Tertiary**
serum PTH and Ca^{2+}	↑ PTH; ↑ Ca^{2+}	↑ PTH; normal or ↓ Ca^{2+}	↑ PTH; ↑ Ca^{2+}
aetiology	adenoma hyperplasia carcinoma	chronic renal failure malabsorption osteomalacia and rickets pregnancy and lactation	adenoma resulting from overstimulation of glands in secondary hyperthyroidism
predominant effects	hypercalcaemia	increased bone resorption	hypercalcaemia and increased bone resorption

Fig. 11.13 Comparison of primary, secondary, and tertiary hyperparathyroidism.

Hypoparathyroidism

Hypoparathyroidism is a condition of reduced or absent PTH secretion, resulting in hypocalcaemia and hyperphosphataemia.

The causes of hypoparathyroidism are:
- Removal or damage of the parathyroid glands during thyroidectomy: commonest cause of hypothyroidism resulting from inadvertent damage, e.g. by interference with their blood supply, or deliberate removal during surgery of the thyroid gland.
- Autoimmune parathyroid disease: usually occurs in patients who have another autoimmune endocrine disease, e.g. Hashimoto's disease or Addison's disease.
- Congenital deficiency (DiGeorge syndrome): rare, congenital disorder caused by arrested development of the third and fourth branchial arches, resulting in an almost complete absence of the thymus (see Chapter 14) and parathyroid gland.

The effects of hypoparathyroidism are:
- $\downarrow$ release of Ca^{2+} from bones.
- $\downarrow Ca^{2+}$ reabsorption but $\uparrow Po_4^{3-}$ reabsorption by kidney.
- $\downarrow$ 1-hydroxylation of 25-hydroxyvitamin D by kidney.

Most symptoms of hypoparathyroidism are those of hypocalcaemia:
- Tetany: muscular spasm provoked by lowered plasma Ca^{2+}.
- Convulsions.
- Paraesthesiae.
- Psychiatric disturbances, e.g. depression and irritability.
- Rarely: cataracts, alopecia, brittle nails.

Management is by treatment with large doses of oral vitamin D; the acute phase requires intravenous calcium and calcitriol (1,25-dihydroxycholecalciferol, i.e. activated vitamin D).

Multiple endocrine neoplasia (MEN) syndromes

These are syndromes in which patients develop tumours in a number of different endocrine organs. Patients are younger than those who develop single sporadic tumours and usually have a strong family history of multiple endocrine tumours with autosomal dominant inheritance.

There are three main types of MEN syndrome:
- MEN I (Werner's) syndrome.
- MEN IIa (Sipple's) syndrome.
- MEN IIb (sometimes called MEN III) syndrome.

MEN I (Werner's) syndrome

Patients usually show a combination of hyperparathyroidism (usually chief cell hyperplasia), pituitary adenomas, and pancreatic tumours (gastrin and insulin producing). Rarely, there may also be thyroid tumours and adrenal cortical adenomas.

MEN IIa (Sipple's) syndrome

Patients have a combination of phaechromocytoma (50% bilateral) and medullary carcinoma of the thyroid (often bilateral and multinodular). Rarely there may also be hyperparathyroidism due to parathyroid hyperplasia.

MEN IIb (MEN III) syndrome

Patients have all of the features of MEN IIa with additional features of:
- Neuromas and ganglioneuromas in the dermis and submucosal regions throughout the body.
- Marfanoid body habitus with poor muscle development.
- Skeletal abnormalities, e.g. kyphosis, pes cavus and high arch palate.

The facial appearance is characteristic with thick, bumpy lips, broad-based nose, everted eyelids and grossly abnormal dental enamel.

- ○ **State the actions of PTH.**
- ○ **Define primary, secondary and tertiary hyperparathyroidism.**
- ○ **Describe the aetiology and clinical effects of primary hyperparathyroidism.**
- ○ **What are the causes of secondary hyperparathyroidism?**
- ○ **Describe the aetiology and clinical effects of hypoparathyroidism.**
- ○ **Define the multiple endocrine neoplasia syndromes, and name the organs involved in each type.**

DISORDERS OF THE ADRENAL GLAND

Hormones of the adrenal gland
The adrenal gland has two distinct endocrine components derived from different embryonic tissue: the cortex and the medulla.

Cortex
This is the outer part of the gland, derived from the mesoderm, which synthesizes, stores and secretes various cholesterol-derived hormones, namely:
- Glucocorticoid hormones, e.g. hydrocortisone.
- Mineralocorticoid hormones, e.g.aldosterone.
- Sex steroids.

Medulla
This is the inner part of the gland derived from the neuroectoderm, forming part of the sympathetic nervous system. It synthesizes and secretes the vasoactive amines adrenaline and noradrenaline.

Hyperfunction of the adrenal cortex
Cushing's syndrome
The symptoms and signs are associated with prolonged inappropriate elevation of free corticosteroid levels (Fig. 11.14).

Clinical features—The main effects of sustained elevation of glucocorticoid secretion are:

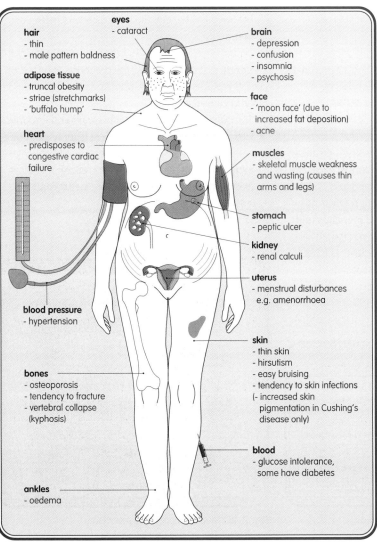

Fig. 11.14
Systemic effects of Cushing's syndrome.

eyes
- cataract

hair
- thin
- male pattern baldness

adipose tissue
- truncal obesity
- striae (stretchmarks)
- 'buffalo hump'

heart
- predisposes to congestive cardiac failure

blood pressure
- hypertension

bones
- osteoporosis
- tendency to fracture
- vertebral collapse (kyphosis)

ankles
- oedema

brain
- depression
- confusion
- insomnia
- psychosis

face
- 'moon face' (due to increased fat deposition)
- acne

muscles
- skeletal muscle weakness and wasting (causes thin arms and legs)

stomach
- peptic ulcer

kidney
- renal calculi

uterus
- menstrual disturbances e.g. amenorrhoea

skin
- thin skin
- hirsutism
- easy bruising
- tendency to skin infections
(- increased skin pigmentation in Cushing's disease only)

blood
- glucose intolerance, some have diabetes

227

The aetiology and clinical features of Cushing's syndrome are common topics in MCQs.

- Central obesity and moon face.
- Plethora and acne.
- Menstrual irregularity.
- Hirsutism and hair thinning.
- Hypertension.
- Diabetes.
- Osteoporosis: may cause collapse of vertebrae, rib fractures.
- Muscle wasting and weakness.
- Atrophy of skin and dermis: paper thin skin with bruising tendency, purple striae.

Aetiopathogenesis—Patients with Cushing's syndrome can be classified into two groups on the basis of whether the aetiology of the condition is ACTH-dependent or independent (Fig. 11.15).

ACTH-dependent aetiology:
- Pituitary hypersecretion of ACTH (Cushing's disease): bilateral adrenal hyperplasia secondary to excessive secretion of ACTH by the pituitary gland (p. 214).
- Ectopic ACTH or CRH production by non-endocrine neoplasm, e.g. oat cell carcinoma of bronchus and some carcinoid tumours. In cases of malignant bronchial tumour, the patient rarely survives long enough to develop any physical features of Cushing's syndrome.

Non-ACTH-dependent aetiology:
- Iatrogenic steroid therapy: commonest cause of Cushing's syndrome.
- Adrenal cortical adenoma: well-circumscribed yellow tumour usually 2–5 cm in diameter. Extremely common as an incidental finding in up to 30% of all post-mortem examinations. Colour is due to stored lipid (mainly cholesterol) from which hormones are synthesized. Vast majority have no clinical effects (i.e. they are non-functioning adenomas), with only a small percentage producing Cushing's syndrome.
- Adrenal cortical carcinoma: rare and almost always associated with the overproduction of hormones, usually glucocorticoids and sex steroids. Patients usually have features of Cushing's syndrome mixed with androgenic effects which are particularly noticeable in women. Tumours are usually large and yellowish-white, and local invasion and metastatic spread are common.

Irrespective of the aetiology, the diagnosis is based on clinical features and the demonstration of a raised plasma cortisol level.

The aetiology of the disorder is elucidated through:
- Dexamethasone suppression test (suppression of cortisol levels in Cushing's disease due to suppression of pituitary ACTH secretion).
- MRI and CT scan visualization of pituitary and adrenal glands.

Classification of Cushing's syndrome	
Type	**Cause**
ACTH-dependent	iatrogenic (ACTH therapy) pituitary hypersecretion of ACTH ectopic ACTH syndrome (benign or malignant non-endocrine tumour)
non-ACTH-dependent	iatrogenic, e.g. prednisolone adrenal cortical adenoma adrenal cortical carcinoma

Fig. 11.15 Classification of Cushing's syndrome.

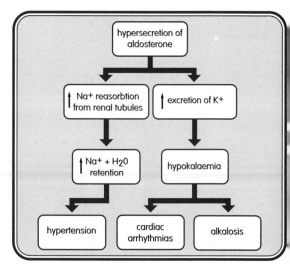

Fig. 11.16 Effects of hyperaldosteronism.

- Analysis of blood ACTH (high = pituitary adenoma or ectopic ACTH source; low = primary adrenal tumour).

Treatment of the underlying cause is essential as untreated Cushing's syndrome has a 50% 5 year mortality rate.

Hyperaldosteronism

Excessive production of aldosterone by the zona glomerulosa of the adrenal cortex results in increased Na^+ retention and increased K^+ loss.

The aetiology is as follows:

- Primary hyperaldosteronism: autonomous hypersecretion of aldosterone which is almost invariably caused by adrenal cortical adenoma (Conn's syndrome).
- Secondary hyperaldosteronism: hypersecretion of aldosterone secondary to an increased production of angiotensin II following activation of the renin–angiotensin system. May be precipitated by congestive cardiac failure, cirrhosis, nephrotic syndrome, hypertension. This is more common than primary form of disorder.

The effects of hyperaldosteronism are shown in Fig. 11.16.

Clinical features are:

- Hypertension: often the only presenting feature. Commonly occurs in the younger age group.
- Hypokalaemia: usually accompanies hypertension and may give rise to polyuria,

nocturia, polydipsia, paraesthesia, muscle weakness or paralysis.

Secondary hyperaldosteronism also has additional features of underlying disease.

Biochemical diagnosis:

- $\uparrow Na^+$, $\downarrow K^+$.
- $\uparrow$ Aldosterone.
- Plasma renin: $\downarrow$ in Conn's syndrome but $\uparrow$ in secondary hyperaldosteronism.

Radiological diagnosis is by visualization of adrenal cortical adenoma by CT scan or MRI.

Management:

- Primary hyperaldosteronism: surgical removal of the affected adrenal.
- Secondary hyperaldosteronism: treatment of the underlying cause.

Congenital adrenal hyperplasia

This rare, autosomal recessive disorder is caused by a deficiency of the enzyme 21-hydroxylase, required for the synthesis of both cortisol and aldosterone. Failure of cortisol production produces an increase in ACTH secretion by the pituitary and hyperplasia of adrenal cortex.

Production of androgens by the adrenal cortex does not require 21-hydroxylase, thus adrenal hyperplasia causes excessive secretion of androgens resulting in masculinization of females and precocious puberty in males. Also, aldosterone deficiency is serious, causing a life-threatening salt loss unless replacement therapy is given.

Hypofunction of the adrenal cortex
Addison's disease

This rare condition of chronic adrenal insufficiency is due to a lack of glucocorticoids and mineralocorticoids. Its estimated prevalence in the developed world is 0.8 cases per 100 000 population.

The clinical features outlined in Fig. 11.17 are a result of glucocorticoid deficiency together with mineralocorticoid insufficiency, loss of adrenal androgen production and increased ACTH secretion.

Aetiology—Autoimmune destruction of the cortex of both adrenals is the commonest cause of Addison's disease. It is often associated with autoimmune thyroid disease, autoimmune gastritis and other endocrine organ autoimmune diseases.

Clinical features of Addison's disease	
Hormonal abnormality	**Clinical features**
glucocorticoid insufficiency	vomiting and loss of appetite weight loss lethargy and weakness postural hypotension hypoglycaemia
mineralocorticoid insufficiency	$\downarrow$ serum Na^+, $\uparrow$ serum K^+ chronic dehydration hypotension
increased ACTH secretion	brownish pigmentation of skin and buccal mucosa
loss of adrenal androgen	decreased body hair, especially in females

Fig. 11.17 Clinical features of Addison's disease.

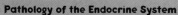
Adrenal insufficiency is also a well-recognized complication of patients with AIDS and may result from a variety of causes, including bilateral adrenal tuberculosis and fungal infections.

Other rarer causes of Addison's disease are adrenal destruction by tumour, haemochromatosis, and amyloidosis.

Biochemical diagnosis:
- Measurement of plasma ACTH and cortisol: ↑ ACTH, ↓ cortisol.
- ACTH stimulation test: ACTH is administered and plasma cortisol levels are monitored. Failure of cortisol levels to rise indicates Addison's disease.
- Plasma electrolytes: ↓ Na⁺, normal or ↑ K⁺, ↑ urea.
- Blood glucose: usually low.
- ↑ Plasma renin activity and normal or ↓ aldosterone.

Management is by glucocorticoid replacement therapy, and usually mineralocorticoid therapy.

Primary acute adrenocortical insufficiency (adrenal crisis)

This may occur as a result of:
- Iatrogenic: abrupt cessation of prolonged high-dose therapeutic corticosteroids (prolonged corticosteroid therapy produces lowered endogenous steroid production, leading to atrophy of the adrenal cortex).
- Bilateral adrenal haemorrhage: caused by Gram-negative (usually meningococcal) septicaemia (Waterhouse–Friderichsen syndrome) and adrenal vein thrombosis secondary to retroperitoneal haemorrhage.
- Complication of chronic adrenal failure: addisonian crisis.

Clinical features are:
- Profound hypotension.
- Vomiting.
- Diarrhoea.
- Abdominal pain.
- Pyrexia.

An adrenal crisis is a medical emergency and requires intravenous hydrocortisone and intravenous fluid. The precipitating cause should be sought and if possible treated.

Secondary adrenocortical insufficiency

This adrenocortical insufficiency is caused by adrenal atrophy secondary to:
- Hypothalamic or pituitary disease (tumours or surgical destruction), which produces lowered ACTH, hence lowered endogenous glucocorticoids and aldosterone.
- Glucocorticoid therapy which produces lowered ACTH (suppression), hence lowered endogenous glucocorticoids and aldosterone.

The adrenal medulla
Phaeochromocytoma

This is a rare tumour of the adrenaline- and noradrenaline-secreting cells (chromaffin cells) of the adrenal medulla (see Chapter 6).

Tumours of extra-adrenal paraganglia
Neuroblastomas

These rare tumours are derived from neuroblasts. Affected sites are the adrenal medulla, the mediastinum (usually in association with the sympathetic chain), and the coeliac plexus.

They are almost exclusively tumours of children, but very rare above 5 years of age, although adult cases do very occasionally occur. The tumour is highly malignant and usually inoperable.

Ganglioneuroma

A benign tumour derived from sympathetic nerves, this is most common in the posterior mediastinum, but 10% of casesarise in the adrenal medulla.

- **Describe the aetiology and features of Cushing's disease.**
- **Describe the aetiology and features of hyperaldosteronism.**
- **What are the clinical effects of congenital adrenal hyperplasia?**
- **Name the diseases associated with hypofunction of the adrenal cortex.**
- **What clinical effects are associated with Addison's disease?**
- **Name the tumours that can affect the adrenal medulla.**

DISORDERS OF THE ENDOCRINE PANCREAS

Diabetes mellitus (DM)

This multisystem disease of an abnormal metabolic state is characterized by hyperglycaemia due to inadequate insulin action/production. DM can be classified into primary and secondary.

Primary DM

A primary disorder of insulin production/action, this accounts for 95% of diabetic cases.

Secondary DM

In 5% of cases diabetes may be secondary to:
- Pancreatic diseases, e.g. chronic pancreatitis or haemochromatosis.
- Hypersecretion of hormones which antagonize the effects of insulin, e.g. glucocorticoids in Cushing's syndrome, growth hormone in acromegaly, adrenaline in phaeochromocytomas.

Primary DM is by far the most important cause of diabetes, and is further classified into:
- Type I, also known as insulin-dependent DM (IDDM) or juvenile onset diabetes.
- Type II, also known as non-insulin-dependent DM (NIDDM) or mature onset diabetes.

The basic features of these two types of diabetes are described in Fig. 11.18.

Type I diabetes mellitus

Aetiology and pathogenesis—Type I diabetes mellitus is an organ-specific, autoimmune-induced disorder characterized by the antibody-mediated destruction of the endocrine cell population of the islet cell of the pancreas.

Two main factors are thought to predispose to autoimmunity:
- Genetic predisposition: patients with type I diabetes are usually HLA-DR3 or HLA-DR4 positive, a feature which is also shown by other organ-specific autoimmune diseases.
- Viral infection: viral infection may trigger the autoimmune reaction; viruses implicated include mumps, measles and Coxsackie B.

One postulated mechanism is that viruses induce mild structural damage to the islet cells thereby altering their antigenicity, and that certain individuals with the genetic predisposition to organ specific autoimmune disease then mount an autoimmune response against the damaged insulin-secreting cells.

Histologically, the pancreas shows lymphocytic infiltration and destruction of insulin-secreting cells of islets of Langerhans. Destruction of insulin-secreting cells results in insulin deficiency with hyperglycaemia and other secondary metabolic complications.

Type II diabetes mellitus

Aetiology and pathogenesis—The precise aetiopathogenesis of type II diabetes is unclear but the following factors are thought to be involved:
- Genetic factors: familial tendency with >90% concordance rate amongst identical twins. However, there are no HLA associations and inheritance is considered to be polygenic.
- Relative insulin deficiency: reduced secretion compared to amounts required, possibly related to islet cell ageing.

Table comparing type I and type II diabetes mellitus (DM)	
Type I	**Type II**
childhood/adolescent onset	middle-aged/elderly onset
1/3 of primary diabetes	2/3 of primary diabetes
females = males	females > males (by 4:1)
acute/subacute onset	gradual onset
thin	obese
ketoacidosis common	ketoacidosis rare
plasma insulin absent or low	plasma insulin normal or raised
insulin sensitive	insulin insensitive (end-organ resistance)
autoimmune mechanism (islet cell antibodies present)	non-autoimmune mechanism (no islet cell antibodies)
genetic predisposition associated with HLA-DR genotype	polygenic inheritance

Fig. 11.18 Table comparing type I and type II diabetes mellitus (DM).

- Insulin resistance: tissues are unable to respond to insulin due to an impairment of the function of insulin receptors on the surface of target cells.

Diagnosis of DM

Irrespective of aetiology, the diagnosis of DM depends on the finding of hyperglycaemia. However, the distribution curve of blood glucose concentration for whole populations is unimodal with no clear division between normal and abnormal values.

Diagnostic criteria (Fig. 11.19) are therefore arbitrary, and in general diabetes mellitus is indicated by either:

- Fasting venous blood glucose level of >7.8 mmol/L.
- Random venous blood glucose level of >11.1 mmol/L.

A distinction is made between diabetes mellitus and impaired glucose tolerance in cases where fasting or random blood sugar level is borderline; in this case, the response to an oral load of glucose can be assessed via a glucose tolerance test.

Complications of DM

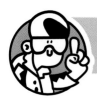

The complications of DM is a common essay question.

Acute complications of DM

Diabetics are particularly prone to several types of coma. These are (in decreasing order of frequency) due to:

- Hypoglycaemia: complication of overtreatment with insulin.
- Ketoacidosis: common in type I diabetes due to ↑ breakdown of triglycerides → ↑ production of ketone bodies → ketoacidosis → impaired consciousness.
- Hyperosmolarity (aketotic or non-ketotic coma): ↑ plasma glucose concentration → ↑ plasma osmolarity → cerebral dehydration → coma. More common in type II diabetes.
- Lactic acidosis: increased concentrations of lactic acid (produced as an end product of glycolysis instead of pyruvate) may cause coma.

Chronic complications of DM

In recent years, with the advent of insulin therapy and various oral hypoglycaemic agents, morbidity and mortality associated with DM are more commonly the result of the chronic rather than the acute complications of the disorder (Fig. 11.20).

The most important chronic complications of diabetes are:

- Vascular disease: atherosclerosis and diabetic microangiopathy.
- Renal disease: diabetic nephropathy.
- Eye disease: diabetic retinopathy.
- Predisposition to infections.
- Peripheral nerve damage: diabetic neuropathy.

Vascular disease

Atherosclerosis—Diabetics suffer from an increased severity of atherosclerosis than non-diabetics of the same age and gender, probably due to the increased plasma levels of cholesterol and triglycerides.

The main clinical sequelae of this are seen in:

- Heart → ischaemic heart disease.
- Brain → cerebral ischaemia.
- Legs and feet → gangrene: ischaemia of toes and areas on the heel is a characteristic feature of diabetic gangrene.
- Kidney → chronic nephron ischaemia, an important component of the multiple renal lesions in diabetes.

Diagnostic criteria for diabetes mellitus using an oral glucose tolerance test		
Diagnosis	**Venous whole blood glucose**	
	fasting sample	2 hours after 75 g glucose load
normal	<5.6 mmol/l	<6.7 mmol/l
impaired glucose tolerance	<6.7 mmol/l	6.7–10 mmol/l
diabetes mellitus	>6.7 mmol/l	>10.0 mmol/l

Fig. 11.19 Diagnostic criteria for diabetes mellitus using an oral glucose tolerance test.

Diabetic microangiopathy—Small arterioles and capillaries show a characteristic pattern of wall thickening, which is due to a marked expansion of the basement membrane termed hyaline arteriolosclerosis.

Abnormality is widespread and contributes to ischaemic changes which are symptomatic in the kidney, the retina, the brain and peripheral nerves.

Diabetic nephropathy

Diabetes is now one of the most common causes of end-stage renal failure. Associated renal disease can be divided into three forms:

- Complications of diabetic vascular disease: atherosclerosis (atheroma affecting aorta and renal arteries → ischaemia); diabetic microangiopathy (glomerular capillary basement membrane thickening [hyaline arteriolosclerosis] → ischaemic glomerular damage).
- Diabetic glomerulosclerosis (diffuse and nodular types): ↑ leakage of plasma proteins through capillary wall into glomerular filtrate → proteinuria and progressive glomerular hyalinization with eventual chronic renal failure.
- Increased susceptibility to infections → papillary necrosis. Acute pyelonephritis is a common

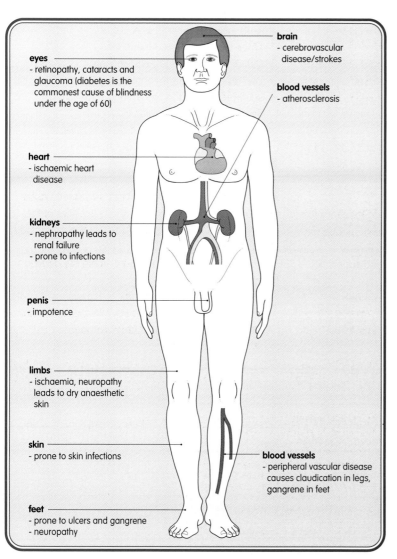

Fig. 11.20 Chronic complications of diabetes mellitus.

brain
- cerebrovascular disease/strokes

eyes
- retinopathy, cataracts and glaucoma (diabetes is the commonest cause of blindness under the age of 60)

blood vessels
- atherosclerosis

heart
- ischaemic heart disease

kidneys
- nephropathy leads to renal failure
- prone to infections

penis
- impotence

limbs
- ischaemia, neuropathy leads to dry anaesthetic skin

skin
- prone to skin infections

blood vessels
- peripheral vascular disease causes claudication in legs, gangrene in feet

feet
- prone to ulcers and gangrene
- neuropathy

complication of diabetes mellitus and occurs as a result of the relative immune suppression seen in diabetics together with reduced neutrophil function.

Eye disease

Diabetes is the commonest cause of acquired blindness in the Western world, and can affect the eyes in five main ways:

- Background retinopathy: small vessel abnormalities in retina leading to hard exudates, haemorrhages and microaneurysms. Does not usually affect acuity.
- Proliferative retinopathy: extensive proliferation of new capillaries in the retina. Sudden deterioration in vision may result from vitreous haemorrhage from the proliferating new vessels or the development of retinal detachment.
- Maculopathy: caused by oedema, hard exudates or retinal ischaemia and causes marked reduction in acuity.
- Cataract formation: greatly increased incidence in diabetics.
- Glaucoma: increased incidence in diabetics due to neovascularization of the iris (rubeosis iridis).

Predisposition to infections

Patients with diabetes have an increased tendency to develop infections, usually of a bacterial or fungal nature. The main target organs are:

- Skin: folliculitis, erysipelas, cellulitis and superficial fungal infections.
- Oral and genital mucosae: especially with *Candida*.
- Urinary tract: increased predisposition to acute

pyelonephritis, often associated with recurrent lower urinary tract infections.

Diabetic neuropathy

This is possibly due to a disease of the small vessels supplying the nerves (see Chapter 6, p. 65).

Management of DM

The primary aim of treatment is to maintain a normal or near normal blood glucose level at all times. The closer the blood glucose concentration is kept to normal, the more normal the body's total metabolic profile and the lower the incidence of vascular disease. Regardless of the aetiology, the type of treatment required is determined by the circulating plasma insulin concentration.

Three methods of treatment are:

- Diet alone: 50% of diabetic patients.
- Diet and oral hypoglycaemic drugs, e.g. sulphonylureas and biguanides—20–30% of diabetic patients.
- Diet and insulin: 20–30% of diabetic patients.

Islet cell tumours

These tumours are rare compared to those of the exocrine pancreas, and occur most commonly in the 30–50 year age group.

Insulinomas

The commonest islet cell tumours, these are derived from pancreatic β-cells:

- Produce hypoglycaemia through hypersecretion of insulin.
- May produce permanent brain damage.

Summary of islet cell tumours		
Islet cell tumour	Occurrence	Clinical features
insulinoma	70–75%	hypoglycaemia
gastrinoma	20–25%	Zollinger–Ellison syndrome: gastric hypersecretion, multiple peptic ulcers and diarrhoea
VIPoma	rare	watery diarrhoea, hypokalaemia and achlorhydria
glucagonoma	rare	secondary diabetes mellitus, necrolytic migratory erythema and uraemia
somatostatinoma	rare	diabetes mellitus, cholelithiasis and steatorrhoea

Fig. 11.21 Summary of islet cell tumours.

- Majority are solitary, non-metastasizing lesions (10% are multiple and 10% are malignant).

Zollinger–Ellison syndrome

This syndrome of gastric hypersecretion, multiple peptic ulcers and diarrhoea is caused by the gastrin-secreting tumour (gastrinoma) of the pancreatic G-cells. Tumours are multiple in 50% of cases, and are often malignant, with 10–20% occurring in other sites, e.g. the duodenum.

It may also be part of the MEN I syndrome, with adenomas also present in other endocrine glands (see p. 226).

Other islet cell tumours

For a summary of islet cell tumours see Fig. 11.21.

VIPomas

These produce vasoactive intestinal polypeptide (VIP), resulting in a syndrome of watery diarrhoea, hypokalaemia and achlorhydria (WDHA).

Glucagonomas

These glucagon-secreting tumours are derived from pancreatic α-cells and produce secondary diabetes mellitus (usually mild), necrolytic migratory erythema (skin rash) and uraemia.

Somatostatinomas

These somatostatin-producing tumours derived from pancreatic δ-cells are associated with diabetes mellitus, cholelithiasis and steatorrhoea.

- **Compare the pathogenesis and features of type I and type II diabetes mellitus.**
- **What are the causes of secondary diabetes mellitus?**
- **What are the diagnostic criteria for diabetes mellitus?**
- **List the acute and the chronic complications of diabetes mellitus.**
- **Name the types of islet cell tumours, and describe their clinical features.**

DISORDERS OF THE VULVA, VAGINA, AND CERVIX

Infections of the lower genital tract
Bartholin's cyst
This common, benign, mucus-secreting cyst is on the vulva derived from Bartholin's glands (mucus-secreting glands in the posterior part of the labia majora). Frequently there is superimposed infection—Bartholin's abscess.

Viral infection
Viral infections of the vulval skin are typically due to either herpes simplex virus (HSV) or human papillomavirus (HPV).

HSV
HSV infection of the vulva (herpes vulvitis) produces initially painless blisters, which subsequently break down to form a painful, sore, eroded area. Infection is acquired through sexual contact and disease is more common in young women.

HPV
This sexually transmitted disease may present with a thickening of the vulval skin and mucosa (flat condyloma) in the labia minora, or as multiple protuberant warts (condylomata acuminata) which may be either sessile or pedunculated. There is a strong link between HPV infections of the vulva and intra-epithelial neoplastic change in both the vulva (see below) and cervix.

Bacterial and protozoal infections
Gardnerella vaginalis
This Gram-negative coccobacillus is often associated with other sexually spread infections. The patient complains of a foul-smelling discharge, which is thin, greyish and sometimes shows bubbles. Examination confirms both the discharge and the odour.

Chlamydia trachomatis
The main feature of this disease is the production of painful superficial groin nodes (lymphogranuloma venereum) which may rupture through the skin. It is preceded by a painless vulval ulceration which is often overlooked. Later, chronic lymphatic obstruction leads to non-pitting oedema of the external genitalia.

Trichomonas vaginalis
This sexually transmitted flagellated protozoan organism is typically asymptomatic in men, but in women it often produces an intensely irritating vaginal discharge with inflammation of the vulva, vagina and cervix. The discharge is often frothy and offensive.

Treponema pallidum
A sexually transmitted spirochaetal bacterium responsible for syphilis, this disease typically involves three stages (primary, secondary, and tertiary):
- Primary: small indurated lesions (chancres) develop at the site of entry of the organism (vulva, vagina, glans of penis, or perianal area).
- Secondary: characterized by multiple, moist, warty, vulvovaginal and perineal lesions (condylomata lata). There is often a papular eruption on the trunk, limbs, palms and soles with generalized lymphadenopathy.
- Tertiary: involves the CNS (see Chapter 6).

Fungal and yeast infection
Fungal infections are usually caused by either superficial dermatophytes or *Candida albicans*. There is usually associated fungal vaginitis presenting with a copious vaginal discharge and vulval reddening and soreness.

Candida albicans
This is a normal commensal of the vagina, but its proliferation is usually suppressed by normal vaginal flora. (*Candida* was formerly known as *Monilia*.)
Conditions that predispose to candidial overgrowth are:
- Pregnancy/oestrogen contraceptives: high concentration of oestrogens in the blood.
- Immunosuppressive therapy, e.g. cytotoxic drugs and corticosteroids.

- Glycosuria, e.g. diabetes, pregnancy (due to lowering of the renal threshold for sugar).
- Antibiotic therapy: destruction of normal commensal bacteria.
- Chronic anaemia: iron stores are needed to maintain an adequate immune reaction.

The organism can also be sexually transmitted.

Macroscopically, white plaques of fungal hyphae develop on inflamed vaginal mucosa, and vaginal discharge is associated with severe vulval irritation. Infections are often severe in diabetics.

Dermatophytes

Infection of vulval skin with dermatophytic fungi produces a similar superficial inflammation and soreness.

Both candida and dermatophytes can be treated with fungicidal pessaries or systemic therapy.

Fig. 12.1 shows a table of the organisms that cause infections of the lower genital tract.

Dysplastic and neoplastic disorders of the vulva and vagina

Tumours of the vulva

Squamous cell carcinoma

This typically occurs in elderly women, and may show extensive local invasion and metastases in inguinal lymph nodes. The majority of cases appear to arise *de novo*, but some arise in epithelium in which there is severe dysplasia amounting to carcinoma in-situ, known as vulval intraepithelial neoplasia.

Organisms that cause infections of the lower genital tract	
Infection	**Organism**
viruses	HPV HSV
bacteria	*Gardnerella vaginalis* *Chlamydia trachomatis* (lymphogranuloma venereum) *Treponema pallidum* (syphilis)
protozoa	*Trichomonas vaginalis*
fungi and yeast	dermatophytes, *Candida albicans*

Fig. 12.1 Organisms that cause infections of the lower genital tract.

Vulval intra-epithelial neoplasia (VIN)

This is generally seen in patients younger than those with invasive tumours. There is often coexistent evidence of HPV warty change in the affected and adjacent epithelium. Although invasive carcinoma and VIN do occasionally coexist in elderly women, it is thought that progression of VIN to invasive carcinoma is not common.

Tumours of the vagina

Dysplastic

Vaginal intra-epithelial neoplasia (VAIN)

This is rare compared to cervical intra-epithelial neoplasia (CIN). Most cases are found in women previously treated for CIN or invasive cervical cancer.

Neoplastic

Primary malignant tumours of the vagina are extremely rare, but include squamous cell carcinomas and adenocarcinomas.

Secondary tumours are more common, particularly from malignant tumours of the cervix, endometrium and ovary. Vaginal bleeding after hysterectomy for uterine or ovarian malignancy should always be investigated and biopsied because of the frequency of metastatic tumour in the residual vaginal vault.

Inflammation of the cervix

Acute and chronic cervicitis

Acute cervicitis

There is acute inflammation of the cervix with erosion. It is occasionally seen in herpes simplex infection, typically with herpetic disease of the vulva and vagina.

Chronic cervicitis

This chronic inflammation of the cervix is typically caused by the same organisms responsible for infective vaginitis: *Trichomonas, Candida, Gardnerella*, and the gonococci. It is characterized by a heavy plasma cell and lymphocytic infiltrate.

Endocervical polyps

These common abnormalities derived from the endocervix affect about 5% of women. Polyps protrude from the cervix through the external os, and may cause intermenstrual bleeding from erosion and ulceration.

Macroscopically, these are smooth, rounded or pear-shaped polyps about 1–2 cm in diameter.

Microscopically, they are composed of endocervical stroma and glands. The surface of the polyp may show ulceration and inflammation and, if long standing, there may be surface squamous metaplasia.

Neoplasia of the cervix
Cervical intra-epithelial neoplasia (CIN)
This is the preneoplastic (dysplastic) proliferation of the metaplastic epithelium of the transformation zone of the cervix.

Aetiology—There is a strong association with HPV infection.

Risk factors are:
- Sexual intercourse: there is a very low incidence in virgins.
- Early age at first intercourse: there is a higher incidence in girls who have intercourse before the age of 17.
- Sexually transmitted diseases: there is a higher incidence in women with a history of sexually transmitted diseases.
- Smoking: there is a higher risk in women who smoke tobacco.
- Human papillomavirus: coexistence of HPV with CIN and invasive carcinoma in cone biopsy and colposcopy specimens suggests a link. DNA from HPV types 16, 18 and 33 has been identified in over 60% of cervical carcinomas. Proteins produced by HPV are thought to inactivate products of tumour suppressor genes thereby facilitating tumour development.
- HIV infection: carcinoma of the cervix is predisposed by immunosuppression and has increased in incidence as a consequence of AIDS.

Classification
Three grades of severity are recognized dependent upon what proportion of the thickness of the cervical epithelium is replaced by atypical cells.
- CIN I (mild dysplasia): upper two-thirds of epithelium normal, basal third atypical cells.
- CIN II (moderate dysplasia): upper half of epithelium normal, atypical cells occupy the lower half.
- CIN III (severe dysplasia): corresponds to carcinoma in-situ. Atypical cells extend throughout the full thickness of the epithelium with minimal differentiation and maturation on the surface.

Progression of CIN
CIN is associated with a risk of progression to an invasive carcinoma, the risk for CIN I being lowest, and for CIN III being highest.

The natural history of CIN is important as it determines how often screening is required to detect progression of the disease.

Screening for CIN
The aim of screening is to detect atypical cells in the preinvasive stage of the disease by cytological examination of a smear of surface epithelial cells removed from the cervix. It has been suggested that smears repeated every three years are adequate for the purposes of population screening.

Management is by the local destruction of abnormal epithelium by cryotherapy, laser therapy or cone biopsy following histological confirmation of its nature.

Cervical intra-epithelial neoplasia is the classic example of a preneoplastic condition that can be identified by screening and managed effectively to prevent development of invasive cervical carcinoma.

Squamous cell carcinoma
The vast majority of cervical carcinomas are squamous cell carcinomas arising from the transformation zone or ectocervix.

Incidence is 3800 new cases of cervical cancer each year in England and Wales, with about 2000 deaths per year. This type of carcinoma occurs in all ages from late teens onwards, but the average age is 50 years.

The carcinoma is preceded by the preinvasive phase of CIN (see above). Risk factors are as for CIN.

Macroscopically, tumours demonstrate the following features:
- Early: areas of granular irregularity of the cervical epithelium, progressive invasion of the stroma causing abnormal hardness of the cervix.
- Late: fungating ulcerated areas, which destroy the cervix.

Microscopically, lesions fall into three histological patterns:

- Keratinizing, large cell squamous carcinoma (40%).
- Non-keratinizing, large cell squamous carcinoma (50%).
- Non-keratinizing, small cell squamous carcinoma (10%).

The common presenting symptom is vaginal bleeding in the early stages, but advanced neglected tumours may cause urinary obstruction due to bladder involvement.

Invasive carcinomas are managed according to the degree of local invasion and survival is related to the stage of the disease (Fig. 12.2).

Invasive carcinoma is usually managed by radical surgery and/or radiotherapy and/or chemotherapy depending on the stage of the disease.

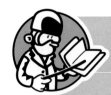

- Name the common infections of the lower genital tract.
- What conditions predispose to candidal overgrowth?
- Name the tumours of the vulva and vagina.
- What are the causes of acute and chronic cervicitis?
- List the risk factors for CIN and squamous cell carcinoma of the cervix.
- Describe the histological criteria for the grading of CIN I to III.

DISORDERS OF THE UTERUS AND ENDOMETRIUM

Inflammatory disorders
Chronic endometritis
An inflammation of the endometrium, this is typically associated with menstrual irregularities and often found in women who are being investigated for infertility.

Microscopically, there is lymphoid and plasma cell infiltration of the endometrium.

Risk factors—The majority of cases are associated with a definite clinical risk factor for developing inflammation:

- Recent pregnancy, miscarriage or instrumentation (50% of cases).
- Pelvic inflammatory disease, e.g. salpingitis (25% of cases).
- Previous use of intrauterine contraceptive devices (about 20% of cases).
- Gonococcal or chlamydial infection or TB (5% of cases).

Disorders of the endometrium
Adenomyosis
A condition in which the endometrium grows down to develop deep within the myometrium. This may cause enlargement of the uterus and is sometimes associated with menstrual abnormalities and dysmenorrhoea.

Macroscopically there are small, irregular, endometrial lesions, some of which are cystic, which can be seen within the affected myometrium. Involvement of the myometrium may be diffuse (more common) or focal with deep nodules of endometrium (nodular adenomyosis).

Microscopically, islands of endometrium are found deep within muscle but in continuity with surface endometrium.

Endometriosis
There is ectopic growth of the endometrium outside the uterus which still responds to cyclical hormonal stimulation. Phases of proliferation and breakdown are associated with the development of the fibrous adhesions

Stages and prognosis for carcinomas of the cervix		
Stage	5-year survival (%)	Degree of local invasion
I	90	confined to cervix
II	75	invasion of upper part of vagina or adjacent parametrial tissues
III	30	spread to pelvic side wall, lower vagina or ureters
IV	10	invasion of rectum, bladder wall or outside pelvis

Fig. 12.2 Stages and prognosis for carcinomas of the cervix.

and accumulation of haemosiderin pigment. This affects 1 in 15 women of reproductive age. There are numerous sites:

- Common: ovaries, fallopian tubes, round ligaments, pelvic peritoneum.
- Less common: intestinal wall, bladder, umbilicus, laparotomy scars.
- Rare: lymph nodes, lung, pleura.

Theories of origin

The aetiopathogenesis of endometriosis remains unclear, but there are three main theories.

Retrograde menstruation

During menstruation, fragments of endometrium migrate along the fallopian tubes into the peritoneal cavity. In normal women, the immune system destroys this material. However, in women susceptible to endometriosis the immune surveillance is absent, and ectopic endometrium implants within the peritoneal cavity.

Metaplasia of peritoneal epithelium

This sees the differentiation of peritoneal epithelium into endometrium. It may also cause the development of a fallopian tube-type epithelium, causing the related condition of endosalpingosis. The stimulus for such metaplasia remains uncertain.

Metastatic spread of endometrium

Endometrium found in the nodes, pleura, lungs and umbilicus is spread by the lymphatics or blood vessels.

None of these hypotheses alone explains endometriosis in all of its manifestations and it is likely that all three mechanisms are operative to differing degrees.

Macroscopically, the foci of endometriosis appear as cystic and solid masses, which are characteristically dark brown due to accumulated iron pigment from repeated bleeding.

Microscopically, solid masses of endometriosis are composed of endometrial glands and stroma, fibrosis, and macrophages containing iron pigments.

Endometriosis may present with cyclical pelvic pain, dysmenorrhoea and infertility.

The complications are:

- Infertility (about 30% of cases): may be due to inability of the ovaries to ovulate; ovulation occurring into closed off areas of fibrosis; damage to tubal fimbria; kinking of tubes by adhesions; blockage of tube by deposits of endometriosis in the wall.
- Bowel obstruction: ectopic endometrial tissue stimulates fibrosis and may cause fibrous adhesions between adjacent organs.
- Chocolate cysts: whole of fallopian tube and ovary may be converted into a cystic mass containing brown, semi-liquid material.

Endometriosis is dependent on oestrogen for continued growth and proliferation, with the disease becoming inactive after oophorectomy or onset of the menopause. Thus, induction of the hypo-oestrogenic state by suppression of the hypothalamic–pituitary–ovarian axis with analogues of gonadotrophin-releasing hormone is effective in many cases.

Functional endometrial disorders
Anovulatory cycle

A menstrual cycle which is not associated with the development and release of the ovum from the ovary, this is normal and common at both the start and end of reproductive life. Several follicles may start to develop and for a time produce hormones. However, the attempt ends in atresia and the atretic follicle is absorbed.

It is associated with irregular menstruation, although the effects of excessive oestrogen stimulation are manifest in the endometrium as the proliferation of glands.

Other causes of anovulation are listed in Fig. 12.3.

Inadequate luteal phase

The irregular ripening of a follicle is associated with infertility. This may be caused by failure of the production of progesterone by the corpus luteum or by defective receptors for progesterone within the endometrium. Examination of the endometrium in the second half of the menstrual cycle shows inadequate or absent development of secretory changes.

Effects of oral contraceptives

Oral contraceptive pills cause changes in the structure of the endometrium, which is greatly reduced in bulk.

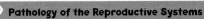

Glands become small and inactive with poor development of stroma.

Menopausal changes

The menopause is the cessation of menstruation which normally occurs between 45 and 56 years. It occurs as a result of a lack of primordial follicles because all have been used, and because of a more refractory receptor function in the granulosa and thecal cells.

Associated endometrial changes

The endometrial glands are lined by inactive cuboidal cells and may form large cystic spaces. There is no evidence of mitotic activity, reflecting a lack of oestrogenic stimulation. The uterus becomes smaller and is less supported due to atrophy of the cardinal, uterosacral and uteropubic ligaments.

Endometrial hyperplasia

Hyperplasia of the endometrium typically occurs in the third and fourth decades, in response to oestrogenic stimulation. It presents with haemorrhage, but the severity or frequency is not related to the degree of pathological change.

Fig. 12.4 shows the different types of endometrial hyperplasia.

Non-physiological causes of anovulation		
Type	**Cause**	**Clinical feature**
primary ovarian dysfunction	genetic	e.g. Turner's syndrome, autoimmune
secondary ovarian dysfunction	disorders of gonadotrophin regulation	hyperprolactinaemia
	gonadotrophin deficiency	pituitary tumour pituitary infarction pituitary ablation
	functional	weight loss exercise
	polycystic ovary syndrome	–

Fig. 12.3 Non-physiological causes of anovulation.

Types of endometrial hyperplasia			
Degree of hyperplasia	**Morphological features**	**Progression to adenocarcinoma (%)**	**Time taken (years) to develop into adenocarcinoma**
mild (most common)	cystic glandular hyperplasia with characteristic appearance of 'Swiss cheese'. (Previously known as metropathia haemorrhagica.) Cells show no cytological atypia	1	10
moderate	crowding of glands in a back-to-back fashion. Epithelium is stratified and mitoses are relatively frequent. Cells show no cytological atypia	5	7
severe	cellular atypia is prominent, glands are distorted by intraglandular polypoid formations, and mitosis are frequent	30	4

Fig. 12.4 Types of endometrial hyperplasia.

The importance of endometrial hyperplasia is that it is associated with an increased risk of the development of endometrial adenocarcinoma, i.e. it is thought to be preneoplastic.

Neoplastic disorders

Benign

Endometrial polyps

These localized overgrowths of endometrial glands and stroma are very common and are typically seen in the perimenopausal age range. They are thought to be caused by over-proliferation of glands in response to oestrogenic stimuli.

Macroscopically, they are found in the uterine fundus; their size is variable but they are usually 1–3 cm in diameter and have a firm, smooth, nodular appearance within the endometrial cavity, but occasionally prolapse through the cervical os. They may develop ulceration or undergo torsion.

Microscopically, they are cystically dilated endometrial glands in a vascular stroma.

Clinical features are associated with menstrual abnormalities and dysmenorrhoea.

Fibroids (leiomyomas)

These benign, smooth muscle tumours arise in the muscle wall of the uterus. They are the commonest of all pelvic tumours, affecting over half of all women over the age of 30, usually becoming symptomatic in the decade before the menopause. Their cause is unknown but risk factors include:

- Age: rare under 30 years.
- Race: more common in Afro-Caribbean populations.
- Parity: more common in nulliparous and women with low fertility.
- Genetic: often a family history.

Leiomyomas have the following features:

- Oestrogen sensitive.
- Fast growing in pregnancy.
- Shrink: at menopause or with antigonadotrophic hormone therapy.

Sites within the uterus (Fig. 12.5) are:

- Subserous: just beneath the peritoneum on the outer uterine surface.
- Interstitial (most common): surrounded by smooth muscle.
- Submucous: lying immediately below the endometrium.

Macroscopically, they are:

- Rounded, rubbery, pale nodules with whorled appearance on cut surface.
- Well circumscribed with pseudocapsule and may become pedunculated forming polyps.
- Size is variable. Most common are 2–4 cm (but range from <1 cm up to 20–30 cm in diameter).
- Typically multiple.

Remember that fibroids are not fibromas, but are benign tumours of smooth muscle (leiomyomas).

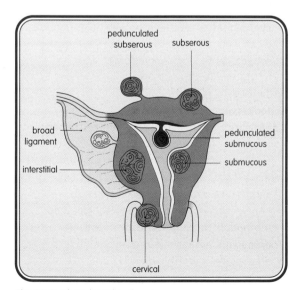

Fig. 12.5 Fibroids within the uterus.

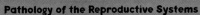

Microscopically, they are seen as:
- Islands of smooth muscle cells with intervening collagenous stroma.
- Lacking cellular atypia and with very few mitoses.
- Several rare histological variants, e.g. myxoid.

Clinical features—Leiomyomas may present with abnormal menstrual bleeding, dysmenorrhoea, and infertility.

Complications are:
- Ischaemic degeneration: uterine fibroids frequently outgrow their blood supply especially in pregnancy. Pedunculated tumours may undergo torsion, developing venous infarction. Lesions become soft and uniformly dark red (so-called 'red degeneration').
- Pregnancy: during pregnancy leiomyomas may cause complications such as spontaneous abortion, premature labour, or obstruction of labour.
- Compression: may cause problems because of their effects as a large abdominal mass, e.g. compressing the bladder.

Investigations are by ultrasound and laparoscopy.

Management is:
- Surgical: women who no longer wish to conceive usually undergo hysterectomy.
- Medical: uterine leiomyomas depend on oestrogen for maintenance of size, thus the treatment of women whose families are incomplete is aimed at inducing shrinkage of fibroids with GnRH agonists, which induce hypo-oestrogenism. Allows easier surgical removal by myomectomy.

Malignant

Endometrial carcinoma

Adenocarcinomas of the endometrium are extremely common tumours, accounting for about 7% of all cancers in women. The mean age of presentation is 56 years, and 80% of women are postmenopausal.

Endometrial carcinoma is associated with:
- Hyperoestrogenic state: obesity, diabetes, late menopause, prolonged use of unopposed oestrogens, oestrogen-secreting tumours.
- Previous pelvic irradiation.
- Lower parity.

There are two main groups—hyperoestrogenic and non-hyperoestrogenic tumours.

Hyperoestrogenic tumours
These are associated with a generally good prognosis and occur in patients close to the menopause, associated with an abnormal oestrogenic stimulation of the endometrium and endometrial hyperplasia. Most tumours are adenocarcinomas (60%) and are graded (I–III) according to the amount of glandular and solid pattern within the tumour. High grade is associated with a worse prognosis.

Non-hyperoestrogenic tumours
These are more often associated with a poor prognosis, occur in older postmenopausal women, and are not associated with oestrogenic stimulation or endometrial hyperplasia.

Macroscopically, there are:
- Small tumours: diffuse, solid areas or polypoid lesions in the endometrium.
- Larger tumours: fill and distend the endometrial cavity with soft, white, friable tissue.

Microscopically, they are seen as:
- Hyperoestrogenic tumours: typically well-differentiated adenocarcinomas composed of hyperplastic endometrial glandular tissue with only superficial myometrial invasion at diagnosis.
- Non-hyperoestrogenic tumours: typically poorly differentiated with deep myometrial invasion.

The condition may present with postmenopausal bleeding, blood-stained discharge, and irregular bleeding of all cases.

The main route of spread is by local invasion to the fallopian tubes, ovaries, bladder or rectum.

If venous and lymphatic invasion occurs, there may be involvement of the vagina and para-aortic nodes. Widespread haematogenous metastasis is uncommon except with papillary serous carcinomas and clear cell carcinomas.

Invasion into the myometrium is closely correlated with the prognosis—those with small invasive depth having a better prognosis than those with deeper involvement.

The prognosis of uterine carcinoma is related to stage (Fig. 12.6).

Clinical staging of endometrial cancer			
Stage	Proportion of cases (%)	Degree of invasion	5-year survival (%)
I	80	Corpus of uterus only	75
II	5	Corpus and cervix	52
III	5	Invasion confined to pelvis	30
IV	10	Invasion outside pelvis or involves bladder or rectal mucosa	10

Fig. 12.6 Clinical staging of endometrial cancer.

- ○ Define 'endometriosis' and 'endometritis'.
- ○ List the clinical features and complications of endometriosis.
- ○ What is endometrial hyperplasia and why is it important?
- ○ Define 'fibroids' and describe their characteristics.
- ○ Name the two groups of endometrial carcinomas.

DISORDERS OF THE OVARY AND FALLOPIAN TUBES

Inflammatory disorders and infections
Salpingitis
This is inflammation of the fallopian tube(s).

Suppurative salpingitis
Aetiology—It is almost always caused by ascending infection from the uterine cavity.

Predisposing factors are:
- Following pregnancy and endometritis.
- Intrauterine contraceptive device (IUCD) use.
- Sexually transmitted disease (*Mycoplasma*, *Chlamydia* and gonococci).
- *Actinomyces*: colonization of the genital tract in association with use of IUCDs.

Macroscopically, tubes are swollen and congested, and the serosal surface appears red and granular due to vascular dilatation.

Microscopically, tubal epithelium shows neutrophil infiltration and the lumen may contain pus.

Chronic inflammation may supervene with sequelae of fibrosis and occlusion of the tubal lumen on resolution.

Complications are:
- Infertility: fibrosis causes distortion of mucosal plicae and occlusion of tubal lumen.
- Pyosalpinx: massive distension of tubal lumen by pus.
- Hydrosalpinx: dilatation of a fallopian tube by clear watery fluid with flattening of the mucosa. Acquired with healing of previous inflammation.

Tuberculous salpingitis
This is a tuberculous infection of the fallopian tubes.

Its aetiology is the haematogenous spread of *Mycobacterium tuberculosis* from a site outside the genital tract.

Tubes develop multiple granulomas in the mucosa and wall, causing adhesions to adjacent tissues (especially ovaries). In advanced cases, tubes may develop into cavities filled with caseous necrotic material.

Pelvic inflammatory disease (PID)
This combined infection of the fallopian tubes, ovaries and peritoneum is typically a result of ascending infection, or less commonly postoperative infection. Predisposing factors are as for suppurative salpingitis (see above).

Neisseria gonorrhoea and *Chlamydia trachomatis* are the most common responsible organisms although anaerobic organisms are often found in pelvic abscesses.

Inflammation is initially acute, and without prompt treatment may progress to chronic PID with associated complications of tubal oedema, development of adhesions within tubes, hydrosalpinx or pyosalpinx (see above).

Clinical features are:
- Symptoms: gradual onset of pelvic pain, irregular bleeding, fever.
- Signs: abdominal tenderness and guarding, extreme tenderness of the vaginal fornices.

Treatment is by the removal of the IUCD (if present) and the use of broad spectrum antibiotics.

Cysts of the ovary and fallopian tubes
Ovarian cysts
Ovarian cystic lesions are extremely common, and can be either neoplastic or non-neoplastic. The majority of non-neoplastic cysts arise from developing Graafian follicles; a minority are derived from surface epithelium.

Follicular cysts
These unruptured, enlarged Graafian follicles are lined by granulosa cells, with an outer coat of thecal cells. Normal ovaries commonly contain one or more small cysts (<5 cm in diameter), which typically disappear by the resorption of fluid. However, multiple follicular cysts are found in:
- Metropathia haemorrhagica: cystic hyperplasia of the endometrium.
- Polycystic ovary syndrome (see below).

Most cysts are clinically insignificant though some may be a cause of hyperoestrogenism.

Luteal cysts (luteinized follicular cysts)
These are similar to follicular cysts, except the thecal coat is luteinized. The cyst is lined by an inner layer of large luteinized granulosa cells and an outer layer of smaller luteinized thecal cells.

Polycystic ovary syndrome (Stein–Leventhal syndrome)
This is a complex adrenal–ovarian disorder in which multiple small follicular cysts develop beneath a thickened, white ovarian capsule as a result of increased secretion of androgens from the adrenal glands or ovaries or both.

Clinical features—Patients have a persistent anovulatory state, high levels of LH and oestrogen, and low levels of FSH with high levels of circulating androgen. There is insulin resistance and hyperinsulinism.

Common presenting symptoms are:
- Menstrual irregularity.
- Infertility.
- Hirsutism.
- Acne.
- Occasional galactorrhoea.

Complications—High oestrogen levels may cause endometrial hyperplasia and increase the risk of the development of endometrial carcinoma.

Cysts of the fallopian tubes
Benign cysts of the fallopian tubes are common. There are two main types:
- Fimbrial cysts: extremely common, small, benign cysts containing clear fluid. Unilocular and typically situated at the fimbrial end of the tube.
- Cysts of Morgagni (paratubal cysts): cystic lesions situated adjacent to the fimbrial ends of the fallopian tubes and thought to be derived from remnants of the Wolffian duct.

Neoplastic disorders of the ovary
Ovarian cancer is responsible for more deaths than any other gynaecological malignancy, largely because it often presents at an advanced stage.

Primary ovarian cancers account for 5% of all malignancies in women. There are several different types.

A logical way of classifying ovarian tumours is according to the normal tissue constituents from which they are derived:
- **Surface epithelial tumours (70% of all cases).**
- **Germ cell tumours (20% of all cases).**
- **Sex cord and stromal tumours (10% of all cases).**

Surface epithelial–stromal tumours

Epithelial tumours of the ovary comprise about 70% of all ovarian tumours and about 90% of malignant tumours. They are typically found in adult life.

The aetiology is uncertain but there is a higher incidence among women of higher social classes, and a decreased risk conferred by pregnancy and the oral contraceptive pill.

Types—Epithelial tumours are derived from surface epithelium which is in turn derived from embryonal coelomic epithelium. Tumours with this origin can differentiate along different pathways into different types of tumours:

- Tubal differentiation: serous ovarian tumours.
- Endometrial differentiation: endometrioid and clear cell ovarian tumours.
- Endocervical differentiation: mucinous ovarian tumours.
- Transitional differentiation: Brenner tumour.

Microscopically, these tumours are classified into benign, malignant, and borderline malignancy (abnormal tissue architecture with atypical cells but no evidence of invasion). The majority behave in a benign fashion, the remainder behaving as low-grade malignant tumours.

Serous tumours of the ovary

These ovarian cystic tumours of tubal differentiation contain a watery fluid; the majority (70%) are benign.

Benign (serous cystadenoma)

Macroscopically, this is a thin-walled, unilocular cystic tumour. It is bilateral in about 10% of cases. Microscopically, it is lined by cuboidal regular epithelium.

Malignant (serous cystadenocarcinoma)

This is the most common form of ovarian carcinoma.

Macroscopically, it is bilateral in about 50% of cases, and may be cystic, mixed solid and cystic, or largely solid.

Microscopically, cystic cavities are lined by columnar and cuboidal cells with papillary proliferations of cells and solid areas. Cells are pleomorphic and mitoses are seen. Invasion of the ovarian stroma occurs, confirming the malignant character.

Prognosis—It is associated with an overall 20% 5 year survival.

Borderline serous tumours

Macroscopically, these are bilateral in 30% of cases, and either cystic or mixed solid and cystic.

Microscopically, they are similar to serous cystadenocarcinomas but invasion of the ovarian stroma does not occur, despite the presence of cellular atypia.

Prognosis—The y are associated with an overall 75% 10 year survival.

Mucinous tumours of the ovary

These multilocular cystic ovarian tumours of endocervical differentiation contain gelatinous material.

Benign (mucinous cystadenomas)

Macroscopically, multilocular cystic lesions contain glutinous, viscid, mucoid material. They are bilateral in only 5% of cases.

Microscopically, cysts are lined by a single layer of columnar, mucin-secreting cells with regular nuclei and no atypical features or mitoses.

Malignant (mucinous cystadenocarcinomas)

These occur in young women, with a median age at diagnosis of 35 years.

Macroscopically, they are identical to benign mucinous cystadenomas, but may grow to a very large size, and solid areas are seen in the walls of some cysts. They are bilateral in 25% of cases.

Microscopically, they are columnar, mucin-secreting cells of the lining epithelium showing pleomorphism and mitoses. Invasion of the ovarian stroma is seen, confirming the malignant nature.

Prognosis—Overall survival is 34% at 10 years.

Borderline mucinous tumours

These resemble mucinous cystadenocarcinomas both macroscopically and microscopically except that there is no evidence of stromal invasion, and they are bilateral in only 10% of cases.

Prognosis—Overall survival is 90% at 10 years.

Endometrioid tumours

These ovarian tumours show endometrial differentiation. The vast majority are malignant (endometrioid carcinomas), accounting for 20% of all ovarian carcinomas.

The clear cell carcinoma is a variant of endometrioid carcinoma characterized by the presence of cells with clear cytoplasm and containing abundant glycogen.

Prognosis—Overall, these carcinomas have 40% 5 year survival rate.

Brenner tumours of the ovary

Tumours composed of nests of epithelium resembling a transitional cell epithelium of the urinary tract, these are associated with a spindle-cell stroma. The epithelial component may be benign, borderline or malignant.

Macroscopically, the lesions are solid and have a firm, yellowish-white cut surface.

Microscopically, the nests of the transitional cell epithelium are separated by a spindle cell stroma.

Germ cell tumours

These account for 20% of ovarian neoplasms occurring from childhood onwards, and may be benign or malignant.

Teratoma

Benign cystic teratomas (dermoid cysts of the ovary)
These account for about 10% of all neoplasms of the ovary.

Macroscopically, the affected ovary is replaced by cystic structures lined by skin and skin appendages, particularly hair. Teeth, bone, respiratory tract tissue, mature neural tissue and smooth muscle are other common elements.

Solid teratomas
These rare but potentially malignant tumours are composed of a variety of tissue components such as squamous epithelium, cartilage, smooth muscle, respiratory mucosa and neural tissue. Lesions are larger and more solid than benign cystic teratomas and are mainly seen in adolescents.

Dysgerminoma

This rare malignant tumour is similar to seminoma of the testis. Tumours predominantly arise in young females, with enlargement of affected ovaries. Normal ovarian tissue is replaced by a soft white tumour, which is highly radiosensitive.

Yolk-sac tumours

Rare, highly malignant tumour, these are usually seen in women under 30 years of age. Lesions typically secrete α-fetoprotein detectable in the blood as a tumour marker. The prognosis is poor without treatment, but there is an improved outlook with combination chemotherapy.

Sex-cord stromal tumours

These ovarian tumours are derived from primitive sex cords of the fetal ovary. Several tumours of this group secrete oestrogen, thus patients may develop endometrial hyperplasia and a predisposition to endometrial neoplasia.

Granulosa cell tumours

These are composed of the granulosa cells derived from follicles. About 75% secrete oestrogen and present with signs of hyperoestrogenism. They are potentially malignant, but if confined to the ovary, then they are associated with an excellent prognosis.

Sertoli–Leydig cell tumours (androblastomas)

Rare, small, benign tumours largely confined to the ovary, these are composed of a mixture of cell types normally seen in the testis. They may cause masculinizing effects from secreted hormones.

Gonadoblastomas

These rare, benign lesions contain derivatives of primitive germ cells and sex-cord stromata. Lesions typically develop in the gonads of phenotypic females carrying a Y chromosome. The germ cell component may undergo a malignant change to form a dysgerminoma.

Steroid cell tumours

These rare, benign tumours are composed of cortical adrenal-like cells containing abundant lipid. Tumours often present with symptoms of virilization due to androgen production.

Fig. 12.7 provides a table of the primary ovarian neoplasms and their origins.

Metastatic

The ovary is a common site of tumour metastasis, typically from the breast and GI tract.

Krukenberg's tumour

This is an enlarged ovary with a metastatic signet ring-cell adenocarcinoma (typically of gastric origin).

Primary ovarian neoplasms and their origins	
Origin	**Neoplasms**
surface epithelial–stromal tumours	serous ovarian tumours mucinous ovarian tumours endometrioid and clear cell ovarian tumours Brenner tumours
germ cell tumours	teratoma: • benign cystic teratomas • solid teratomas dysgerminomas yolk-sac tumours malignant mixed germ cell tumours
sex cord–stromal tumours	granulosa cell tumours Sertoli–Leydig cell tumours (androblastomas) gonadoblastoma steroid cell tumours

Fig. 12.7 Primary ovarian neoplasms and their origins.

Tumours of the fallopian tubes

Tumours of the fallopian tubes are extremely rare, and can be benign or malignant.

Benign
Adenomatoid tumours
These are typically of the mesosalpinx.

Malignant
Malignant tumours of the fallopian tubes can be:
- Primary: adenocarcinomas; typically affect postmenopausal women. Poor prognosis due to late presentation.
- Secondary: endometrial tumours may spread up the tubal lumen, and metastatic disease in the pelvic peritoneum may involve the tubal serosa.

DISORDERS OF THE PLACENTA AND PREGNANCY

Ectopic pregnancies

A fertilized ovum is implanted outside the uterine cavity. This occurs in about 1 in 300 pregnancies. The fallopian tube (especially in the ampulla) is by far the most common site for this; other sites of abnormal implantation are very rare but include the peritoneal cavity, the ovary and the cervix.

The aetiology is uncertain but ectopic pregnancies are possibly the result of some structural abnormality of the fallopian tube, e.g. scarring or adhesions resulting from previous episodes of salpingitis or endometriosis, or previous tubal surgery for contraceptive purposes, i.e. sterilization.

Pathogenesis—Following implantation, the proliferation of trophoblasts erodes the submucosal blood vessels, precipitating severe bleeding into the tubal lumen. The muscular wall of the fallopian tube is unable to undergo hypertrophy or distend, and so tubal pregnancy almost always results in the rupture of the fallopian tube with the death of the fertilized ovum, typically in the early stages of pregnancy and often before the patient is even aware of being pregnant.

- What conditions predispose to the development of salpingitis?
- Name the different types of cystic lesions that affect the ovary and fallopian tube.
- How are ovarian tumours classified?
- Describe the different types of ovarian surface epithelial tumour.
- Name the tumours that may affect the fallopian tubes.

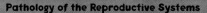
The types of rupture are:

- Into the lumen of the fallopian tube: common in ampullary pregnancy. Conceptus is extruded towards the fimbriated end of the tube. Mild haemorrhage into the peritoneal cavity occurs, which may collect as a clot in the pouch of Douglas.
- Into the peritoneal cavity: occurs most commonly from the isthmus of the tube, either spontaneously or as a result of pressure (e.g. straining at the stool, coitus or pelvic examination). Haemorrhage is likely to be severe.
- Retroperitoneal (rare): rupture occurs into the potential space between the leaves of the broad ligament. Haemorrhage into the site is more likely to be controlled.

Clinical features are:

- Severe lower abdominal pain: usually localized to the side of the ectopic pregnancy, but less localized if the fallopian tube ruptures.
- Vaginal bleeding: occurs after the death of the ovum, and is an effect of oestrogen withdrawal.
- Anaemia: due to internal blood loss.
- Shock may occur if haemorrhage is severe and rapid, e.g. due to large vessel erosion. This is most dangerous and dramatic consequence of tubal pregnancy.

Spontaneous abortion

Many fertilized ova fail to implant successfully, and it has been estimated that more than 40% of all conceptions fail to convert into recognizable pregnancies. Of those that survive this far, 15% terminate in a clinically recognized spontaneous abortion.

Aetiology—Causes of spontaneous abortion differ at different stages of pregnancy, as shown in Fig. 12.8.

Types of spontaneous abortions

Threatened

There is bleeding from the placental site, which is not yet severe enough to terminate the pregnancy. The cervix is closed but there may be a few painful uterine contractions. The pregnancy is likely to continue.

Inevitable

Bleeding is slight but the cervix is usually open. Clinically the patient presents as a threatened abortion but bleeding is retroplacental and the fetus is already dead. Occasionally, products of conception may be felt in the cervical canal.

Incomplete

The fetus and membranes are expelled but the chorionic tissue remains attached and bleeding continues. Abortion must be completed by curettage.

To remember the causes at different stages of pregnancy, learn the following rules of thumb:
- First trimester causes: majority are associated with abnormal fetuses.
- Second trimester causes: mainly due to uterine abnormalities.
- Third trimester causes: mainly the result of maternal abnormalities.

Causes of spontaneous abortion	
Time	**Cause**
first trimester	abnormal chromosomal karyotypes, particularly Turner's syndrome structural developmental abnormalities, e.g. neural tube defects maternal SLE transplacental infection, e.g. *Brucella*, *Listeria*, rubella, *Toxoplasma*, cytomegalovirus and herpes
second trimester	chorioamnionitis rupture of membranes placental haemorrhages structural abnormalities of the uterus, e.g. congenital uterine malformations large submucosal leiomyomas incompetence of the cervix abnormal placentation (but more common in third trimester)
third trimester	uncontrolled hypertension eclampsia placental abnormalities, e.g. placental haemorrhage, abruption and infarction
at any time	endocrine abnormalities: diabetes, hypothyroidism, deficiency of progesterone or luteinizing hormone trauma: surgical operation, blow to abdomen, or hypotensive shock

Fig. 12.8 Causes of spontaneous abortion.

Complete
The products of conception have been passed per vaginum and the uterus is empty. There is little bleeding, the uterus is small and the cervix closed.

Missed abortion
The embryo fails to develop or dies *in utero* but the products of conception are not expelled. The whole pregnancy is gradually absorbed, and often presents gynaecologically as an unexplained amenorrhoea. After about 12 weeks, the formation of a carnous mole (lobulated mass of laminated blood clot) is likely and after 18 weeks a macerated fetus is usually expelled.

Recurrent
This refers to three consecutive spontaneous abortions.

Pre-eclampsia and eclampsia
Pre-eclampsia
This is high blood pressure (>140/90 mmHg) developing during pregnancy in a woman whose blood pressure was previously normal. It occurs in about 10% of all pregnant women. The aetiology is unknown.

Risk factors are:
- Parity.
- Diabetes.
- Hypertension.
- Multiple pregnancies.
- Primigravidae.
- Women over the age of 35.

It is thought to develop due to the failure of the narrow spiral arteries of the placenta to convert into low-resistance vascular sinuses.

Placental ischaemia results in poor fetal growth and the liberation of substances that cause vasoconstriction and promote hypertension.

Endothelial cells of kidney arterioles become swollen, and fibrin deposition occurs in glomeruli leading to proteinuria (Fig. 12.9).

The condition may be mild or severe:
- Mild cases (majority): blood pressure is <100 mmHg diastolic and there is no associated proteinuria.

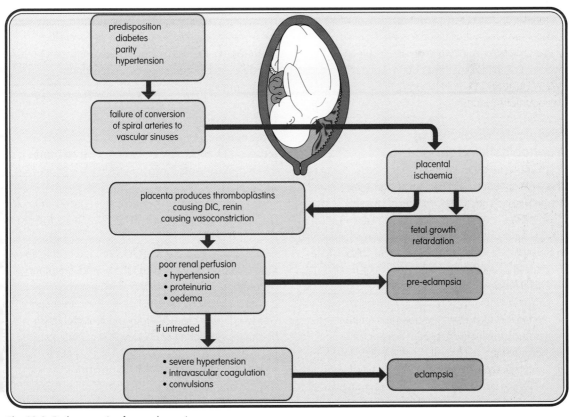

Fig. 12.9 Pathogenesis of pre-eclampsia.

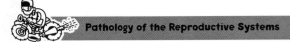

- Severe cases: diastolic pressure is consistently >100 mmHg and there is proteinuria and severe peripheral oedema (pre-eclamptic toxaemia syndrome).

Effects of pre-eclampsia

Reduced placental blood flow causes an increased risk of fetal hypoxia in late pregnancy, particularly during labour, with resultant perinatal mortality. The fetus may also suffer intrauterine growth retardation and have a low birth weight.

Maternal problems are less common, being largely confined to severe pre-eclampsia, which may progress into full-blown eclampsia (see below).

The disease resolves immediately after delivery.

Eclampsia

This is the occurrence of one or more convulsions not caused by other conditions such as epilepsy or cerebral haemorrhage in a woman with pre-eclampsia.

Incidence is rare; only a small proportion of patients with severe pre-eclampsia develop eclampsia.

Clinical features are severe systemic disturbance, i.e. frontal headaches, rapid and sustained rise in blood pressure, shock, anuria and fits.

There is disseminated intravascular coagulation with widespread occlusion of blood vessels, fibrinoid necrosis of vessel walls, and, in fatal cases, widespread microinfarcts in the brain, liver, kidneys and other organs.

Fatal eclampsia is now rare due to treatment of the pre-eclamptic syndrome.

Neoplastic disorders of trophoblastic origin

Hydatiform mole

This is the abnormal development of a gestational trophoblast leading to the formation of a benign mass of cystic vesicles derived from chorionic villi. It occurs in 1 in 2000 pregnancies in the UK and USA, but more frequently in some parts of Asia, South America and Africa.

There are two types:

- Partial: cystic vesicles are found in only a part of the placenta. Fetal parts and some normal placental villi are present along with the abnormal trophoblastic tissue. Low risk of subsequent development of malignancy.
- Complete: mole forms a bulky mass which may fill the uterine cavity. No fetal parts or normal placental villi are present. Low risk of subsequent development of malignancy.

The aetiopathogenesis is unknown.

Clinical features are:

- Amenorrhoea followed by continuous or intermittent vaginal bleeding.
- Other symptoms of pregnancy: vomiting, pre-eclampsia.
- Enlarged soft uterus (often larger than dates would suggest).

Diagnosis is by elevated chorionic gonadotrophin excretion in urine (typically much greater than in normal pregnancies), and by ultrasound for the absence of the fetus.

Treatment is by evacuation of the uterus, with a second aspiration or curettage 2 to 4 weeks later to ensure complete removal of the mole.

Follow-up is by regular estimations of hCG for at least a year. Detection of hCG after one month may suggest incomplete removal and the persistence of trophoblastic disease. Untreated, this carries a risk of The subsequent development of a malignant tumour of trophoblast or choriocarcinoma.

Invasive mole (chorioadenoma destruens)

A hydatidiform mole invades through the decidua into the myometrium and associated blood vessels. Perforation of the uterus may occur, resulting in invasion of the parametrium. True malignant transformation is rare.

Choriocarcinomas

These malignant tumours of trophoblastic tissue with a propensity for invading vessel walls, and blood-borne metastases occur early to many sites, particularly the lung and brain.

They are rare in the UK and USA (at 1 per 50 000 pregnancies) but more common in Asia, South America and Africa.

Aetiology—About 50% develop from a hydatidiform mole and about 20% arise after a normal pregnancy with a variable time lag (a few months to many years).

The prognosis is excellent as the tumours respond well to cytotoxic chemotherapy (particularly if post-treatment monitoring of hCG levels is carried out).

Placental site trophoblastic tumour

This is a rare tumour in which the bulk of the tissue consists of chorionic epithelium but with very few villi. Typically benign, it may undergo malignant change.

- **What is an ectopic pregnancy? Name the types of rupture.**
- **List the causes of spontaneous abortion.**
- **Name the types of spontaneous abortion.**
- **Describe the clinical features of pre-eclampsia and eclampsia.**
- **What is a hydatiform mole?**

DISORDERS OF THE BREAST

Inflammatory disorders and infections
Acute mastitis and breast abscess
These are uncommon, and usually are complications of lactation. The most frequent organism is *Staphylococcus aureus* which gains access through cracks and fissures of the nipple and areola. An abscess may form if drainage is inadequate.

Mammary duct ectasia
There is an abnormal progressive dilatation of the large breast ducts, which accumulate inspissated secretions. The aetiology is unknown and affects older women (perimenopausal age range). Patients develop a firm breast lump, which may mimic a carcinoma. There may also be blood-stained nipple discharge.

Fat necrosis
This is usually caused by trauma. Histology shows necrosis with multinucleated giant cells and later fibrosis. It may cause a discrete lump mimicking a carcinoma.

Fibrocystic changes
Simple fibrocystic change
This is a generic term for a number of benign lesions in the breast which may occur together and may produce a discrete mass mimicking a carcinoma. Peak incidence is around the menopause. Aetiology is unknown.

The histological changes that may be present include:
- Cysts: ranging in size from microscopic to palpable lesions 1–2 cm in diameter. Cytological examination of aspirated fluid is necessary to distinguish them from carcinomas.

- Apocrine metaplasia: epithelial lining of hyperplastic ducts undergoes metaplasia to that of normal apocrine glands.
- Fibrosis: replacement of breast tissue by dense fibrous tissue.
- Sclerosing adenosis: marked proliferation of specialized hormone-responsive stromal tissue and myoepithelial cells forming localized areas of irregular stellate, collagenous sclerosis in which epithelial elements are also present. Difficult to distinguish from some patterns of invasive carcinoma.
- Papillomatosis.

There is no increased risk of a carcinoma unless there is accompanying epithelial hyperplasia (see below).

Epithelial hyperplasia
This describes the proliferation of epithelial cells within ducts or lobules (ductal hyperplasia and lobular hyperplasia respectively). There are two types:
- Hyperplasia of the usual type: normal cytology and tissue architecture with no signs of malignancy.
- Hyperplasia of atypical type: biological spectrum between some abnormalities of cytology/architecture and carcinoma in-situ.

The risk of subsequent invasive breast carcinoma is increased in individuals with florid usual hyperplasia, further increased in subjects with atypical hyperplasia and almost certain in those with some types of carcinoma in-situ (comedo).

Epithelial hyperplasia can only be diagnosed by a pathologist looking at excised breast tissue microscopically.

The following benign pathologies may cause discrete breast lumps or nipple discharge which mimic carcinomas:
- **Duct ectasia.**
- **Fat necrosis.**
- **Fibrocystic disease (fibrosis, sclerosing adenosis, papillomatosis).**
- **Intraduct papilloma.**
- **Fibroadenoma.**

Neoplasms of the breast

Fibroadenoma

This common benign tumour with a proliferation of both stroma and epithelium, occurs in young women (most frequently the 25–35 age group). It produces discrete but mobile breast lumps typically 1–4 cm in size.

Phyllodes tumour

A tumour composed of both a stroma and epithelium, where the stroma is more cellular than fibroadenomas, this is less common than the latter and occurs in the older age group (peak incidence being 45 years). Clinically, the tumour presents as a breast lump.

Macroscopically, there are rubbery white lesions consisting of a whorled pattern of slit-like spaces and solid areas.

Microscopically, there is a variable appearance, classified into benign (90% of cases), or of borderline malignant potential or definitely malignant.

There is the potential for local recurrence with increasing aggressiveness and the tumour may eventually metastasize.

Intraductal papilloma

Epithelial proliferation within ducts produces papillary structures. These occur in older women and may produce a blood-stained nipple discharge. Papillomas are usually solitary with no increased risk of a carcinoma. However, there is a rare condition of multiple intraduct papillomas which is premalignant.

Carcinoma

Incidence—20% of all cancers in women and the commonest cause of death in the 35–55 year age group of women, increasing with age steeply to 45 years and continuing to increase less steeply thereafter.

There is a 200-fold female preponderance, with the highest rates in America, western Europe, and the Antipodes, and the lowest rates in Africa and Southeast Asia.

Predisposing factors are:
- Atypical epithelial proliferation.
- Mutations of BRCA 1 and 2 genes.
- Long interval between menarche and menopause.
- Older age at first pregnancy.
- Obesity.
- High-fat diet.
- Ionizing radiation.

Macroscopic features—A discrete lump with tethering to the skin or surrounding connective tissue.

Microscopic features—Adenocarcinoma of one of the following histological subtypes:
- Ductal (commonest).
- Lobular.
- Tubular.
- Medullary.

Spread is as follows:
- Direct: skin and muscles of the chest wall.
- Lymphatic: axillary lymph nodes, internal mammary lymph nodes.
- Blood: lungs, then anywhere.
- Transcoelomic: pleural cavities and pericardium.

Prognosis—Related to tumour grade and type (tubular—best prognosis), size of the tumour, lymph node status, and oestrogen receptor status (usually responds to tamoxifen if positive).

Figs 12.10–12.12 give the type, spread and TNM staging of breast carcinoma respectively.

Screening for breast carcinoma

There is no direct screening method equivalent to the cytology of the uterine cervix. The primary screening modality is mammography which is more effective in older women with less radiodense breast tissue. Abnormalities seen on mammograms include calcification and soft tissue deformity. Diagnosis of screen-detected lesions is by aspiration cytology or tissue

Types of breast carcinoma	
Character	**Neoplasm**
non-invasive	ductal carcinoma *in situ* lobular carcinoma *in situ*
invasive	invasive ductal carcinoma (85%) invasive lobular carcinoma (10%) mucinous tubular medullary

Fig. 12.10 Types of breast carcinoma.

biopsy. In Britain there is a National Health Service Breast Screening Programme with 3 yearly mammography for all women over the age of 50. Results are awaited to see if this reduces the mortality from breast carcinoma.

The male breast
Gynaecomastia
This is the benign enlargement of breast tissue.

Aetiology—Hormonal influences including increased oestrogen production or receptor sensitivity. It is associated with liver disease, stilboestrol therapy for prostate carcinoma and drugs such as chlorpromazine.

Carcinoma
Less than 1% of breast carcinomas occur in men. The condition is associated with Klinefelter's syndrome. and is usually of the ductal type; the lobular type has not been described.

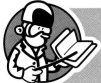

- List the pathologies that may cause a breast lump.
- List the predisposing factors for the development of breast carcinoma in females.
- Describe the rationale for a breast screening programme.

DISORDERS OF THE MALE REPRODUCTIVE SYSTEM

Disorders of the penis
Inflammation and infection
Viral infection
Common viral infections of the penis include genital herpes and genital warts (condyloma acuminatum).

Genital herpes
This is an acute infection of the penile mucosa by the herpes simplex virus with the formation of typical herpetic vesicles on the glans penis. The vesicles soon burst to produce shallow painful ulcers.

The virus may remain latent for many years. Recurrent herpes infections are caused by reactivation of the virus and may be precipitated by a febrile illness, immune suppression, emotional stress or UV light.

Condyloma acuminatum (genital warts)
These cauliflower-like warts are seen on the penis and around the perineum and caused by one of the human papillomaviruses.

Spread of breast carcinoma	
Spread	**Area**
direct	skin
lymphatic	axillary lymph nodes internal mammary lymph nodes supraclavicular lymph nodes
haematogenous	liver lung opposite breast bone brain

Fig. 12.11 Spread of breast carcinoma.

TNM staging of breast carcinoma		
Tumour	**Nodes**	**Metastases**
T1 tumour 20 mm or less; no fixation or nipple retraction	N0 node negative	M0 no distant metastases
T2 tumour 20–50 mm, or less than 20 mm with fixation	N1 axillary nodes mobile	M1 distant metastases present
T3 tumour 50–100 mm, or less than 50 mm with fixation	N2 axillary nodes fixed	
T4 greater than 100 mm, or chest wall invasion	N3 supraclavicular nodes positive or arm oedema	

Fig. 12.12 TNM staging of breast carcinoma.

Bacterial infection

Inflammation of the glans (balanitis) and prepuce (posthitis) can be caused by a variety of bacterial organisms, the most common of which are staphylococci, coliforms, gonococci and *Chlamydia*.

The appearance is that of marked congestion and oedema with exudate on the surface of the glans. Ulceration with chronic scarring may occur if untreated.

Syphilis—primary chancre

A solitary, firm papule (typically painless) later ulcerates to form a shallow, clean-based depression with extensive surrounding induration and inguinal lymphadenopathy. The responsible organism is *Treponema pallidum*.

The commonest sites are the glans and the inner side of the prepuce but occasionally also the shaft.

The condition heals spontaneously in about 2 months, or more rapidly with treatment. Untreated, it will progress to secondary and tertiary syphilis.

Lymphogranuloma venereum (lymphogranuloma inguinale)

This venereal disease is characterized by granulomatous lesions and caused by *Chlamydia trachomatis*.

Clinical features are:

- Small primary lesion: develops at site of inoculation, usually transient and often unnoticed.
- Unilateral lymphadenopathy (primarily inguinal): occurs 1–2 weeks postinfection. Nodes are at first discrete, but later coalesce.

The disease follows a chronic course varying from weeks to months. Healing occurs with fibrosis resulting in lymphatic blockage.

Late complications are external genitalia elephantiasis or rectal strictures due to lymphatic obstruction.

Fungi

Infection with *Candida albicans* is common in men with diabetes mellitus.

Neoplastic disorders

Benign

Condyloma acuminatum

This is described above.

Malignant

Carcinoma in situ (erythroplasia of Queyrat)

Penile carcinoma *in situ* is restricted to the glans and resembles non-specific balanitis with single or multiple, flat, red, glistening areas. There is a spectrum of changes from dysplasia to carcinoma *in situ* grouped together as penile intra-epithelial neoplasia. Many cases are associated with HPV infection.

The condition leads to invasive cancer unless treated vigorously with local irradiation or 5-fluorouracil cream.

Squamous cell carcinoma

This is a well-differentiated, keratinizing, invasive tumour usually seen in elderly men, occurring most commonly in uncircumcised men, and thought to be associated with a previous infection with human papillomavirus.

It presents as a warty, cauliflower-like growth that bleeds easily. It is typically slow growing but is often neglected because of patient embarrassment.

Disorders of the testis and epididymis
Congenital abnormalities and regression
Cryptorchidism

This is a condition caused by maldescent of the testes, affecting about 5% at birth, although many descend by the first birthday.

In embryo, the testes develop from the genital ridge high on the posterior wall.

At about 7 months' gestation, the testes migrate

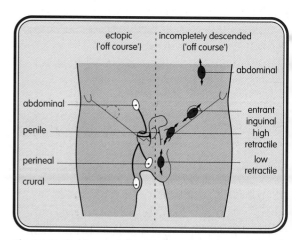

Fig. 12.13 Maldescended testes showing common sites of arrest. (Adapted with permission from *Lecture Notes On Urology*, 5th edn, by J. Blandy, Blackwell Science, 1998.)

down the posterior abdominal wall and are guided by a cord (the gubernaculum) through the inguinal ring into the scrotum.

Occasionally, migration fails to occur and one (75% of cases) or both (25% of cases) testes become arrested somewhere along the route (Fig. 12.13). There are three versions of this type of problem:
- Abdominal testicle: usually found just inside the internal ring.
- Inguinal testicle: in the inguinal canal.
- Retractile testicles (most common): high retractile testicle—rides up and down from the external ring to the upper part of the scrotum; low retractile testicle—can be persuaded to reach the bottom of the scrotum. Usually settles at puberty and does not need an operation.

The complications are:
- Infertility: temperature of aberrant locations is higher than in scrotum, and prevents normal germ cell development. The testis remains small and incapable of producing effective spermatozoa.
- Malignancy: more common in an undescended testis; about one in ten of all testicular tumours arise in association with cryptorchidism.
- Inguinal hernia: there is nearly always a patent tunica vaginalis which predisposes to the development of an inguinal hernia.
- Torsion of the testicle (see below).

Management is by detection and correction of testicular maldescent. This is important because of the increased risk of testicular carcinoma. Some restoration of function may be achieved by 'orchidopexy' at an early stage (the testis is surgically pulled down into the scrotal sac).

Abnormalities of the tunica vaginalis
The tunica vaginalis and tunica albuginea are invested with mesothelial cells and may be the site of fluid accumulation, inflammation or (uncommonly) tumour formation.

Hydrocele
Fluid accumulates in the cavity bounded by the tunica vaginalis. This is the most common cause of swelling within the scrotum.

The aetiology is as follows:
- Congenital patency of the processus vaginalis often with continuity into the peritoneal cavity.

- Secondary to tumours, epididymitis, mumps or acute orchitis.

Haematocele
Blood accumulates of in the cavity bounded by the tunica vaginalis.

Aetiology—Trauma, torsion of the testis, haemorrhage into pre-existing hydrocele, generalized bleeding disorders, or rarely due to the extension of the testicular tumour through the tunica vaginalis.

Chylocele
Obstruction to the lymphatic drainage of the tunica and cord occurs.

Hernias
Indirect inguinal hernias (described in Chapter 9) typically occur as a result of patent processus vaginalis.

Trauma and vascular disturbances
Torsion
There is twisting of a testicle on its pedicle with obstruction of venous return such that blood continues to enter the testis, but cannot leave. The testis becomes swollen and painful and eventually becomes infarcted (venous infarction). In advanced torsion, the testis is almost black as a result of vascular congestion.

Early detection and surgical relief are required to save testicular viability. Surgical removal is necessary for advanced disease.

Varicocele
Variceal dilatation of the veins of the pampiniform plexus of the spermatic cord occurs.

Neoplastic disorders
Tumours of the testis, although relatively uncommon, are important since many occur in young men, and are the commonest form of malignancy in this age group.

Their incidence is uncommon (only affecting 1–2%), but with an increasing incidence in many Western countries, especially Denmark.

Typically they are seen in early adult life and particularly significant in those aged between 20 and 45.

Their aetiology is unknown; maldescent of the testis is the only known risk factor.

Clinical presentations are:
- Painless unilateral enlargement of testis (majority).
- Secondary hydrocele.

- Symptoms of metastases: especially in malignant teratoma, e.g. haemoptysis from lung deposits, hepatomegaly or retroperitoneal mass due to metastasis to para-aortic lymph nodes.
- Endocrine effects: gynaecomastia, precocious puberty (typically from Leydig or Sertoli cell tumours).

There are two main groups of testicular tumours:
- Germ cell tumours (97% of cases): derived from multipotential germ cells of the testis arising as teratomas and seminomas.
- Non-germ cell tumours (3% of cases): derived from specialized and non-specialized support cells of the testis.

Germ cell tumours

Germ cell tumours are subdivided into:
- Seminomas: tumours showing spermatogenic differentiation.
- Teratomas: tumours retaining their totipotentiality for differentiation.
- Combined tumours: mixture of both seminomatous and teratomatous differentiation.

Seminoma

The most common malignant testicular tumour, this accounts for about 50% of all malignant germ cell tumours.

Histological types of seminoma are:
- Classic seminoma (most common subtype): characteristic feature is the presence of fibrous septa with lymphocytic infiltrate.
- Spermatocytic seminoma: larger tumour cells with some small cells resembling spermatocytes.

- Anaplastic seminoma: cells show marked pleomorphism and increased mitotic activity.
- Seminomas with trophoblastic giant cells: associated with increased blood levels of human chorionic gonadotrophin secreted by trophoblastic cells.

Teratoma

This tumour of germ cell origin is composed of several types of tissue representing endoderm, ectoderm, and mesoderm. These are more aggressive tumours than seminomas.

Teratomas are classified according to their histological pattern. There are two separate classification systems, the British system and the WHO system. These are compared in Fig. 12.14 and are basically defined as follows:
- Differentiated teratoma: a rare type of teratoma in which tissues are well differentiated and fully matured so that a wide range of organoid structures (e.g. skin, hair, cartilage, and bone) can be identified. Lesions are usually seen in young children and behave in a benign fashion.
- Malignant teratoma intermediate: partly solid and partly cystic tumour. Mixture of well differentiated areas (resembling differentiated teratoma) and areas of malignancy with cellular pleomorphism and necrosis.
- Malignant teratoma undifferentiated: completely undifferentiated tumour with marked nuclear pleomorphism and a high mitotic rate. There is usually extensive tumour necrosis.
- Malignant teratoma trophoblastic: tumour contains areas of syncytiotrophoblast and cytotrophoblast arranged in a villous pattern. Often haemorrhagic

Comparison of the British and WHO classifications of teratomas		
Type of differentiation	British	WHO
somatic	differentiated teratoma	mature teratoma
	malignant teratoma intermediate	immature teratoma or mixed teratoma and embryonal carcinoma
none	malignant teratoma undifferentiated	embryonal carcinoma
extra-embryonic	yolk sac tumour	yolk sac tumour
	malignant teratoma trophoblastic	choriocarcinoma

Fig. 12.14 Comparison of the British and WHO classifications of teratomas.

due to vascular invasion (blood-borne metastases common); hCG and α-fetoprotein are useful markers and may be measured in serum or demonstrated in syncytiotrophoblast by immunocytochemistry.

- Yolk sac tumour (orchioblastoma) is a highly malignant tumour derived from germ cells, and comes in two types:
  - Pure form: more common in children especially in the first 3 years of life.
  - Mixed form: most commonly mixed with undifferentiated germ cells. Presence of yolk sac elements in association with other elements confers a worse prognosis.

The tumour makes α-fetoprotein, which can be detected in the serum or by immunohistochemical detection.

Combined germ cell tumour
Between 10 and 15% of germ cell tumours consist of a mixture of seminomatous and teratomatous elements.

Prognosis of germ cell tumours
The prognosis of testicular teratomas has improved greatly with the use of cytotoxic chemotherapy and is related to histological type, as well as to tumour stage. In general, germ cell tumours containing trophoblastic, yolk sac and undifferentiated elements have the worst prognosis.

Non-germ cell tumours
Non-germ cell tumours are subdivided into:
- Sex cord and stromal tumours: interstitial (Leydig) cell tumour, Sertoli cell tumour.
- Others: mainly malignant lymphomas and metastatic tumours.

Interstitial (Leydig) cell tumour
This rare tumour arises from the interstitial or Leydig cells of the testis. It may produce androgens, oestrogens, or both, causing precocious development of secondary sexual characteristics in childhood or loss of libido/gynaecomastia in adults.

The majority of such tumours are benign but those over 5 cm in diameter and those with mitoses may behave in a malignant fashion.

Sertoli cell tumour (androblastoma)
This well-circumscribed tumour is composed of cells resembling normal Sertoli cells of the tubules. Most lesions are benign.

Malignant lymphomas
The non-Hodgkin's-type lymphoma is usually a poorly differentiated B cell lymphoma with a diffuse pattern. These comprise about 7% of testicular tumours with a peak incidence between 60 and 80 years.

Metastatic tumours
The spread of other tumours to the testis may occasionally occur, particularly in acute leukaemia.
Fig. 12.15 provides a summary of testicular tumours.

Disorders of the prostate
Benign prostatic hyperplasia
Non-neoplastic enlargement of the prostate is the most common disorder of the prostate affecting almost all men over the age of 70, but it is found with increasing frequency and severity from about 45 years onwards.

The aetiopathogenesis is uncertain but believed to be a result of androgen–oestrogen imbalance. A periurethral (central) group of prostatic glands (not the

Summary of testicular tumours	
Germ cell tumours (97% of cases)	
seminomas	classic seminoma spermatocytic seminoma anaplastic seminoma seminomas with trophoblastic giant cells
teratomas	differentiated teratoma malignant teratoma intermediate malignant teratoma undifferentiated malignant teratoma trophoblastic yolk sac tumour
combined	mixture of seminomatous and teratomatous elements
Non-germ cell tumours (3% of cases)	
sex-cord and stromal tumours	interstitial (Leydig) cell tumour Sertoli cell tumour
others	malignant lymphomas metastatic tumours

Fig. 12.15 Summary of testicular tumours.

Many testicular tumours have useful cell markers:
- **Trophoblastic germ cell tumours:↑ hCG.**
- **Yolk sac tumours: ↑ α-fetoprotein.**
- **90% of patients with malignant teratoma undifferentiated: ↑ α-fetoprotein, ↑ hCG or both.**
- **50% of patients with malignant teratoma intermediate: ↑ α-fetoprotein, ↑ hCG or both.**
- **10% of patients with seminoma: ↑ hCG.**

true prostatic glands at the periphery) are hormone sensitive and undergo hyperplasia. Their continuing enlargement compresses peripheral true prostatic glands leading to their collapse, leaving only fibrous supporting stroma (Fig. 12.16).

Affected lobes are:
- Two lateral lobes (majority of cases).
- Posterior lobe (uncommon) causing an obstruction of the urinary outflow tract at the internal urinary meatus at the bladder neck.

Macroscopically:
- Nodular pattern of hyperplastic glandular acini separated by fibrous stroma.
- Some nodules are cystically dilated and contain a milky fluid.
- Other nodules contain numerous calcific concretions (corpora amylacea).

Microscopically, the epithelium of hyperplastic acini (larger than normal) are lined by tall columnar epithelial cells, and may form irregular papillary folds.

Infarction causes necrotic areas with a haemorrhagic margin. There is often muscular hypertrophy particularly in the region of the bladder neck.

Clinical presentation—Compression of the prostatic

urethra by the enlarged prostate causes difficulties with micturition, mainly a delay in starting to pass urine, a poor or intermittent stream, and dribbling at the end of micturition.

Complications—Prolonged prostatic obstruction can lead to several complications which are outlined in Fig. 12.17.

Neoplastic disorders
Prostatic carcinoma
This is an adenocarcinoma of the prostate and is shown in Fig. 12.18. It is the second most common type of cancer in males, and its incidence is increasing. It is rare before 55 years with a peak incidence between 60 and 85 years.

Its aetiology is uncertain but there is probably hormonal involvement (reduced androgens).

It arises in the true prostatic glands at the periphery of the prostate, and is therefore often well established before the development of symptoms of difficulty with micturition due to urethral obstruction. Indeed, some tumours may remain silent even in the presence of widespread metastases.

Types are divided into three groups on the basis of their behaviour:

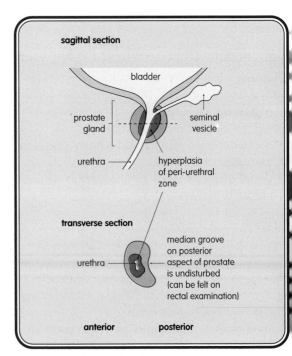

Fig. 12.16 Benign prostatic hyperplasia.

- Latent: small foci of well-differentiated carcinoma, frequently an incidental finding in prostatic glands of elderly men. Remain confined to prostate for a long period.
- Invasive: invade locally and metastasize.
- Occult: not clinically apparent in primary site but present as metastatic disease.

Macroscopically, there are diffuse areas of firm, white tissue merging into fibromuscular prostatic stromal tissues. Distortion and extension outside the prostatic capsule is common producing a firm, craggy mass that can be palpated on rectal examination.

Microscopically, the majority have a differentiated glandular pattern (good prognosis); a minority have poorly differentiated sheets of cells with no acinar pattern (poor prognosis).

Spread is:
- Direct: to the base of the bladder and adjacent tissues. May cause obstruction of the urethra (difficulty in micturition) and may block the ureters, causing hydronephrosis.
- Lymphatic: to pelvic and para-aortic nodes.
- Haematogenous: most commonly to bone, but also to the lungs and liver. Bone metastases are typically sclerotic with bone production (dense on radiograph) rather than lytic with bone destruction.

Clinical features are:
- Urinary symptoms (delay in starting to pass urine, poor stream, terminal dribbling).
- Hard, craggy prostate on rectal examination.
- Bone metastases: pain (especially back pain), fracture, anaemia.
- Lymph node metastases.

Diagnosis is by:
- Imaging: ultrasound, X-ray, isotope bone scan.
- Biopsy: immunohistochemical detection of prostate-specific antigen (PSA) and prostate-specific acid phosphatase (PSAP) in biopsy material.
- Serology: PSA and PSAP may also be used as serum markers for disease, levels being particularly raised when there is metastatic disease.

Treatment—Many prostatic carcinomas are dependent on testosterone for growth, and about 75% of patients benefit from a treatment which reduces androgen levels, e.g. orchidectomy or treatment with oestrogenic drugs, or agonists of luteinizing hormone-releasing hormone may induce tumour regression.

Complications of benign prostatic hyperplasia	
bladder wall	hypertrophy of smooth muscle trabeculation: due to prominent bands of thickened smooth muscle diverticula: protrude between trabeculae
bladder size	dilatation: due to failure of bladder wall compensatory mechanisms
ureteric changes	dilatation of ureters
urinary infection (cystitis)	bladder fails to empty completely after micturition, and residual urine is liable to infection
kidney disease	pyelonephritis: from ascending infection impaired renal failure hydronephrosis calculi

Fig. 12.17 Complications of benign prostatic hyperplasia.

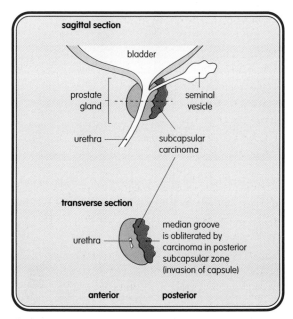

Fig. 12.18 Prostatic carcinoma.

- Name the common infections of the penis.
- Describe the malignant tumours of the penis.
- Explain the pathogenesis of cryptorchidism.
- Define hydrocele, haematocele and varicocele.
- Explain the classification of testicular carcinomas.
- Describe the pathology of benign prostatic hyperplasia.

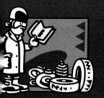

13. Pathology of the Musculoskeletal System

Achondroplasia
This hereditary disorder of endochondral ossification results in dwarfism due to short limbs.

Incidence—The commonest cause of dwarfism occurring in about 1 per 10 000 births.

Aetiology—Autosomal dominant, but there is a high incidence of spontaneous mutation accounting for its sudden appearance in a child with normal parents (increased incidence with paternal age).

Pathogenesis—Normal column formation of cartilage cells at epiphyseum during bone growth does not occur, resulting in diminished lengthening of cartilage bones (e.g. long bones, base of the skull and pelvis). Periosteal bone formation is normal. Cartilage bones are therefore shortened but thick and strong. Membranous bone (such as the vault of the skull) is not affected.

The appearance is as follows:
- Long bones: approximately two-thirds the normal length. More marked in proximal segment (thigh or arm). Bow-leg is characteristic.
- Spine: lumbar lordosis.
- Pelvis: reduced in all diameters.
- Head: as child develops, vault of skull (membrane bone) increases in size, but base of skull and face (cartilage bone) do not develop to the same extent.

> **Achondroplasia results in non-proportional dwarfism, i.e. trunk is of normal size, but arms and legs are much shorter than normal.**
>
> **Other common types of dwarfism (e.g. pituitary hormone deficiency or malnutrition) are typically proportional, with all bones being affected equally.**

Head becomes enlarged with prominent forehead and a depressed bridge of the nose.

Treatment—Excessive bowing may require operative correction.

Prognosis—Heterozygous condition is compatible with normal survival and life-span.

Disorders of the bone matrix
Osteogenesis imperfecta
This heterogeneous group of rare congenital disorders is characterized by abnormal collagen formation with unusually brittle and fragile bones.

Aetiology—Mutation of gene coding for type I collagen resulting in abnormal collagen formation in osteoid. The pattern of inheritance can be either dominant or recessive.

Appearance—There is a marked variation in severity, but the following abnormalities are generally present:
- Bones: slender with thin trabeculae but normally mineralized. Widespread weakness of bone results in multiple fractures frequently leading to severe deformity.
- Other: formation of the teeth is also affected and the collagen of the sclera of the eye is poorly formed giving rise to characteristic physical sign of pale blue sclerae.

There are three types:
- Fetal type: intrauterine fractures and delayed ossification of the skull. Stillbirth is common.
- Infantile type: less severe form. Fractures are less numerous but prognosis for life is still very limited.
- Adolescent type: normal at birth but tendency to develop fractures later. Fractures become less common as child gets older.

Prognosis—In severe cases, the prognosis for life is poor.

Osteoporosis
Slowly progressive disorder characterized by reduced bone mass as a result of a relative increase in bone erosion which is not adequately counteracted by new bone formation.

Incidence—The commonest metabolic bone disease. Widespread in the elderly, it is an important cause of morbidity and even mortality, the weakened bone being particularly predisposed to fracture with minimal trauma (Fig. 13.1).

Macroscopically—Bones are lighter in weight, less dense on radiography (Fig. 13.2) and show thinning of the cortex. Lumbar vertebral bodies are more biconcave than normal such that the intervertebral disc space appears more spherical. Similar shaped vertebral bodies are seen in fish and consequently they are referred to as 'fish vertebrae'.

Microscopically—Bone trabeculae are thinner and reduced in number, and there is a decrease in the number of osteoblasts. Mineralization is not affected.

Complications are:

- Bone pain: especially in back due to compression of vertebral bodies. Multiple compressions lead to overall loss of height which may be compounded by uneven compression of vertebrae leading to anteroposterior bending of the spine (kyphosis).
- Fractures: reduced bone mass leads to increased fractures following minimal trauma, especially of neck of femur and wrists.

Management—Emphasis is on prevention rather than treatment, namely avoidance of risk factors, physical exercise, and adequate calcium intake.

Hormone replacement therapy (HRT) should be considered in women with low bone mass following menopause.

Mucopolysaccharidoses

This group of autosomal recessive disorders of mucopolysaccharide (glycosaminoglycans, such as dermatan sulphate and heparin sulphate) metabolism results in abnormal substrate accumulation in cells of the brain and other tissues.

The main disorders are Hurler's syndrome (gargoylism) and Hunter's syndrome, both of which are associated with a wide variety of clinical features including stiff joints and short stature.

Disorders of osteoclast function
Osteopetrosis (marble bone disease; Albers–Schönberg disease)

This rare inherited disorder is characterized by increased density of all cartilagenous bones, especially the vertebrae, pelvic bones and ribs.

Pathogenesis—Increased bone density is thought to be secondary to defective resorption of bone by osteoclasts.

Appearance—There is no discernible differentiation of cartilagenous bones into cortex and medulla, the cortical compact bone extending into the medulla which is thus devoid of cancellous bone.

Type and associated risk factors for osteoporosis	
Type	**Risk factors**
idiopathic	female early menopause small stature thin physique family history advanced age nulliparity
secondary-generalized	**m**etabolic: low calcium intake, impaired supply of protein (e.g. nephrotic syndrome or cirrhosis of liver), scurvy **a**ssorted endocrine disorders: thyrotoxicosis, panhypopituitarism and Cushing's syndrome **s**teroid therapy **c**igarette smoking **a**lcohol abuse **r**educed physical activity **a**luminium antacids
secondary-localized	disuse atrophy: especially in neurological limb paralysis or post fracture

Fig. 13.1 Type and associated risk factors for osteoporosis.

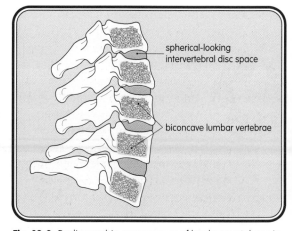

Fig. 13.2 Radiographic appearance of lumbar vertebrae in osteoporosis.

Effect—Bones are excessively dense, yet extremely brittle and prone to fracture. In addition to increased predisposition to fractures, the condition causes depression of marrow function and compression of cranial nerves within the base of the skull.

Paget's disease of the bone (osteitis deformans)

This chronic disease of excessive uncontrolled resorption and deposition of bone particularly affects the skull, backbone, pelvis and long bones. It is rare before 40 years, but increases in incidence with age thereafter, with males more affected than females.

Aetiology—Unknown, but recent evidence suggests a paramyxovirus infection of the osteoclasts.

Pathogenesis—Large, abnormal, multinucleated osteoclasts cause excessive bone erosion with destruction of trabecular and cortical bone. Each wave of bone destruction is followed by a vigorous but uncoordinated osteoblastic response, producing new osteoid to fill the defects left by the osteoclasts. However, both osteoclastic erosion and osteoblastic deposition are random, haphazard and unrelated to functional stresses on the bone, resulting in greatly distorted bone architecture.

Morphology—Bone shows a characteristic woven, non-lamellar pattern indicative of rapid reparative deposition. There are often well marked 'cement lines' visible producing the characteristic 'mosaic' or 'crazy-paving' appearance.

Although bone bulk is often increased, it is typically weaker than normal and more prone to fractures. X-rays reveal patchy sclerosis.

Disruption of bone architecture is followed by progressive increased vascularity in the spaces between the thickened bone trabeculae.

The effects of Paget's may be widespread (affecting many bones) or localized (confined to one area in a single bone—monostotic Paget's disease).

Most patients present with one or both of the following features:

- Bone pain: usually localized to site of most active disease.
- Bone deformity: seen only where there is extensive involvement of an entire bone or series of bones, most commonly enlargement of skull or thickening, enlargement and bowing of tibia.

Complications—Some patients occasionally present with the complications of Paget's disease:

- Nerve compression symptoms: usually seen in association with Paget's disease of the skull, in which enlargement of the pagetic bone can lead to cranial nerve palsies. Vertebral disease may cause kyphosis, shortening of trunk and compression of nerves in intervertebral foramina.
- Pathological fracture: bone is increased in bulk but is weaker than normal and more likely to fracture with trivial trauma.
- Cardiac hypertrophy: due to increased vascularity of bones.
- Malignant tumour (1% of cases): usually osteosarcoma, which may develop in areas of long-standing active Paget's disease.

Investigations are:

- Serology: normal calcium and phosphate, increased alkaline phosphatase.
- Urine: increased urinary excretion of hydroxyproline.
- Abnormal isotope bone scans.
- X-ray: localized bone enlargement, altered trabecular pattern and alternating areas of rarefaction and increased density.

Management is by analgesia for bone pain, and calcitonin or bisphosphonates for severe bone pain not controlled by analgesics. The latter cause inhibition of bone resorption.

Hyperparathyroidism

Elevated secretion of PTH stimulates osteoclastic bone resorption and inhibits osteoblastic bone deposition. This is described in more detail in pp 224–225.

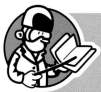

- Name the bones that are commonly affected in achondroplasia.
- Describe the aetiology of osteogenesis imperfecta.
- List the risk factors for osteoporosis.
- What are the complications of osteoporosis?
- Define 'osteopetrosis' and describe the pathogenesis.
- Describe the morphology of affected bone in Paget's disease.

INFECTIONS AND TRAUMA

Pyogenic osteomyelitis

This infection of bone typically affects the cortex, medulla and periosteum, and is most commonly encountered in children under the age of 12. The most common causative organisms are *Escherichia coli* (particularly in infants and the elderly), and *Salmonella* (particularly in patients with sickle-cell disease).

Infective organisms gain access to the medullary cavity of bone by two main routes:

- Direct access through an open wound, particularly when open fractures are involved. Also important in postoperative patients who have had surgery on bones (particularly prosthetic joint replacements).
- Blood-borne spread: following bacteraemia from a focus of sepsis elsewhere.

Clinical features—Abrupt onset of severe pain at the site of bone infection accompanied by fever and malaise.

Complications and sequelae:

- Resolution: with appropriate antibiotic therapy.
- Pathological fracture: purulent acute inflammatory exudate formed in closed compartment of marrow cavity causes compression of vessels with necrosis of medullary bone trabeculae, resulting in increased predisposition to fractures.
- Adjacent sepsis: destruction of cortical bone may lead to discharge of pus into extraosseous connective tissue, and infection may track through to skin surface producing a chronic discharging sinus.
- Chronicity: inflammation tends to become chronic because of localization of infection to confined space of marrow cavity. Organisms may remain viable within marrow cavity for many years. Chronicity results in extensive bone destruction, marrow fibrosis and recurrent focal suppuration (Brodie's abscess). There is also reactive new bone formation, particularly around inflamed periosteum, leading to a thickened and abnormally shaped bone.
- Amyloidosis: long-standing chronic bone infection is a significant cause of secondary AA amyloidosis (see Chapter 14).

Diagnosis is by blood culture and isotope scan.

Management is by antibiotic therapy with surgical exploration and decompression if there is not an immediate response to the antibiotics.

Tuberculous osteomyelitis and Pott's disease

In tuberculous osteomyelitis the marrow cavity contains rapidly enlarging caseating granulomas which destroy trabecular and cortical bone.

The mode of infection is usually by haematogenous spread from a lung focus in children or the elderly. Vertebral bodies (Pott's disease) are the commonest site (affected in 50% of cases) but long bones, fingers and joints are also involved.

Healing occurs with antituberculous chemotherapy firstly by fibrosis and subsequently by new bone formation.

Skeletal syphilis

Two types, both of which are now rare:

- Congenital: osteochondritis and periostitis.
- Acquired: periostitis and gummas.

Fractures

A fracture is a break in the continuity of bone. Note that any break, even of only one cortex, constitutes a fracture. Fractures are the commonest abnormality of bone and are caused by physical trauma.

There are several ways of classifying fractures, e.g. according to causation, according to pattern of fracture or according to their relation to surrounding tissues. The latter is the simplest method.

Types of fracture

Fractures can be classified into two main types according to their relation to surrounding tissues:

- Simple: without contact with external environment, i.e. skin or mucous membrane overlying bone is intact. Less likely to become infected.

- Compound: with direct contact between fracture and external environment, e.g. a fracture of the tibia with laceration of overlying skin. More likely to become infected.

Other descriptive terms for fractures are:
- Comminuted: more than two fragments present.
- Complicated: involvement of nerve, artery or viscus.
- Pathological: fracture occurring in abnormal bone.
- Stress: fracture resulting from repeated application of minor force.
- Greenstick: only one cortex of bone is fractured.

Processes of healing
Bone fractures heal by granulation tissue formation with fibrous repair followed by new bone formation in the fibrous granulation tissue.

The sequence of events in healing of a simple undisplaced fracture is illustrated in Fig. 13.3.

Complications of healing
Bones show great capacity for healing, but certain complications can occur:
- Malunion: poor anatomical alignment of fractures results in deformity, angulation or displacement.
- Delayed union: common and is said to have occurred when a fracture has not united in a reasonable time (defined as 25% longer than the average time taken for that particular type of fracture to unite).
- Non-union: if union has not occurred within one year, then terminology is changed from one of 'delayed union' to one of 'non-union'. Defect is typically filled with fibrous tissue—fibrous ankylosis.

Causes of complications
Efficient healing of fractures requires optimal conditions. Factors that prevent efficient healing are:
- Poor apposition of fractured bone ends.
- Inadequate immobilization.
- Interposition of foreign bodies or soft tissues.
- Infection.
- Corticosteroid therapy.
- Poor general nutritional status.
- Poor blood supply.

Avascular necrosis (osteonecrosis)
Ischaemic necrosis of cortical and trabecular bone is caused by:
- Fractures that interfere with blood supply to certain bones (most important cause) especially affecting femoral and humeral heads, scaphoid and talus.
- OA or inflammatory joint disease: osteonecrosis is seen in approximately 20% of femoral heads removed from patients who have had total hip arthroplasties.
- Vasculitis affecting extraosseous arteries.
- Obliteration of intraosseous sinusoids by thrombi, sickled erythrocytes, fat and nitrogen emboli.
- Idiopathic: osteonecrosis occurs without obvious associated disease at a number of well-defined regional bone sites (femoral head, metatarsal head, tarsal navicular, lunate, medial femoral condyle).

Investigation is by plain radiograph, isotope bone scan with ^{99}Tc diphosphonate, and CT/MRI scan.

Management is by avoiding weight bearing, analgesia for pain relief, and NSAIDs for anti-inflammatory.

Surgery:
- Bone decompression.
- Osteotomy to reduce mechanical stresses on affected bone segments.
- Joint replacement is often required in patients with more advanced disease and secondary OA.

- **What are the complications of pyogenic osteomyelitis?**
- **Explain what is meant by simple and compound fractures.**
- **Describe the healing of a simple fracture.**
- **Name the factors that prevent efficient healing.**
- **List the causes of avascular necrosis.**

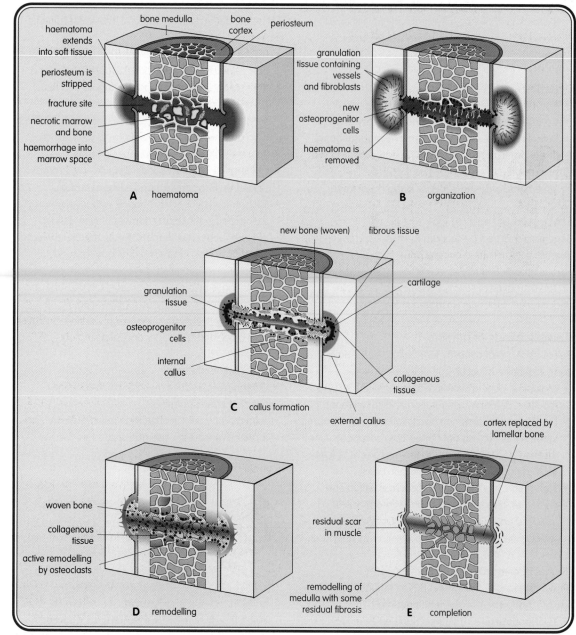

Fig. 13.3 Healing of a simple fracture. (A) Haematoma formation, due to tearing of medullary blood vessels. (B) Organization—migration of neutrophils and macrophages into fracture with organization of haematoma within about 24 hours. Capillaries and fibroblasts proliferate forming fibrovascular granulation tissue. New osteoprogenitor cells (derived from mesenchymal precursor cells) mature into osteoblasts and migrate into granulation tissue. (C) Callus formation—osteoblasts deposit large quantities of osteoid collagen in a haphazard way producing a woven bone pattern. Fracture is bridged on outside by external callus (may contain cartilage) and is bridged in medullary cavity by internal callus (rarely contains cartilage). However, direct ossification may occur between fractured ends if they are closely apposed. (D) Remodelling—about 3 weeks post fracture, callus is well established and undergoes remodelling. Osteoclastic resorption and osteoblastic osteoid synthesis removes surplus calcified callus, replacing bulky, woven bone with compact, organized, lamellar bone. Process takes several months. (E) Completion—formation of new lamellar trabecular bone is complete. Bone is orientated in a direction determined by stresses to which it is exposed with mobilization. However, even after remodelling, cortical irregularities and minor marrow space fibrosis persist at site of fracture.

TUMOURS OF THE BONES

Metastatic disease of the skeleton
Most common tumours in bone are blood-borne metastases from other primary sites, and tumours of haemopoietic cells located within the marrow spaces of bones, particularly myeloma.

Secondary tumours of bone are more common in adults than children, whereas primary tumours of bone are generally more common in children than adults.

Carcinomas
There are five common carcinomas that have a predilection for metastasizing to bone:
- Adenocarcinoma of the breast.
- Carcinoma of bronchus (particularly small-celled, undifferentiated carcinoma).
- Adenocarcinoma of the kidney.
- Adenocarcinoma of the thyroid.
- Adenocarcinoma of the prostate.

Metastases occur most commonly to parts of the skeleton that contain vascular marrow, especially vertebral bodies, ribs, pelvis and upper ends of the femur and humerus.

Osteolytic versus osteosclerotic metastases
Most metastatic tumour cells within bone marrow spaces lead to erosion of bone (osteolytic metastases). However, prostatic carcinoma (and very rarely breast carcinoma) produces metastatic deposits in which there is stimulation of new bone formation (osteosclerotic metastases) particularly in the lumbosacral vertebrae.
Clinical features:
- Bone pain: usually localized to site of deposits.
- Fractures: erosion of trabecular bone either directly, or through osteoclast-stimulated bone erosion (osteolytic metastases) → bone weakness → increased predisposition to pathological fractures.

Complications are:
- Leukoerythroblastic anaemia: a result of extensive replacement of bone marrow.
- Symptoms of hypercalcaemia: caused by release of calcium from bone by osteolytic process.
- Nerve and spinal compression: particularly in vertebral metastases.

Haematopoietic malignancies
Haematopoietic malignances found in bone (e.g. myelomas, lymphomas, leukaemias, etc.) are discussed in Chapter 14.

Bone-forming tumours
Primary tumours derived from cells involved in bone formation and modelling are relatively rare.

Osteoma
Benign, smooth, rounded bone tumour is seen on the surface of long bones or skull bone. Apart from visible or palpable swelling, there are usually no symptoms.

Ivory osteoma
This cortical bone tumour is composed of densely compact bone with haversian systems. It occurs most frequently in the vault of the skull and is usually asymptomatic.

Cancellous osteoma (exostosis)
This cancellous bone tumour forming an outgrowth from the end of a long bone usually rises to a point.

Osteoid osteoma and osteoblastoma
Osteoid osteoma
Rarely causing severe bone pain, this typically arises between the ages of 10 and 30 years. Most commonly it affects long bones of the lower leg, but it may occur in any bone except the skull. Tumours are composed of active osteoblasts which deposit large, irregular masses of osteoid collagen in a haphazard manner.
   Radiographs characteristically show a central dense area surrounded by a halo of translucency. Excision is usually curative and lesions do not recur.

Osteoblastoma (giant osteoid osteoma)
This large tumour with similar histological features to osteoid osteoma mainly affects the bones of the hands, feet and vertebrae. Tumours are typically more locally aggressive and can recur after incomplete excision.

Osteosarcoma

This malignant tumour of osteoblasts occurs most often in adolescent children. The majority arise around the knee (the lower end of the femur or upper end of the tibia) and a minority in other long bones such as the upper end of humerus or femur.

Symptoms are bone pain increasing gradually with tumour growth, but the tumour is often well-advanced at the time of diagnosis.

Spread—The tumour grows rapidly within the medullary cavity, eventually eroding through the cortical plate into soft tissue. Metastasis occurs early via the bloodstream, usually to the lung.

Tthe prognosis is poor (5–10% 5 year survival) but has improved with the adoption of earlier surgical treatment combined with radiotherapy/chemotherapy.

Osteosarcoma in adults is largely confined to elderly patients with a long history of active Paget's disease of the bone.

Cartilage-forming tumours
Osteochondroma

This benign tumour grows as an exophytic nodule from metaphyses of long bones. It is also known as a 'cartilage-capped exostosis' as it is composed of protruberant bone covered with a cap of cartilage and an outer layer of perichondrium.

Lesions are found most commonly in the humerus, femur and the upper end of the tibia, and they may be solitary or multiple (typically autosomal dominant condition, hereditary multiple exostoses). Chondrosarcomatous change is rare in solitary lesions but more common in hereditary multiple lesions.

Chondroma

The most common benign tumour of cartilage-forming tissue, this is composed of a scattering of benign chondrocytes embedded in a cartilaginous matrix.

Tumours are thought to originate from residual nests of cartilage cells left behind in metaphysis as bone growth proceeds. They are found most commonly in small bones of hands and feet.

They may be single ('solitary enchondroma') or multiple ('enchondromatosis'). (The term 'enchondroma' is used to indicate that the tumour arises and grows within bone as opposed to osteochondroma which grows as a nodular exophytic lesion.) A solitary chondroma rarely undergoes malignant change, but occasionally happens in multiple enchondromatosis.

Chondrosarcoma

This slow-growing malignant tumour often reaches a large size, eventually breaking through the periosteum into surrounding soft tissue, but usually maintaining a clearly defined border.

Macroscopically, there is a glistening white appearance, similar to that of normal cartilage.

Microscopically:
- Majority are low-grade, well-differentiated tumours that metastasize very late, and are histologically similar to benign cartilaginous tumours. Radical local surgery may be curative.
- Minority are high-grade, poorly differentiated tumours with marked pleomorphism, high mitotic activity and grow rapidly with early blood-borne metastases.

Chondroblastoma (Codman's tumour)

A rare tumour derived from chondroblasts, this typically occurs in males aged 20 years or younger. Typically it affects epiphyseal bone, especially of the knee or upper end of the humerus.

Microscopically, cells frequently show mitosis and 'giant' cells (smaller than those seen in giant cell tumour). Some areas of cartilage may calcify or show bone formation.

Despite increased mitoses, tumours are usually benign. Occasional cases are locally aggressive and rarely some metastasize without showing any significantly different histological features.

Chondromyxoid fibroma

This rare benign tumour is composed of lobules of fibrous tissue separated by myxomatous tissue containing cells in lacunae (thus mimicking the appearance of cartilage).

Typically it occurs below the age of 30 years, arising at the epiphyseal line (especially upper end of the tibia and small bones of the hands and feet) but sparing the epiphysis. Microscopically, cells are often atypical, and may result in an incorrect histological interpretation as a chondrosarcoma.

Fibrous and fibro-osseous tumours
Fibroma

A benign tumour, this is composed of inactive, acellular, fibrous tissue. Stroma may ossify to form an ossifying fibroma. The main complication is pathological fracture.

Fibrous dysplasia

This condition results from the disorganization of tissue differentiation and the modelling of diaphyses. Shafts are usually thickened and may be painful. It may affect one bone (monostotic) or many (polyostotic) and deformity may be severe. Pathological fractures often occur, but they have normal healing potential. Prognosis of life is not affected.

Fibrosarcoma and malignant fibrous histiocytoma

Fibrosarcoma

This malignant tumour of fibroblasts can be classified into two types:

- Endosteal fibrosarcoma: arises within bones and gives rise to destructive lesions as it grows out. Metastasis is to both local lymph nodes and lungs. Associated with a poor prognosis.
- Periosteal fibrosarcoma: seldom invades bone or metastasizes to distant sites. Treatment is by local excision.

Malignant fibrous histiocytoma

This high-grade malignant bone tumour contains a mixture of spindle-shaped fibroblasts with histiocytic cells, many of which are multinucleated. Fibroblasts are characteristically arranged in a cartwheel-like formation (storiform pattern).

Other tumours

Ewing's sarcoma

A highly malignant bone tumour derived from marrow endothelium, this affects children between the ages of 5 and 15. Areas of osteolytic bone destruction surrounded by layers of new periosteal bone give the tumour a characteristic 'onion skin' appearance on X-ray. Pain, swelling and tenderness may be associated with fever and leukocytosis (thus tumours are sometimes mistaken for osteomyelitis). Five-year survival is virtually nil despite radiotherapy and amputation.

Giant cell tumour (osteoclastoma)

Osteolytic lesions arise in the epiphyses of long bones, typically in young and middle-aged adults, and are generally more common in women.

The tumour is composed of a mass of large multinucleated giant cells resembling large osteoclasts

embedded in a supporting spindle-celled stroma. There is a gradual expansion of lesions into the metaphysis and the erosion of cortical bone, yet penetration of the periosteum or articular cartilage is rare.

Osteoclastoma is generally classed as benign but can recur after local removal. About 10% of cases are malignant and metastasize to the lung via the blood stream.

See Fig. 13.4 for a summary of bone tumours.

Summary of bone tumours		
Type	**Tumour**	**Clinical features**
metastatic (secondary)	carcinoma of bronchus (esp. small cell) adenocarcinomas of the breast, kidney and thyroid prostate	metastases occur most commonly to vertebral bodies, ribs, pelvis and upper ends of femur and humerus
primary	bone-forming tumours	osteoma osteoid osteoma osteoblastoma osteosarcoma
	cartilage-forming tumours	osteochondroma chondroma chondroblastoma (Codman's tumour) chondrosarcoma chondromyxoid fibroma
	fibrous and fibro-osseous tumour	fibroma fibrous clysplasia fibrosarcoma malignant fibrous histiocytoma
	others	Ewing's sarcoma giant cell tumour (osteoclastoma)

Fig. 13.4 Summary of bone tumours.

- List the five common carcinomas that metastasize to bone.
- Name the skeletal sites to which carcinomas normally metastasize.
- Name the bone-forming tumours.
- Describe the different cartilage-forming tumours.
- What is Ewing's sarcoma?

DISORDERS OF THE NEUROMUSCULAR JUNCTION

Overview

Several diseases of muscle have been shown to be due to disorders affecting transmission at the neuromuscular junction (NMJ).

Clinical presentation of NMJ dysfunction:

- Fatiguability: primarily affecting proximal limb muscles, extraocular muscles (causing ptosis or diplopia) and muscles of mastication, speech and facial expression.
- Periodic paralysis: sudden reversible attacks of paralysis and flaccidity.

Disorders can be classified into two types, pre- and postsynaptic abnormalities, depending on which of the synaptic membranes is affected.

Presynaptic abnormalities
Botulism

This rare form of food poisoning is caused by ingestion of a toxin produced by the bacterium *Clostridium botulinum*, found in imperfectly treated tinned food or preserved fish contaminated with the microbe.

Pathogenesis—The toxin binds irreversibly to those presynaptic nerve terminals of axons whose impulse transmission is acetylcholine (Ach)-mediated, which include NMJ, autonomic ganglia and parasympathetic nerve terminals. Binding of the toxin prevents the release of Ach.

Clinical symptoms are chiefly vomiting and pareses of skeletal, ocular, pharyngeal and respiratory muscles. Antitoxin is available but has no effect once the toxin is bound. Recovery of transmission is achieved by terminal axonal sprouting and the formation of new synaptic contacts. Mortality can be high.

Lambert–Eaton myasthenic syndrome

This autoimmune disorder is characterized by abnormal fatiguability and is often found in patients with lung cancer. Autoantibodies bind to presynaptic voltage-dependent calcium channels at motor nerve terminals to cause functional loss. This in turn causes the reduced release of acetylcholine in response to nerve stimulation. Small cell lung carcinoma cells express calcium channels suggesting that autoantibody production is triggered by these tumour antigens.

Postsynaptic abnormalities
Myasthenia gravis

This autoimmune disease is characterized by a progressive failure to sustain a maintained or repeated contraction of striated muscle. Prevalence is about 1 in 30 000. The disease usually appears between the ages of 15 and 50 years and females are more often affected than males.

Aetiology—Autoantibodies are produced by B lymphocytes which are defectively controlled by T lymphocytes, a result of a disorder of the thymus gland. About 25% of cases have a thymoma (see Chapter 14, pp. XX–XX), others having thymic gland hyperplasia.

Other associations are thyrotoxicosis, DM, RA, and SLE.

Pathogenesis—Autoantibodies bind to the Ach receptor located in the postsynaptic membrane of muscle motor endplates. These antibodies prevent synaptic transmission by blocking the receptor sites.

Presentation:

- Early symptoms: intermittent ptosis or diplopia, weakness of chewing, swallowing, speaking or of moving the limbs. Movement is initially strong, but rapidly weakens.
- Later symptoms: respiratory muscles may be involved and respiratory failure is not an uncommon cause of death. Asphyxia occurs readily as the cough may be too weak to clear foreign bodies from the airways. Muscle atrophy may occur in long-standing cases.

The disease runs a remitting/relapsing course, and relapses may be precipitated by emotional disturbances, infections, pregnancy or severe muscular effort.

Investigations:

- Tensilon test: administration of a therapeutic trial of a short-acting, anticholinesterase drug that increases Ach concentrations in the synaptic cleft and allows transmission.
- Autoantibody screen: elevated Ach receptor antibody if found in 80% of cases.
- Thyroid function tests: to screen for associated autoimmune disease of thyroid gland.
- PA and lateral chest radiograph/CT scan of thorax to identify thymomas.
- EMG may show a characteristic decremental response.

Management:
- Medical: anticholinesterase drugs (prevent breakdown of Ach at NMJ); immunological treatment—plasma exchange (removal of antibody from the blood), intravenous immunoglobulin, immunosuppressant treatment.
- Surgical: thymectomy (may improve myasthenia in a proportion of cases).

The prognosis is variable. If the disorder is confined to eye muscles, then the prognosis for life is normal and disability slight. A prognosis of myasthenia associated with thymoma is markedly worse.

- **Name the presynaptic abnormalities of the NMJ.**
- **How is botulism transmitted?**
- **Define 'Lambert–Eaton myasthenic syndrome'.**
- **What is myasthenia gravis?**
- **Describe the pathogenesis and clinical presentation of myasthenia gravis.**

THE MYOPATHIES

Definition
Myopathy is any condition that primarily affects muscle physiology, structure or biochemistry.

Inherited myopathies
X-linked muscular dystrophy
This inherited disease of muscle is characterized by the progressive degeneration of single muscle cells over a prolonged period of time, with fibre regeneration and the development of fibrosis.

Dystrophy is a term used to describe inherited degenerative muscle diseases.

Duchenne muscular dystrophy
The pattern of inheritance is X-linked recessive, hence the disorder is almost exclusively seen in males. This is the most common form of muscular dystrophy in childhood, affecting 1 in 3000 male births.

The disorder is due to a mutation of the gene coding for dystrophin, a protein that normally anchors the actin cytoskeleton of muscle fibres to the basement membrane via a membrane glycoprotein complex (Fig. 13.5). Lack of this protein renders fibres liable to tearing with repeated contraction.

Different degrees of severity of Duchenne dystrophy result from different mutations within the dystrophin gene:
- Severe Duchenne dystrophy: complete failure to produce dystrophin as a result of mutations causing gene frameshifts.
- Moderate to severe forms of Duchenne dystrophy: dystrophin is produced but anchorage is inefficient due to mutations in binding sites for either membrane glycoprotein complex or actin cytoskeleton.
- Mild form of Duchenne dystrophy (Becker's dystrophy): mutation in middle rod region still allows anchorage of muscle to basement membrane.

Morphological features—Muscle changes associated with Duchenne are illustrated in Fig. 13.6.

Clinical features—Childhood onset of muscle weakness with a high serum creatinine kinase level (caused by muscle necrosis) and calf hypertrophy due to fatty replacement of muscle (Fig. 13.6). Cardiac

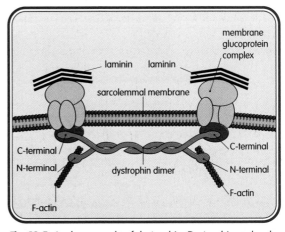

Fig. 13.5 Anchorage role of dystrophin. Dystrophin molecule is a long, rod-shaped protein, one end binding to membrane glycoprotein, the other to actin, with middle rod region.

muscle is also affected leading to cardiomyopathy (see Chapter 7, pp. 90–91).

The prognosis depends on the degree of severity; for severe Duchenne it is very poor, most affected individuals dying in their late teens.

Myotonic disorders
Myotonic disorders are diseases in which there is a continuing contraction of muscle after voluntary contraction has ceased.

Myotonic muscular dystrophy
This autosomal dominant disorder is characterized by muscle weakness, myotonia (inability to relax muscles), and several non-muscle features including cataracts, frontal baldness in males, cardiomyopathy and low intelligence.

This is the most common inherited muscle disease of adults, affecting 1 in 8000.

The molecular basis is a gene located on chromosome 19 coding for cAMP-dependent protein kinase. Mutation is an unstable trinucleotide repeat sequence which shows features of anticipation (see Chapter 5). The mechanism through which this mutation causes myotonia is unknown.

Microscopically, affected muscles show abnormalities of fibre size with fibre necrosis, abundant

internal nuclei and replacement by fibrofatty tissue.

The disorder usually becomes apparent in adolescence or early adulthood with facial weakness and distal weakness in the limbs.

Prognosis—Death is commonly due to involvement of respiratory muscles in middle-age.

Acquired myopathies
Idiopathic inflammatory myopathies
There is primary inflammation of muscle with resulting fibre necrosis. The inflammatory infiltrate is mainly composed of T lymphocytes and monocytes as part of an abnormal autoimmune response. There are three main types of inflammatory myopathies, as follows.

Polymyositis
This inflammatory muscle disorder is characterized by weakness, pain and swelling of proximal limb muscles and facial muscles, often with ptosis and dysphagia. It is the commonest inflammatory muscle disorder, though still relatively rare, affecting 2 per 10 million per year worldwide. It occurs most frequently in adults, with females more than males by 3:1.

Aetiology—A cell-mediated autoimmunity but the mechanism of sensitization is unknown.

Associations:
- Increased predisposition in people with HLA-B8/DR3.
- Connective tissue diseases such as SLE, rheumatoid disease or scleroderma.
- Dermatomyositis: muscle disease is accompanied by a characteristic skin rash.
- Malignancy: particularly in association with bronchial, breast, ovarian, gastric and nasopharyngeal carcinoma.

Microscopically, there is a lymphocytic infiltration of muscle with fibre necrosis.

Clinical features—An insidious onset in the third to fifth decade with a weakness of the pelvic and shoulder girdle muscles. Progression is typically slow but may eventually involve pharyngeal, laryngeal and respiratory muscles leading to dysphagia, dysphonia and respiratory failures. Spontaneous remissions with the return of muscle strength may also occur.

Investigations—Blood: increased muscle enzymes, tests for rheumatoid factor and antinuclear factor are

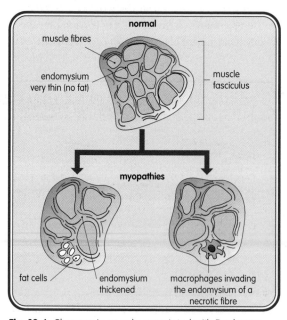

Fig. 13.6 Changes in muscle associated with Duchenne muscular dystrophy.

often positive. EMG: useful for differentiating polymyositis from peripheral myopathies. Muscle biopsy: muscle necrosis and regeneration in association with inflammatory cell infiltrate. MRI: non-invasive detection of active myositis.

Treatment—It may respond to immunosuppressive treatment such as corticosteroids and azathioprine.

Dermatomyositis
Polymyositis is accompanied by periorbital oedema and a characteristic purple 'heliotrope' rash on the upper eyelids. Often, there is an erythematous, scaling rash on the face, shoulders, upper arms and chest with red patches over the knuckles, elbows and knees.

Inclusion body myositis
This slowly progressive inflammatory muscle disorder is clinically similar to polymyositis, but occurs mainly in the elderly. By light microscopy histological features are also similar to polymyositis, but with electron microscopy vacuoles containing filamentous inclusion bodies can be seen within fibres.

Endocrine myopathies
There is a weakness and wasting of muscle associated with endocrine disease. The main causes are:
- Corticosteroid-induced myopathy: either therapeutic or in Cushing's disease.
- Myopathies of thyroid dysfunction: associated with both hyper- and hypothyroidism.
- Myopathy of osteomalacia: painful myopathy often without much wasting or weakness.

Changes are usually reversible with appropriate therapy.

Toxic myopathies
Muscle damage may by incurred by a wide variety of drugs, the most common of which is alcohol. Damage to muscle is usually reversible on withdrawal of the toxic agent.

Ethanol
This may cause a spectrum of muscle diseases varying from mild, proximal weakness to severe muscle necrosis. Biopsy shows selective atrophy of type 2b fibres, which is reversible in the early stages.

Cholesterol-lowering agents
Diazocholesterol, a drug once used in the treatment of hypercholesterolaemia, causes muscle spasms and weakness with myotonia.

Chloroquine
This drug is used principally in the treatment of malaria associated with myopathy and mild peripheral neuropathy. Damage is reversible on drug withdrawal, but recovery is slow.

L-tryptophan
Eosinophilia myalgia has been reported with tryptophan-containing products.

- **Define the terms 'myopathy', 'dystrophy' and 'myotonia'.**
- **Explain the molecular basis and clinical details for Duchenne muscular dystrophy.**
- **What are the characteristics of myotonic muscular dystrophy?**
- **Describe the three types of idiopathic inflammatory myopathies.**
- **Which hormones can cause endocrine myopathies?**
- **Name two toxins that can induce myopathy.**

ARTHROPATHIES

Osteoarthritis (OA)
This degenerative disease of articular cartilage. is associated with secondary changes in underlying bone resulting in pain and impaired function of affected joint.

It is extremely common—80% of the elderly population show radiographic evidence of OA, although only around 25% of these are symptomatic.

Females are affected more than males, and the disease is often more severe in older women. It is increasingly common above 60 years of age, but may also occur in younger age groups following any form of mechanical derangement.

OA affects joints that are constantly exposed to wear and tear, typically large weight bearing joints, e.g. those of the hip and knee, but also small joints in the hands, particularly the thumb.

The aetiology is as follows:
- Primary: no obvious causes or predisposing factors (majority of cases).
- Secondary: arising as a complication of other joint disorders, mainly inflammatory joint disease, congenital joint deformities, trauma to joints, avascular necrosis of bone.

Secondary OA is also an important component of occupational joint disease, e.g. OA of the fingers in typists and of the knee in professional footballers.

Risk factors for the development of OA are:
- Ageing.
- Abnormal load on joints.
- Crystal deposition.
- Joint inflammation.

Pathological changes

Pathological changes involve cartilage, bone, synovium and joint capsule with secondary effects on muscle (Fig. 13.7).

Early stage:
- Erosion and destruction of articular cartilage: degenerate cartilage splits along lines of fibres to produce fronds of degenerate cartilage (fibrillation). Narrowing of joint space can be seen on radiography.
- Inflammation and thickening of joint capsule and synovium.

Later stages:
- Sclerosis of subarticular bone: caused by constant friction of naked bone surfaces (eburnation).
- Osteophytes form around periphery of joint by irregular outgrowth of bone. Some may break off to form loose bodies within joint. In distal interphalangeal joints of fingers, osteophytes appear as small nodules (Heberden's nodes). In proximal interphalangeal joint, they are Bouchard's nodes.
- Small cysts may develop in areas where bone is not thickened as a result of synovial fluid accumulation in underlying bone.
- Reactive thickening of synovium and joint capsule due to inflammation caused by bone and cartilage debris.
- Atrophy of muscle caused by disuse following immobility of diseased joint.

OA can be classified according to the main presenting features as follows:
- Primary generalized OA: usually associated with development of Heberden's nodes on fingers and is most common in postmenopausal women.
- Erosive inflammatory OA: form of OA in which there is severe inflammation and erosion of cartilage, with rapid progression.
- Hypertrophic OA: florid osteophyte formation and bone sclerosis but with slow progression and relatively good prognosis.

The main symptoms of OA are pain and a limitation in movement of affected joint sometimes associated with visible swelling (partly due to osteophytes and partly to fluid accumulation in joint cavity and synovial fibrosis).

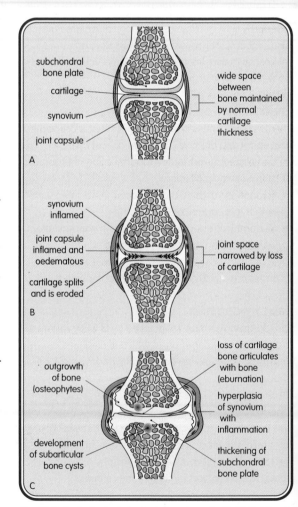

Fig. 13.7 Pathological changes in osteoarthritis (OA). (A) Normal joint. (B) Early stages of OA. (C) Later stages of OA.

In OA of cervical vertebrae (cervical spondylosis), osteophytes compressing emerging spinal nerves are responsible for much of the symptomatology.

Diagnosis—Recognized on X-ray by:
- Narrowing of joint space due to loss of cartilage.
- Presence of osteophytes, producing irregularities at bone margins.
- Cystic appearance just beneath articular surface.
- Sclerosis: increased bone density immediately adjacent to joint space.

Treatment:
- Lifestyle: reduction of pressure across joint, e.g. by weight loss and/or use of walking stick in OA of the hip.
- Medical: analgesics and anti-inflammatories for pain relief, intra-articular or periarticular corticosteroid injections may also be helpful, especially with OA of knee.
- Surgical: corrective and prosthetic surgery for advanced hip or knee disease.

Rheumatoid arthritis (RA)

This inflammatory joint disease is caused by a multisystem connective tissue autoimmune disorder, rheumatoid disease (see Chapter 14). It affects about 1% of the UK population, females more than males by about 3:1. Onset is typically between 35 and 45 years, but follows a normal distribution curve, and no age group is exempt.

Rheumatoid arthritis mainly affects peripheral synovial joints such as the fingers and wrists, but can also affect the knees and more proximal joints.

The aetiology is autoimmune, and there is an association with HLA-DR4 haplotype in most ethnic groups. The condition is characterized by the presence of circulating autoantibody 'rheumatoid factor' (seropositive arthritis) which distinguishes it from several other inflammatory joint diseases (seronegative arthritis).

Pathological changes

There are three main pathological changes (Fig. 13.8):
- Rheumatoid synovitis.
- Articular cartilage destruction.
- Focal destruction of bone.

Rheumatoid synovitis

The synovium becomes swollen and shows a villous pattern. Chronic inflammatory cells (mainly lymphocytes and plasma cells) increase in number within the synovial stroma, often forming an exudate which effuses into the joint space. Fibrin is deposited on the surface of the synovium. Soft tissue swelling from synovial inflammation may be marked.

Articular cartilage destruction

Vascular granulation tissue grows across the surface of the cartilage (pannus) from the edges of the joint. The articular surface shows the loss of cartilage beneath the extending pannus, most marked at joint margins.

Focal destruction of bone

Osteolytic destruction of bone occurs at the edges of the joint. Bone 'erosions' can be seen on radiography, and

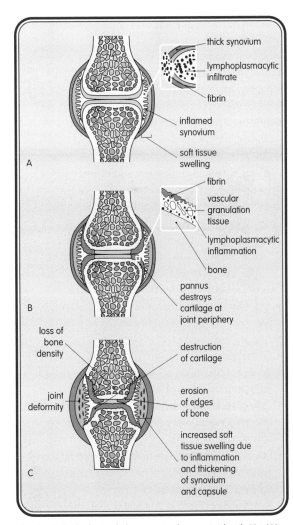

Fig. 13.8 Pathological changes in rheumatoid arthritis. (A) Rheumatoid synovitis. (B) Articular cartilage destruction. (C) Focal destruction of bone.

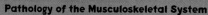
are associated with joint deformity. There is also increased soft tissue swelling due to inflammation and thickening of the synovium and capsule.

Clinical features

Symmetrical polyarthritis

The insidious onset of arthritis first attacks finger joints (mainly metacarpophalangeal and proximal interphalangeal joints) followed by metatarsophalangeal joints and joints of the ankles, wrists, knees, shoulders, elbows and hips (in decreasing order of frequency). However, the disease may also affect joints such as the temporomandibular joint and the synovial joints of the spine (particularly the upper cervical spine). Affected joints become swollen, painful and warm, often with redness of overlying skin.

Joint deformities

As the disease progresses, muscle atrophy and joint destruction result in limitation of joint motion, joint instability, subluxation and deformities. There are also flexion contractures of small joints of the hands and feet, knees, hips and elbows.

Subluxation, a characteristic feature of RA, is a term used to describe a partial dislocation of any joint such that bone ends still make contact, but are misaligned.

Of the hands:

- Anterior subluxation of metacarpophalangeal joints with ulnar deviation of fingers.
- 'Swan neck' deformity: hyperextension of proximal interphalangeal joint with fixed flexion at distal interphalangeal joints.
- Boutonnière (buttonhole) deformity: fixed flexion of proximal interphalangeal joint and extension of the terminal interphalangeal joint.
- Z deformity of thumbs: fixed flexion at metacarpophalangeal joint and hyperextension at interphalangeal joint.

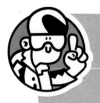
In the hands, rheumatoid arthritis tends to affect MCP and PIP joints whereas osteoarthritis tends to affect PIP and DIP joints.

In the wrists there is often a fixed flexion deformity with a prominent, tender ulnar styloid process and pain on pronation/supination.

In the knees, Baker's cyst (cystic swelling in the popliteal fossa) is seen.

In the cervical spine there is atlantoaxial subluxation.

Deformities are initially correctable but permanent contractures eventually develop such that joints become completely disorganized.

Rheumatoid nodules

Joint changes are often associated with development of subcutaneous rheumatoid nodules, usually located over the extensor aspect of the forearm but occasionally found overlying other bony prominences. Nodules are composed of extensive areas of degenerate collagen surrounded by a giant cell granulomatous reaction.

Other

Other features seen in systemic rheumatoid disease are discussed in Chapter 14. Complications are:

- Secondary osteoarthritis as a result of loss of articular surface particularly in weight-bearing joints such as the knee.
- Septic arthritis: infection of joint secondary to invasion from an ulcerated nodule or infected skin lesion.
- Amyloidosis: found in 25–30% of RA patients at autopsy.
- Carpal tunnel syndrome.
- Ruptured extensor tendons of hand.

Investigations and diagnosis:

- Radiography: periarticular osteoporosis, loss of articular cartilage (joint space), erosions, subluxation and ankylosis.
- Serology: rheumatoid factors (IgG- or IgM- type immunoglobulins which react with the Fc portion of IgG).

- Synovial fluid analysis: useful in the differential diagnosis of inflammatory and degenerative arthropathies.

Diagnosis of RA is made with four or more of the following criteria (American Rheumatism Association, 1988 revision):
- Morning stiffness (>1 hour), of at least six weeks' duration.
- Arthritis of three or more joint areas, of at least six weeks' duration.
- Arthritis of hand joints, of at least six weeks' duration.
- Symmetrical arthritis, of at least six weeks' duration.
- Rheumatoid nodules.
- Rheumatoid factor.
- Radiological changes.

Treatment:
- Anti-inflammatories.
- Immunosuppression: penicillamine, gold, azathioprine, salazopyrine.
- Surgery for advanced painful disease in any joint.

Prognosis—The course of RA is variable:
- 25% remain fit for all normal activities.
- 40% have moderate impairment of function.
- 25% are quite badly disabled.
- 10% become wheelchair patients.

The worst prognosis is associated with high titres of rheumatoid factor, early appearance of erosions, rheumatoid nodules, systemic manifestations and HLA DR4.

Juvenile form of RA
This accounts for approximately 15% of cases of juvenile chronic arthritis. It may begin before 16 years of age. Clinical features are identical to those of adults, and tests for rheumatoid factor are positive. Prognosis is worse than for adults.

Sjögren's syndrome
This autoimmune disorder is characterized by dryness in both eyes and mouth due to impaired tear and saliva production caused by chronic inflammatory infiltrates in both lacrimal and salivary glands. The disorder is present in 15% of all RA cases.

Ankylosing spondylitis
This inflammatory arthritic disorder is characterized by a rigid spine due to ossification of the spinal joints and ligaments. The condition begins in the lumbar vertebral spine and sacroiliac joints, extending upwards to involve thoracic and cervical vertebrae. There may also be involvement of peripheral joints, mainly the hips and knees.

It affects 1% of the population in the UK, typically presenting in late adolescence and young adults (age 15–30 years), and in males more than females by 2:1.

The aetiology is unknown but more than 90% of men with ankylosing spondylitis have the HLA B27 antigen (less than 10% of the normal population have this antigen), which suggests an autoimmune disorder.

Morphological changes—Chronic inflammation of vertebral ligaments slowly heals by dense fibrosis and ossification to form a rigid shell which links the periphery of the vertebral bodies. Eventually the vertebral column becomes fused, inflexible and rigid ('bamboo spine').

Symptoms are typically an insidious onset of recurring episodes of low back pain and stiffness sometimes radiating to the buttocks or thighs. Symptoms are characteristically worse in early morning and after inactivity.

Systemic manifestations include aortic valve incompetence (as a result of rheumatoid aortitis), recurrent iritis and chronic inflammatory bowel disease.

On investigation, the ESR is raised or normal, serology is negative for rheumatoid factor, and X-ray shows typical bamboo spine.

The disease progresses slowly but unremittingly. Management is by:
- Life style: regular physiotherapy and exercise (e.g. non-contact sports like swimming) to maintain as full mobility as possible and prevent deformity.
- Medical: NSAIDs (for symptomatic relief); radiotherapy (if response to drug therapy is unsatisfactory, but carries small risk of leukaemia).
- Surgery for associated hip disease.

Fig. 13.9 shows a table comparing joint diseases.

Comparison of joint diseases			
	Osteoarthritis	Rheumatoid disease	Ankylosing spondylitis
affected age group	elderly	any age	onset usually before 30 years
rheumatoid factor	negative	positive	usually negative
sex	females > males	females > males	males > females
HLA association	none known	HLA DR4	HLA B27
hands	Heberden's nodes (DIP) Bouchard's nodes (PIP)	ulnar deviation of MCP joints swan neck deformity boutonnière deformity Z thumbs prominent ulnar styloid process	–
affected joints	mainly hip, knees and spine	any	mainly spine
joint pathology	erosion of cartilage osteophytes	destruction of joints	bony ankylosis
synovial pathology	slight synovial hyperplasia	florid synovial hyperplasia; pannus	–
associated diseases	–	rheumatoid disease Sjögren's syndrome interstitial lung fibrosis	aortic valve incompetence uveitis inflammatory bowel disease

Fig. 13.9 Comparison of joint diseases. DIP = distal interphalangeal; PIP = proximal interphalangeal.

Arthritis in association with other systemic disease

Reiter's syndrome

This inflammatory syndrome is characterized by the triad of arthritis, urethritis and conjunctivitis. It complicates 0.8% of urethral infection in males, and 0.2% of cases of dysentery. It occurs in males more than females by 20:1, and the usual age of onset is 20–40 years.

Classification is on the basis of aetiology:

- Genital type: usually follows non-specific (non-gonococcal) urethritis, or, less commonly, cystitis or prostatitis.
- Intestinal or postdysenteric type: in some parts of the world may follow dysentery or occasionally non-specific diarrhoea, occurring 10–30 days after intestinal manifestations.

The underlying pathological mechanism is unknown but probably autoimmune.

Clinical features are:

- Arthritis, usually affecting knee or ankle. Clinically and histologically, arthritis resembles rheumatoid

arthritis with chronic inflammatory synovitis.
- Dysuria and penile discharge.
- Conjunctivitis (in 30% of cases).

Prognosis—The first attack typically resolves spontaneously within 6 months. However, 50% of patients relapse and some have continued relapsing of chronic arthritis with attacks recurring at regular intervals, causing disability but seldom deformity. In a minority of cases there is development of severe spondylitis and features very similar to ankylosing spondylitis

Psoriatic arthritis

About 5% of psoriasis patients develop arthropathy which characteristically involves the distal interphalangeal joints (see Chapter 15).

Arthritis associated with GI disease

Bacterial gastroenteritis

This arises post infection with *Salmonella*, *Yersinia* or *Campylobacter*. HLA B27 antigen is present in 80% of affected patients.

Inflammatory bowel disease

Arthritis is seen at some stage in up to 20% of patients with ulcerative colitis and Crohn's disease. Typically it involves knee joints, but occasionally also ankles, elbows and small digital joints. Sacroiliitis and ankylosing spondylitis are also much more frequent in patients with inflammatory bowel disease.

Behçet's syndrome

This syndrome of unknown aetiology is characterized by the triad of oral ulceration, genital ulceration and iritis but is also accompanied by arthritis in 60% of cases.

Arthritis may be chronic or episodic and is usually polyarticular. It most commonly affects the knees and ankles, but occasionally affects the elbows, wrists, and small joints of the hands or feet.

Others

Neuropathic (Charcot's) joint disease

This joint disease occurs secondary to the loss of pain and position sense within the joint which is swollen and deformed, but not painful. Possible causes of loss of joint sensation include diabetic neuropathy, tabes dorsalis, syringomyelia, leprosy and cauda equina lesions (e.g. myelomeningocele).

Sarcoid arthritis

Arthritis occurs in 10% of patients with sarcoidosis, with onset typically in the first year of the disease. It may be of two types:
- Early acute transient type: polyarticular symmetrical arthritis typically affecting knees and ankles, and usually associated with erythema nodosum.
- Chronic persistent type: polyarticular associated with chronic sarcoidosis.

Chronic haemodialysis

There is an increased predisposition to septic arthritis (see below).

Crystal arthropathies

These diseases are characterized by deposition of crystals in joints and soft tissues. Affected patients usually present with an episode of acute arthritis, inflammation being caused by the deposition of the crystals, sometimes called a 'chemical arthritis'. With time, inflammatory changes lead to the development of chronic arthritis with features of osteoarthritis (secondary osteoarthritis).

Nomenclature

The term 'gout' is used as a clinical description of joints affected by crystal deposition. This term is then refined by demonstrating the type of crystal involved. There are two main types of crystal arthropathies: urate gout ('true gout' or just 'gout') and calcium pyrophosphate gout ('pseudogout').

Gout

This acute inflammatory crystal arthropathy is caused by the deposition of urate crystal in joints and soft tissues as a result of hyperuricaemia. It affects 0.3% of the population in the UK and is largely confined to men (90%) although some women develop the condition post menopausally. It can present at any time between the ages of 20 and 60 years.

Aetiology—Uric acid is normally derived from the breakdown of purines and is excreted in the urine. Increased concentrations of serum uric acid (hyperuricaemia) can result in gout.

There are two main causes of hyperuricaemia:
- Underexcretion of uric acid (most common): of uncertain origin but clinically associated with hyperlipidaemia, renal failure, lactic acidosis (alcohol, exercise, starvation, vomiting) and thiazide diuretics.
- Overproduction of uric acid (least common): a result of either high cell turnover (e.g. leukaemia, chemotherapy, severe psoriasis, post trauma, surgery or severe systemic illness), or rare congenital enzyme defects of purine metabolism.

However, it should be noted that the majority of patients who have a raised blood uric acid level will never develop gout or any of its complications. The condition has a familial tendency and is believed to be polygenically inherited.

Pathogenesis—Gout affects the joints, soft tissues and kidney, as follows.

Joints—Urate crystals are deposited in certain joints, forming white powdery deposits on the surface of articular cartilage, beneath which degenerative changes can be seen. Crystal deposition stimulates an acute inflammatory reaction leading to the excruciating pain, oedema and redness seen in the acutely inflamed joint. Microscopically, neutrophil polymorphs can be seen to phagocytose urate crystal in the joint fluid.

Soft tissues—Uric acid crystals are also deposited in the soft tissues around joints, where their presence excites a foreign body, giant cell reaction. These soft tissue masses may enlarge to produce a palpable mass composed of white chalky material (tophi), especially around the pinna of the ear.

Kidney—Urate crystals deposited in the kidney may lead to an interstitial nephritis and to renal calculi composed of uric acid. Precipitation of urates in renal tubules may produce acute tubular necrosis and acute renal failure in leukaemic patients with massive purine release after chemotherapy.

Characteristics of gout are:
- Intermittent attacks of excruciating pain, oedema and redness (acute gouty arthritis).
- Monoarthropathy (90%); polyarthropathy (two or more affected joints) (10%).
- Metatarsophalangeal joint of big toe is most commonly affected (75%) but gout occasionally affects the ankle, or less commonly the knee and hip.

Recurrent attacks affecting the same joint eventually lead to articular cartilage destruction, chronic synovial thickening and secondary osteoarthritis—chronic gouty arthritis.

Diagnosis:
- Clinical features (as above).
- Raised serum urate level (>0.42 mmol/L in adult males; >0.36 mmol/L in adult females).
- Presence of crystals of sodium urate in aspirated synovial fluid from joint (detected with polarizing light).

Management—Analgesia for acute attacks: NSAIDs, e.g. indomethacin, and colchicine. Preventative measures are required for patients with recurrent attacks of gouty arthritis or associated renal disease, thus:
- Allopurinol: suppresses uric acid synthesis by inhibiting xanthine oxidase.
- Uricosuric agents, e.g. probencid.
- Diet: excessive purine intake and over-indulgence in alcohol should be avoided.

Prognosis—Some patients have only a single attack or suffer another only after an interval of many years. More often there is a tendency towards recurrent attacks which increase in frequency and duration so that eventually attacks merge and that patient remains in a prolonged state of subacute gout.

Pseudogout

This acute inflammatory crystal arthropathy is caused by deposition of calcium pyrophosphate crystals in articular cartilage and joint spaces. It is most common in the elderly. and in males more than females.

The aetiology can be sporadic, metabolic, or familial.

Sporadic

In the vast majority of cases, the cause of pyrophosphate deposition is unknown but is probably an age-related phenomenon.

Metabolic

In patients under the age of 60, the disease is often associated with hyperparathyroidism, haemochromatosis or other less common metabolic or endocrine disorders.

Familial

In a minority of patients, the disease is inherited as an autosomal dominant disorder.

Pathogenesis crystals are deposited in the articular cartilage of joints (chondrocalcinosis) where they often remain entirely asymptomatically. However, if crystals are shed into the joint space, patients develop an acute arthritis similar to that seen in urate gout. This shedding of crystals may be precipitated by trauma, intercurrent illness, or may be spontaneous.

With time, damage to cartilage leads to the development of secondary osteoarthritis.

Clinical features—As with gout, the affected joint becomes suddenly painful, warm, swollen and tender. However, the most commonly affected joint is the knee (>50% of cases), followed by the wrist, shoulder and ankle. The duration of the attack can vary from days to weeks, and recurrent attacks are uncommon.

Diagnosis is by X-ray—cartilaginous calcification is usually obvious on X-ray—and by the presence of calcium pyrophosphate dihydrate crystals in aspirated synovial fluid from the joint (detected with polarizing light).

Intra-articular corticosteroids are the most effective treatment for acute pseudogout (anti-inflammatory drugs and colchicine are less effective than in true gout).

Infective (septic) arthritis

This inflammation of a joint is caused by infection, typically bacterial. This may affect any age group, but children and young adults are the most commonly affected. In older adults, most cases are associated with penetrating injury. Males are affected more often than females by 2:1. The knee and hip are the most common sites.

Aetiology—A wide range of bacteria may be responsible, but *Staphylococcus aureus*, streptococci and *Haemophilus* are the most important.

Risk factors are DM, RA, joint puncture or surgery and immunosuppressive treatment.

Bacteria gain access to a joint by:

- Local trauma: well-recognized complication of penetrating injury such as open fractures, insertion of surgical prosthesis and non-sterile, intra-articular infection of steroids for established autoimmune arthritis.
- Spread from adjacent infective foci.
- Bloodstream: less common but an important route in gonococcal infective arthritis in teenagers and young adults. IV drug users are particularly likely to develop septic arthritis associated with Gram-negative bacteraemia.

Clinical features—There is an abrupt onset of severe pain, tenderness, swelling and erythema. The majority of cases affect a single joint only, but some cases of gonococcal arthritis and arthritis in IV drug abusers may affect more joints.

Complications—Untreated, it proceeds rapidly to joint destruction often with osteomyelitis, sinus formation, ankylosis, and dislocation of the hip.

Diagnosis—Radiographs are normal at first, but useful to exclude fractures or other bony injury. Later in the course of the disease, features of periarticular osteoporosis, joint space narrowing, periostitis and articular erosions may become apparent. Examination and culture of aspirated joint space fluid is essential for identification of the causative organism.

Treatment is by antibiotic therapy (i.v. or i.m.).

The prognosis for recovery without joint damage is directly related to the speed with which antibiotic therapy is instituted.

Other types of infective arthritis

Tuberculous arthritis

Now rare, this is the result of bloodstream spread from pulmonary TB. It produces a persistent arthritis with typical caseating granulomatous lesions. The hip and knee are most commonly involved in children, whereas in adults the vertebral column is most often affected.

Infective arthritis in syphilis and brucellosis is now rare.

Lyme disease

This arthritis is due to the spirochaete *Borrelia burgdorferi*. It occurs in outbreaks in the USA and Europe. (For more on Lyme disease, see Chapter 15.)

Virus-associated arthritis

Many different viral infections are associated with a transient arthritis or at least distinct pain within joints. Examples include rubella, viral hepatitis and infectious mononucleosis.

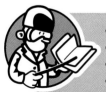

- Define 'osteoarthritis' (OA) and 'rheumatoid arthritis' (RA).
- State the four radiographical diagnostic features of OA.
- Compare the pathological joint changes that occur in OA with those of RA.
- What is ankylosing spondylitis? Describe the morphological changes that occur in the spine.
- Name the types of crystals involved in gout and pseudogout.
- What are the risk factors for the development of infective arthritis?

14. Pathology of the Blood and Immune Systems

AUTOIMMUNE DISEASE

Systemic disease

Autoimmune diseases that cause damage in many tissues and organs, involving a number of systems, are termed 'multisystem' or 'systemic' autoimmune diseases (Fig. 14.1).

Systemic lupus erythematosus (SLE)

This inflammatory disorder of connective tissues is associated with autoantibodies to DNA and other nuclear components. Many tissues are affected, but synovial joints, skin, kidneys and the brain are the major target organs (Fig. 14.2).

SLE affects 30 per 100 000 of the UK population, and presents most commonly in the young and middle-aged with peak incidence between 20 and 30 years of age. Females are more affected than males by about 8:1.

Incidence is higher in Black people and Asians than in Caucasians.

The aetiology is unknown but there is a strong familial tendency. Drugs (hydralazine, phenytoin, procainamide), chemicals, and unidentified viral infections have all been postulated as the sensitizing stimulus to autoantibody production.

Pathogenesis—Antibodies are produced against components of both nucleic acids and cytoplasmic phospholipids:

- Anti-dsDNA: antibody against double-stranded DNA (most frequently detected).
- Anti-ssDNA: antibody against single-stranded DNA.
- Anti-DNA histone: antibody to a protein (histone) packaged with DNA in chromosomes.
- Antiphospholipid (cardiolipin): causes thrombotic tendency, recurrent abortions, false positive test for syphilis.
- Red cell antibodies: cause autoimmune haemolytic anaemia.
- Rheumatoid factors: antibodies directed against self-IgG antibodies.
- Cell- or organelle-specific antibodies (mitochondrial, smooth muscle, gastric parietal cell, etc.).

None of these antibodies is specific for SLE, and most have been detected in other connective tissue disorders or in diseases with an immunological basis.

Microscopically, fibrinoid necrosis is typically seen in vessels of affected organs, especially small arteries, arterioles and capillaries.

Summary of systemic autoimmune diseases			
Disorder	**Sex ratio**	**Type of autoimmunity**	**Clinical features**
SLE	8F:1M	antibodies directed against components of nucleic acids and cytoplasmic phospholipids	skin rashes, neurological disorders, glomerulonephritis, haematological disorders, etc.
rheumatoid disease	3F:1M	rheumatoid factors: autoantibodies directed against native IgG	chronic polyarthritis, subcutaneous nodules, vasculitis, interstitial pulmonary fibrosis, splenomegaly, etc.
polymyositis and dermatositis	3F:1M	cell-mediated autoimmunity	weakness, pain and swelling of proximal limb muscles and facial muscles ptosis and dysphagia dermatomyositis (= additional features of erythematous, scaling rash)

Fig. 14.1 Summary of systemic autoimmune diseases.

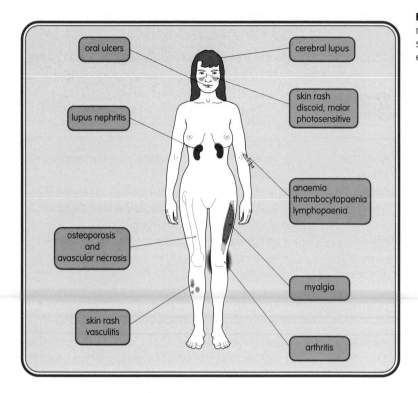

Fig. 14.2 Multisystem manifestations of systemic lupus erythematosus (SLE).

The disease commonly presents with malaise, weight loss, fever, marked musculoskeletal symptoms and a rash. However, the range of features that may occur is vast as demonstrated in the list below.

The American Rheumatism Association's list of diagnostic criteria for SLE

This is listed in order of specificity:

- Discoid skin rash: round ('discoid'), red, scaly, telangiectatic plaques, usually on the face and scalp and less commonly on the hands.
- Neurological disorder: most common feature is non-organic psychiatric disorder of unknown cause, which on autopsy is often found to be associated with either acute neutrophilic or lymphocytic vasculitides in the brain. A variety of symptoms (e.g. grand mal epileptic seizures) are due to infarction and neuronal loss, a result of vascular occlusion attributed to the action of antiphospholipid antibodies on platelet aggregation.
- Malar skin rash: symmetrical erythematous rash on the cheeks and the bridge of the nose (butterfly rash).
- Skin photosensitivity: development of rash of either malar or discoid patterns in sun-exposed areas.

Caused by immune complex deposits on the dermal side of the basement membrane.

- Oral ulceration: red erosions closely resembling oral lichen planus.
- Renal abnormality (lupus nephritis): severity varies from minor abnormalities such as asymptomatic proteinuria to severe glomerular disease leading to renal failure (see Chapter 10).
- Evidence of immunological disorder.
- Haematological disorders: normocytic hypochromic anaemia, autoimmune haemolytic anaemia, reduced peripheral white cell count (usually due to lymphopenia), thrombocytopenia (sometimes associated with antiplatelet antibodies), predisposition to thrombosis (especially if there are anticardiolipin/lupus anticoagulant antibodies).
- Serosal inflammation: pleurisy, pericarditis.
- Presence of antinuclear antibodies: cluster of antibodies that are aimed against nuclei (see above).
- Arthritis, bone disease and/or myalgia: often misdiagnosed as rheumatoid arthritis, beginning in the fingers, wrists and knees. Bone disease usually presents as disproportionately severe osteoporosis for the patient's age. Myalgia in the form of skeletal

muscle pain is common, and is thought to be caused by a lymphocytic vasculitis.

Diagnosis is based on a combination of clinical features and the result of laboratory investigation, primarily the identification of autoantibodies, especially those directed against nuclear DNA. The condition is frequently under-diagnosed.

Treatment is by systemic corticosteroid therapy for acute and life-threatening manifestations of SLE. Immunosuppressive drugs are reserved for patients with severe diffuse proliferative glomerulonephritis who are not responding adequately to steroid therapy.

The disorder follows a protracted course of relapses and remissions. Renal, CNS and cardiac lesions are the most important prognostically. With treatment, in excess of 90% of patients can be anticipated to survive for 10 years.

Rheumatoid disease

This multisystem autoimmune connective tissue disease primarily affects the joints (rheumatoid arthritis) but also the skin, lungs, blood vessels, eyes and the haemopoietic and lymphoreticular systems.

It affects about 1% of the UK population. Onset is typically between 35 and 45 years, but follows a normal distribution curve, and no age group is exempt, with females more affected than males by about 3:1.

The aetiology is unknown, although there is a genetic predisposition and an association with the HLA-DR4 haplotype.

Pathogenesis—Circulating autoantibodies termed 'rheumatoid factors' are present which react with the Fc portion of IgG antibodies. The most common type of rheumatoid factor is of the IgM type, which can form pentamer complexes with circulating IgG. Immune complex deposition then leads to complement activation via the classical pathway, which triggers an inflammatory cascade.

Clinicopathological features

Joints

This symmetrical polyarthritis is characterized by the destruction of articular cartilage and its replacement by chronic inflammatory pannus (see Chapter 13 for full coverage).

Rheumatoid arthritis is a common disease and often appears in the clinical examinations as either a long or short case.

Skin

Subcutaneous rheumatoid nodules can often be seen, usually located over the extensor aspect of the forearm but occasionally found overlying other bony prominences. Nodules are composed of extensive areas of degenerate collagen surrounded by a giant cell granulomatous reaction.

Lungs

Pulmonary involvement causes interstitial pneumonitis and fibrosing alveolitis which eventually leads to a pattern of interstitial pulmonary fibrosis. Also, patients may develop lesions similar to the subcutaneous rheumatoid nodule, both within the lungs and on the pleural surfaces. These rheumatoid granulomas are particularly common in patients who already have industrial lung disease due to inhaling various types of silica; the association of coalminer's lung with rheumatoid granulomas in seropositive miners is called Caplan's syndrome.

Blood vessels

There is the development of vasculitis which is either:
- Acute neutrophilic vasculitis, presenting with purpura and occasional foci of ulceration.
- Lymphocytic vasculitis, producing a more low-key erythematous patchy rash.

Eyes

Dry eye syndrome (keratoconjunctivitis sicca) is caused by lymphocytic inflammation of both lacrimal and mucous glands. Lack of tears leads to secondary inflammation of the cornea. In addition, scleritis may occur due to degeneration of collagenous tissue in the eye, and in severe cases this progresses to perforation of the globe—scleromalacia perforans (rare).

Haemopoietic and lymphoreticular systems

Anaemia of chronic disorders is common in rheumatoid disease, and a minority of patients develop hypersplenism or lymphadenopathy. Felty's syndrome describes a syndrome of splenomegaly, lymphadenopathy, anaemia and leucopenia with rheumatoid arthritis. Sepsis is an important and common cause of death in these patients.

Fig. 14.3 shows a diagram of the clinical features of rheumatoid disease.

Diagnosis:
- Clinical features (Fig. 14.3).
- Radiography: periarticular osteoporosis, loss of articular cartilage (joint space), erosions, subluxation and ankylosis.
- Serology: presence of rheumatoid factors. Two tests— Rose–Waaler test (based on the ability of IgM rheumatoid factor to agglutinate sheep red cells that have been coated with rabbit antisheep antibody); and latex agglutination test (rheumatoid factor agglutinates latex particles that have been coated with human IgG; less specific than the Rose–Waaler test).
- Anaemia: normochromic normocytic.
- ESR and CRP levels: both are typically elevated.

Treatment is by:
- Analgesia and anti-inflammatories.
- Immunosuppressive therapy: penicillamine, gold, azathioprine, salazopyrine.
- Surgery for advanced painful disease in any joint.

Treatment for rheumatoid disease may itself cause pathology, i.e. steroid-induced osteoporosis, analgesic-related ulceration of the stomach, and drug-induced renal disease.

Course and prognosis are variable. Studies of patients with disease of such severity as to require hospitalization showed that within 10 years:
- 25% have complete remission.
- 40% have only moderate impairment of function.
- 25% will be more severely disabled.
- 10% will be severely crippled.

Mortality is greatly increased in patients with functional impairment, the 5 year survival for severely disabled RA patients being reduced by 50%.

Organ- or cell-type specific disease
Autoimmune diseases involving a single organ or cell-type are known as organ- or cell-type specific autoimmune diseases (Fig. 14.4).

Hashimoto's thyroiditis
Organ-specific autoimmune disease eventually causes hypothyroidism as a result of antibody-mediated destruction of the thyroid gland (see Chapter 11, p.220).

Graves' disease
An organ-specific autoimmune disorder, this

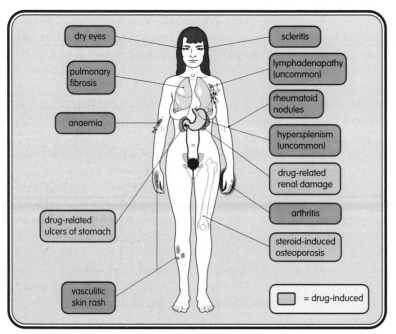

Fig. 14.3 Clinical features of rheumatoid disease.

dry eyes

pulmonary fibrosis

anaemia

drug-related ulcers of stomach

vasculitic skin rash

scleritis

lymphadenopathy (uncommon)

rheumatoid nodules

hypersplenism (uncommon)

drug-related renal damage

arthritis

steroid-induced osteoporosis

= drug-induced

Organ-specific autoimmune diseases		
Disease	**Associated autoantibody**	**Comment**
Graves' disease	LATS (long-acting thyroid stimulator)	hyperthyroidism
Hashimoto's disease	anti-thyroid hormones	hypothyroidism
type I diabetes mellitus	anti-islet β-cell antibody	insulin-responsive hyperglycaemia
Addison's disease	antiadrenal antibodies	hypoadrenocorticalism
autoimmune gastritis	anti-intrinsic factor and antiparietal cell antibodies	pernicious anaemia
vitiligo	–	hypopigmentation
myasthenia gravis	antiacetylcholine receptor antibody	muscle fatigue

Fig. 14.4 Organ-specific autoimmune diseases.

Although organ-specific autoimmune diseases specifically affect one organ, they frequently occur together, e.g. Addison's disease is often associated with autoimmune gastritis, etc.

results in thyrotoxicosis due to overstimulation of TSH receptors of the thyroid gland by autoantibodies (see Chapter 11, p.221).

Type I diabetes mellitus

Type I (insulin-dependent) diabetes mellitus is an organ-specific autoimmune disorder characterized by hyperglycaemia, which is responsive insulin. Disorder is caused by antibody-mediated destruction of the insulin-secreting cell population of the pancreas (see Chapter 11, p.231, for full coverage).

Note that although type I diabetes mellitus is an organ-specific autoimmune disorder (i.e. the autoimmune mechanism attacks only one system—the endocrine pancreas), the effects of hyperglycaemia are multitudinous, affecting many systems, and thus diabetes mellitus is also classified as a multisystem disease.

Addison's disease

This rare condition of chronic adrenal insufficiency is most commonly caused by the autoimmune-mediated destruction of the adrenal cortex (see Chapter 11, p.229). It is often associated with autoimmune thyroid disease, autoimmune gastritis and other endocrine organ autoimmune diseases.

Autoimmune gastritis

Chronic inflammation of the gastric mucosa caused by the autoimmune destruction of gastric parietal cells, with or without intrinsic factor, results in the development of pernicious anaemia.

Vitiligo

The autoimmune destruction of melanocytes causes patchy loss of pigmentation (see Chapter 15, p.346).

Myasthenia gravis

The autoimmune destruction of acetylcholine receptors occurs at the neuromuscular junction (see Chapter 13, p.272).

- List the major target organs of systemic lupus erythematosus.
- Describe the clinical manifestations of systemic lupus erythematosus.
- Define 'rheumatoid disease' and describe its pathogenesis.
- List the major target organs of rheumatoid disease.
- Name the common organ-specific autoimmune diseases.

DISEASES OF IMMUNE DEFICIENCY

Primary immunodeficiencies

Transient physiological agammaglobulinaemia of the neonate

This transient trough in antibody levels, which usually occurs between 3 and 6 months of age, is caused by falling levels of maternally derived IgG prior to the appearance of the infant's own antibody (IgM followed by IgG and IgA); detailed in Fig. 14.5.

It can be more prolonged and more severe in premature infants.

Affected infants are more susceptible to pyogenic infections as they have B cells but lack help from CD4+ T cells (T helper cells) in synthesizing antibodies.

The condition usually resolves by two years but immunoglobulin replacement is sometimes required until normal levels are attained.

X-linked agammaglobulinaemia of Bruton

In this X-linked recessive disorder, affected males present with recurrent infections from between four months and two years of age (maternal IgG protects against earlier infection). It is caused by the inability of

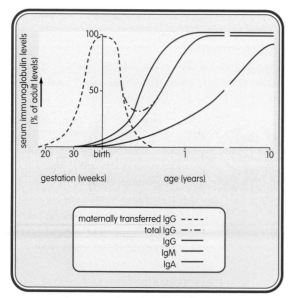

Fig. 14.5 Serum immunoglobulin levels in the neonate. (Adapted with permission from *Introduction to Clinical Immunology*, by M. Haeny, Butterworths, London, 1985).

pre-B cells to differentiate into mature B cells and characterized by:

- Deficiency of B cells and plasma cells.
- Negligible levels of immunoglobulins.
- Small lymph nodes and absent tonsils.

T cells numbers and function are normal, and therefore infections are primarily bacterial.

Treatment is with long-term immunoglobulin replacement therapy and the rigorous use of antibacterial agents.

Common variable immunodeficiency

This acquired form of agammaglobulinaemia is characterized by an increased susceptibility to infections, especially bacterial, presenting most often in the third decade. It is also known as late-onset hypogammaglobulinaemia.

Its aetiology is unknown but may follow viral infection, e.g. Epstein–Barr virus.

Although not hereditary it is commonly associated with MHC haplotypes HLA-B8 and HLA-DR3.

Pathogenesis is variable and can be caused by either.

- Intrinsic B cell defect producing malfunctioning, immature B cells.
- Immunoregulatory T cell imbalance, hence B cells fail to differentiate due to lack of T helper cells or due to overactivity of T suppressor cells.
- Autoantibodies to T or B cells.

The disease is more common and more variable than the X-linked form (hence the name); however, the pattern of infection is similar, chiefly affecting the lungs, sinuses and GI tract.

Treatment is as for X-linked deficiency.

Isolated IgA deficiency

The commonest form of immunodeficiency, this affects 1 in 700 Caucasians (but is very rare in other ethnic groups). Most cases are sporadic but some patients have family members with varied forms of antibody deficiency.

Circulating B cells bearing surface IgA are immature and fail to differentiate into IgA-secreting plasma cells.

Patients are prone to sinopulmonary infections and bowel colonization with *Giardia*, *Salmonella* and other enteric pathogens.

It is associated with an increased incidence of autoimmune diseases and allergies.

DiGeorge syndrome (thymic hypoplasia)

This rare, congenital disorder is caused by the arrested development of the third and fourth branchial arches, resulting in an almost complete absence of the thymus and parathyroid gland.

Immunoglobulin levels are normal but affected individuals have decreased circulating levels of T-lymphocytes, resulting in impaired cell-mediated immunity.

Patients typically develop a triad of infections, namely candidiasis, pneumocystis pneumonia, and persistent diarrhoea.

The syndrome is also characterized by hypocalcaemia (due to hypoparathyroidism) and associated with abnormalities of the great vessels (e.g. transposition or Fallot's tetralogy).

Treatment requires transplantation of thymic tissue.

Severe combined immunodeficiency

This inherited deficiency of lymphocytic stem cells is characterized by:
- Deficiency of both T and B cells.
- Negligible circulating immunoglobulins.
- Greatly reduced cell-mediated immunity.
- Hypoplastic thymus.

The condition can be X-linked or an autosomal recessive disorder. It presents during the first few months of life with a failure to thrive and persistent infections.

Death usually occurs within the first 2 years of life from multiple infections, although a bone marrow transplant can effect a cure in some cases.

Secondary immunodeficiencies

Secondary immunodeficiencies are those that result from extrinsic or environmental causes, as listed in Fig. 14.9 below. The pathologies of most of these diseases are covered in other chapters.

Acquired immunodeficiency syndrome (AIDS)

This syndrome caused by infection with the human immunodeficiency virus (HIV) is characterized by a profound defect in cell-mediated immunity with lymphopenia and diminished T lymphocyte responses.

The usual cause is HIV-1 (Fig. 14.6) although another strain of the virus (HIV-2) has also been associated with AIDS in Africa.

Routes of transmission are threefold: sexual contact, blood-borne (transfusions or contaminated needles), and maternal (placental or via breast milk).

The type of infection associated with diseases of immune deficiency depends on the category of immune disorder:
- B cell deficiencies (defective antibody response): increased susceptibility to opportunistic infections caused by extracellular organisms.
- T cell deficiencies (defective cell-mediated immunity): increased susceptibility to opportunistic infections caused by intracellular organisms.
- Mixed B and T cell deficiencies (defective antibody response and cell-mediated immunity): increased susceptibility to most infections.

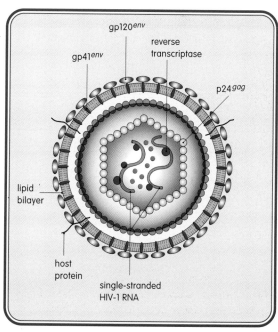

Fig. 14.6 Structure of the human immunodeficiency virus (HIV)-1.

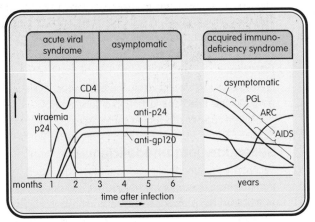

Fig. 14.7 CD4 count, viral antigen (p24) and antibody levels following HIV infection. (p24, nucleocapsid protein; PGL, persistent generalized lymphadenopathy; ARC, AIDS-related complex.)

Pathogenesis

HIV is an enveloped RNA retrovirus that binds to CD4 receptors present on T helper cells and various cells of the monocyte/macrophage system via its cell surface glycoprotein, gp 120.

- Following cell entry, virus loses its coat and utilizes its enzyme, reverse transcriptase, to make viral DNA which is inserted into host chromosome.
- Viral replication is initially repressed by intracellular factors and by cell-mediated immunity mediated by CD8+ cytotoxic T cells, and so the virus can remain latent (i.e. dormant) for months or even years.
- Activation of latently infected T cells triggers viral replication, and infectious virus particles are released, resulting in the infection of more CD4+ cells.

The net result is a depletion of T helper cells, which results in a severely impaired cell-mediated immunity, with a high risk of multiple opportunistic infections.

Correlation of the fall in the CD4 count with increasing viral antigen levels is depicted in Fig. 14.7.

Clinical features—The clinical outcome of HIV infection has been classified into four stages (Fig. 14.8).

The duration of each stage is highly variable—some patients pass directly through stages II and III to AIDS-related conditions or even to fully developed ('full blown') AIDS whilst others remain in the earlier stages for months or years. A small proportion of HIV-infected patients do not develop clinical AIDS.

The reasons for the variations in the course of the disease are not known, and the factors that

Classification of HIV infection	
stage I	initial infection; can be either: • symptomatic seroconversion: mononucleosis-like syndrome, mild meningoencephalitis • asymptomatic seroconversion
stage II	chronic asymptomatic infection: lab tests typically normal but may have anaemia, neutropenia, thrombocytopenia, low CD4 lymphocytes, lymphopenia and hypergammaglobulinaemia
stage III	persistent generalized lymphadenopathy: with or without lab test abnormalities as in stage II
stage IV	AIDS-related complex: generalized lymphadenopathy with persistent fever, weight loss, unexplained diarrhoea, CNS manifestations and haematological abnormalities including thrombocytopenia, leukopenia and anaemia Fully developed AIDS: • wide spectrum of opportunistic infections including *Pneumocystis carinii*, toxoplasmosis, *Cryptococcus*, cryptosporidiosis, atypical mycobacteria, herpes simplex or zoster, oral hairy leukoplakia, histoplasmosis, candidiasis, cytomegalovirus, *Salmonella* • secondary cancers, e.g. Kaposi's sarcoma, non-Hodgkin's lymphoma, squamous carcinoma of the mouth or rectum

Fig. 14.8 Classification of HIV infection.

determine progression from one stage into the next remain unclear.

The prognosis for AIDS patients is very poor: about 90% die within two years of diagnosis.

Treatment is as follows:

- Antimicrobial therapy: aimed at preventing or treating infection, e.g. with prophylactic antibiotics or antifungals.
- Antiviral therapy: reverse transcriptase inhibitors or protease inhibitors (proteases are required for formation of gp120). Success is limited.

Fig. 14.9 gives a summary of immune deficiencies.

AMYLOIDOSIS

Definition and chemical nature of amyloid
Amyloidosis is the deposition of abnormal extracellular fibrillar protein, amyloid, in different tissues. Amyloid is composed of a meshwork of rigid, straight fibrils formed from precursor peptides lined up in an antiparallel, β-pleated sheet structure. It is detected histologically as a bright pink hyaline material and takes up certain stains, the best known being Congo red.

Amyloid formation
Amyloid formation occurs due to the production of either:
- Abnormal amounts of normal precursor peptide

- Describe the life cycle of the human immunodeficiency virus (HIV).
- Describe the stages of HIV infection.
- Which disorders are associated with B cell deficiencies?
- What type of infections are associated with T cell deficiencies?

It is important to note that it is the physical arrangement of the constituent peptides that make a protein an amyloid rather than any specific peptide sequence. There are many different types of amyloid, each being formed from different precursor peptides with the precursors themselves often being fragments of larger proteins.

Fig. 14.9 Summary of immune deficiencies.

Summary of immune deficiencies		
Category	**Deficiency**	**Example**
primary	B cell (antibody deficiency)	transient hypogammaglobulinaemia of infancy X-linked agammaglobulinaemia acquired common variable hypogammaglobulinaemia selective IgA or IgG subclass deficiencies
	T cell	thymic hypoplasia (DiGeorge syndrome)
	mixed B and T cell	severe combined immune deficiency
secondary	B cell (antibody deficiency)	myeloma protein deficiency
	T cell	AIDS Hodgkin's disease non-Hodgkin's lymphoma drugs, e.g. steroids, cyclosporine, azathioprine
	mixed B and T cell	chronic lymphocytic leukaemia post-bone marrow transplantation post-chemotherapy/radiotherapy chronic renal failure splenectomy

(common), e.g. immunoglobulin light chains in multiple myeloma, or serum amyloid A protein in acute phase response. May be due to overproduction, reduced degradation or reduced excretion of protein.

- Normal amounts of abnormal (amyloidogenic) peptide (rare), e.g. due to transthyretin or gelsolin polymorphisms.

Macrophages are then thought to process the precursor proteins to form amyloid fibrils.

Amyloid also contains a serum glycoprotein called serum amyloid P which is thought to assist in its polymerization.

Classification of amyloidosis

Clinically, amyloidosis presents with organ involvement which is either:

- Systemic: may involve many tissues as it is particularly deposited in the blood vessel walls and basement membranes. Usually fatal, death generally occurring from renal or cardiac disease.
- Localized: affects only one organ or tissue. Rarely, may be found without any obvious predisposing cause, the skin, lungs and urinary tract being the most frequent sites.

In both cases, the progressive accumulation of amyloid leads to cellular dysfunction by preventing the normal processes of diffusion through extracellular tissues, and by physical compression of functioning parenchymal cells.

Systemic amyloidosis

Reactive systemic amyloidosis

This amyloid is composed of protein A and is termed the AA type. It is derived from serum amyloid A which is synthesized in the liver and is one of several acute phase reactant proteins, so named because of their increased serum concentration in response to a variety of diseases.

Reactive amyloidosis always has a predisposing cause, which is invariably a chronic inflammatory disorder:

- Chronic infections (e.g. tuberculosis).
- Hodgkin's disease.
- Rheumatoid arthritis.
- Bronchiectasis.
- Chronic osteomyelitis.

AA-type amyloid is deposited in many organs but has a predilection for the liver, spleen and kidney. It results in hepatosplenomegaly with or without renal vein thrombosis and nephrotic syndrome.

Myeloma-associated amyloidosis

This amyloid is composed of immunoglobulin light chains (and/or parts of their variable regions) and is termed AL type. Immunoglobulin light chains are formed by proliferating plasma cells usually in association with:

- Multiple myeloma.
- Waldenström's macroglobulinaemia.
- Heavy chain disease.
- Primary amyloidosis.

Primary amyloidosis is a myeloma-associated amyloidosis which occurs in the absence of any clinically obvious myeloma. It is caused by a clinically occult plasma cell tumour and is accompanied by the presence of a monoclonal immunoglobulin band on serum electrophoresis. It is also known as benign monoclonal gammopathy.

AL-type amyloid is deposited in many organs including the tongue, skin, heart, nerves, kidneys, liver and spleen, and has a predilection for connective tissue within these organs.

Patients may present with heart failure, macroglossia, peripheral neuropathy or carpal tunnel syndrome, or with renal failure.

Haemodialysis-associated amyloidosis

This amyloidosis is associated with long-term haemodialysis for chronic renal failure. Amyloid material deposited in the affected tissues appears to be β_2-microglobulin, and amyloid is termed AH type (H for haemodialysis).

Clinical features include arthropathy and carpal tunnel syndrome.

Hereditary amyloidosis

Hereditary forms of amyloidosis are rare, and include familial Mediterranean fever (AA type) and familial neuropathic forms (AF, prealbumin, type).

Localized amyloidosis

Alzheimer's disease

The commonest example of amyloid deposition occurs in the nervous system, in both Alzheimer's disease and in normal ageing (cerebral angiopathy). The amyloid is composed of peptide fragments termed β-protein or A4 protein, both of which are derived from normal, neuronal membrane protein, Alzheimer precursor protein (APP).

Endocrine amyloidosis

Amyloid material is often found in the stroma of peptide hormone-producing tumours. It is particularly characteristic of medullary carcinoma of the thyroid, a tumour of the calcitonin-producing interfollicular C cells. In this instance, the amyloid contains calcitonin precursor molecules arranged in a β-pleated sheet configuration.

In type II diabetes, the excessive secretion of amylin by the β cells of the pancreas is associated with its deposition as islet amyloid.

Senile amyloidosis

Minute deposits of amyloid usually derived from serum transthyretin (prealbumin) are found in the heart and walls of blood vessels in many organs of elderly people. However, significant signs or symptoms of amyloidosis occur in only a few cases.

- Define 'amyloidosis'.
- Describe the structure of amyloid.
- Describe the formation of amyloid.
- Name the different types of amyloidosis and the main organs that they affect.

DISORDERS OF WHITE BLOOD CELLS AND LYMPH NODES

Leukopenia

Leukopenia is defined as a reduction in circulating leukocytes. The classification of leukocytes is shown in Fig. 14.10.

For a quick revision of leukocyte (white blood cell) classification see Fig. 14.10.

Neutropenia

Neutropenia, a deficiency of neutrophil granulocytes, is the most important form of leukopenia. The lower limit of normal neutrophil count is $2.5 - 10^9$/L (except in Black people and in the Middle East where it is $1.5 - 10^9$/L). Levels of less than these values are classified as neutropenia.

Neutropenia may be selective or part of a general pancytopenia. The causes of both types are listed in Fig. 14.11.

Clinical features depend on the degree of neutropenia:

- Mild: usually asymptomatic.
- Moderate to severe ($<0.5 - 10^9$/L): associated with a progressive increase in risk and severity of infections.
- Levels of $<0.2 - 10^9$/L are associated with a high mortality from overwhelming infections.

Infections are predominantly bacterial and are usually opportunistic, most commonly Gram-positive skin organisms (e.g. *Staphylococcus* and *Streptococcus*) or Gram-negative gut bacteria (e.g. pseudomonads, *E. coli*, *Proteus*, etc.).

They can be either localized (e.g. of the mouth, throat, skin or anus) or generalized (i.e. septicaemias). The latter may be rapidly fatal.

Treatment is of the underlying cause and with antimicrobial therapy.

Reactive proliferation of white cells

Leukocytosis

Leukocytosis is defined as an increase in numbers of circulating white blood cells.

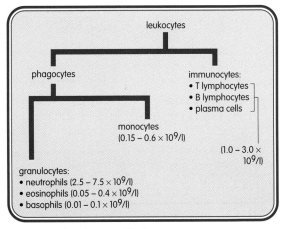

Fig. 14.10 Classification of leukocytes.

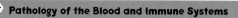

Types of leukocytosis

The types of leukocytosis are:

- Polymorphonuclear leukocytosis (neutrophilia): increased numbers of neutrophils (commonest cause of leukocytosis).
- Monocytosis: increased numbers of the monocyte/macrophage cells.
- Eosinophil leukocytosis (eosinophilia): increased numbers of eosinophils.
- Basophil leukocytosis (basophilia): increased numbers of basophils.
- Lymphocytosis: increased numbers of T and/or B lymphocytes.

Leukocytosis is of two main types:

- Primary: caused by bone marrow disease, e.g. leukaemias, lymphomas, etc. (described later in this chapter).
- Secondary: caused by the normal response of bone marrow to abnormal conditions, e.g. infection. Also known as reactive leukocytosis (Fig. 14.12).

Lymphadenitis

This inflammation of lymph nodes is usually caused by infection and characterized by a painful swelling of the affected nodes as a result of:

- Increased blood flow.
- Macrophage activation and increase.
- Lymphocyte activation and increase.

Additional changes depend on the type of lymphadenitis:

- Acute non-specific lymphadenitis: typically caused by acute infections (e.g. infectious mononucleosis, rubella, pertussis, mumps). Bacterial infection

Causes of neutropenia		
Type	**Cause**	**Clinical features**
selective neutropenia	reduced granulopoiesis	congenital: Kostmann's syndrome—autosomal recessive disease presenting in the first year of life with life-threatening infections cyclical: rare syndrome characterized by recurrent severe but temporary neutropenia with a periodicity of 3–4 weeks nutritional: B_{12} or folate deficiency racial: African races
	accelerated granulocyte removal	immune: • autoimmune • systemic lupus erythematosus • Felty's syndrome • hypersensitivity and anaphylaxis infectious: • viral, e.g. hepatitis, influenza, HIV • fulminant bacterial, e.g. typhoid, miliary tuberculosis
	drug-induced neutropenia	drug-induced damage of either neutrophils or precursor marrow cells can occur via direct toxicity or immune-mediated mechanisms in susceptible individuals; examples of such drugs include: • anti-inflammatory: phenylbutazone, cyclophosphamide • antibacterial: chloramphenicol, cotrimoxazole, sulphasalazine • anticonvulsants: phenytoin • antithyroids: carbimazole • hypoglycaemics: tolbutamide • phenothiazines: chlopromazine, thioridazine • psychotropics and antidepressants: clozapine, imipramine • miscellaneous: gold, penicillamine
part of general pancytopenia	reduced granulopoiesis	bone marrow failure, megaloblastic anaemia
	accelerated granulocyte removal	splenomegaly

Fig. 14.11 Causes of neutropenia.

commonly involves infiltration of node by neutrophils. Most commonly affected lymph nodes are those in the neck associated with tonsillitis.

- Chronic non-specific lymphadenitis: typically caused by chronic infections (e.g. brucellosis, tuberculosis, syphilis, hepatitis). Additional changes include increased plasma cells and granuloma formation.

Neoplastic proliferation of white blood cells

Malignant lymphomas

In this group of lymphoproliferative diseases normal lymphoid tissue is replaced by abnormal cells of lymphoid origin, forming solid malignant tumours of the lymph nodes.

All lymphomas are broadly classified as either Hodgkin's disease or non-Hodgkin's lymphomas.

Causes of reactive leukocytosis	
Cause	**Clinical features**
neutrophilia ($>7.5 \times 10^9$/l)	acute infections haemorrhage/haemolysis inflammation and tissue necrosis metabolic disorders myeloproliferative diseases neoplasia steroid therapy strenuous exercise
monocytosis ($>0.8 \times 10^9$/l)	chronic infections, e.g. tuberculosis brucellosis, malariain flammatory disorders, e.g. rheumatoid disease, SLE, Crohn's disease neoplasia
eosinophilia ($>0.44 \times 10^9$/l)	allergy, e.g. asthma parasites, e.g. tapeworms skin disease, e.g. eczema, psoriasis neoplasia, especially Hodgkin's disease miscellaneous, e.g. polyarteritis nodosa, sarcoidosis
basophilia ($>0.1 \times 10^9$/l)	myxoedema chickenpox myeloproliferative disorders
lymphocytosis ($>3.5 \times 10^9$/l)	acute infections, e.g. infectious mononucleosis chronic infections, e.g. tuberculosis, brucellosis, hepatitis

Fig. 14.12 Causes of reactive leukocytosis.

Hodgkin's disease (HD)

The commonest type of lymphoma, this is characterized by the painless enlargement of one or more groups of lymph nodes, and the presence of large binucleate cells (Reed–Sternberg cells) within them.

It affects 3 per 100 000 in the UK, males more so than females by almost 2:1. It can occur at any age but there are two peaks of incidence—one in young adults (20–30 years old) and the other in late middle-age.

The aetiology of Hodgkin's disease is obscure, as is the origin of the malignant Reed–Sternberg (RS) cells. However, RS cells form only a small percentage of the total population of the affected node, the majority being composed of reactive lymphocytes, plasma cells, histiocytes and eosinophils.

Hodgkin's disease often presents clinically as the enlargement of accessible nodes, most often in the upper half of the body (e.g. cervical or axillary). The disease is initially localized to a single peripheral lymph node region but spreads in a fairly consistent pattern to adjacent nodes via the lymphatics and then, following splenic involvement, to other organs via the bloodstream.

One-third of patients have systemic symptoms, notably weight loss and pyrexia. Symptoms are due to:
- Lymph node enlargement producing mediastinal compression and lymphoedema.
- Haematology: normochromic–normocytic anaemia, neutrophilia, eosinophilia, lymphopenia (advanced disease), raised erythrocyte sedimentation rate (ESR).
- Immunology: depression of T cell function, hence susceptibility to infection.

The stage (extent of spread) of the disease is an important determinant in lymphoma treatment and prognosis. The staging system currently used is known as the Ann Arbor staging system, named after the location at which it was first proposed (Fig. 14.13).

Diagnosis of Hodgkin's disease can only be made on examination of biopsied lymph nodes:
- Macroscopically: affected lymph nodes are enlarged, with a smooth surface, and the lymph node capsule is rarely breached (cf. non-Hodgkin's lymphomas).
- Microscopically: four subtypes of Hodgkin's disease are recognized and classified according to the Rye classification system (Fig. 14.14).

Ann Arbor staging system of Hodgkin's disease	
Stage	**Comment**
I	involvement of single lymph node region (I) or of single extralymphatic organ or site (hence Ie)
II	involvement of two or more lymph node regions, with all lesions confined to the same side of the diaphragm (II), or localized involvement of an extralymphatic site and one or more lymph node regions confined to one side of the diaphragm (IIe)
III	involvement of lymph node regions on both sides of the diaphragm (III) which may also involve the spleen (IIIs), localized extralymphatic sites (IIIe) or both (IIIse)
IV	widespread involvement of extralymphoid sites such as the liver, lung and bone marrow with or without lymph node involvement

Fig. 14.13 Ann Arbor staging system of Hodgkin's disease. Suffix A indicates the absence of systemic symptoms; suffix B indicates the presence of systemic symptoms. For example, stage IIIeB denotes involvement of lymph nodes on both sides of the diaphragm accompanied by localized involvement of an extralymphatic site with systemic symptoms.

Rye classification of Hodgkin's disease	
Type	**Characteristic**
nodular sclerosis (60–70%)	thick bands of collagen encircle abnormal tissue; lacunar cells (variants of Reed–Sternberg—RS—cell) are often numerous; good prognosis
mixed cellularity (15%)	numerous RS cells and intermediate numbers of lymphocytes, plasma cells and eosinophils; poor prognosis
lymphocyte predominant (10%)	numerous lymphocytes, few RS cells and a scattering of unusual Hodgkin's cells—'popcorn' cells (so named due to their excessively lobulated nuclei); increased risk of development of non-Hodgkin's B cell lymphoma; otherwise good prognosis
lymphocyte depleted (2%)	dominance of RS cells but sparse lymphocytes with or without diffuse fibrosis; worst prognosis

Fig. 14.14 Rye classification of Hodgkin's disease.

Treatment is dependent on the stage of the disease, either localized (radiotherapy) or generalized (systemic chemotherapy). Approximately 75% of patients treated for Hodgkin's disease survive for at least five years.

The prognosis of patients with Hodgkin's disease declines with advancing stages and the presence of systemic symptoms.

Non-Hodgkin's lymphomas (NHL)

NHLs include all lymphomas other than Hodgkin's disease. They are predominantly diseases of middle and later life, with males affected more than females.

The aetiology of NHLs is poorly understood but several factors have been implicated:

- Immunosuppression: increased incidence in primary immunosuppressive diseases, e.g. X-linked agammaglobulinaemia.
- Viral infection with lymphotropic viruses, e.g. EBV, HTLV-1, HIV.
- Toxic chemicals.
- Radiation.

Chromosomal translocations are a feature of many types of lymphoma, for example:

- Burkitt's lymphoma: translocation 8;14.
- Follicular B cell lymphoma: translocation 14;18.
- Small or large cell diffuse lymphomas: associated with translocation 11;14.

These translocations cause a neoplastic transformation due to the transfer of an oncogene or oncogene-regulatory gene to an abnormal site resulting in the increased expression of that oncogene.

In malignant lymphomas, the tumour represents a clone of cells whose maturation is fixed at a particular stage of development.

Understanding the normal development of lymphocytes (Fig. 14.15) is essential towards an understanding of the classification of these diseases.

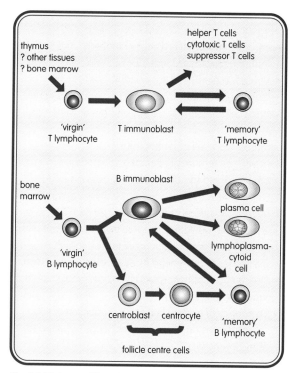

Fig. 14.15 Normal lymphocyte development. (Adapted with permission from *Essential Haematology*, 3rd edn, by V. Hoffbrand and J. Pettit, Blackwell Science, 1993.)

The vast majority (over 90%) of NHLs are B cell lymphomas, which are derived from follicle centre cells. These tumours have either follicular or diffuse architecture.

Clinical manifestations of NHLs are similar to those of Hodgkin's disease but are more varied due to their heterogeneous nature. The majority present with asymmetric painless enlargement of lymph nodes in one or more peripheral lymph node regions. However, extranodal presentation is more frequent than in HD, with 20% of all NHLs originating within extranodal sites.

Common primary extranodal sites include the orbit, nasopharynx, tonsil, GI tract, skin and bone.

Systemic symptoms are less prominent than in HD although fever is a feature of extensive disease.

Classification of NHLs

Several classification systems are used for NHLs.

One relatively simple classification is based on the Kiel system (Fig. 14.16) and considers the following:

- Degree of malignancy: low grade (associated with well-differentiated, relatively inactive cell types—progress over years); high grade (associated with primitive actively proliferating cells—progress over weeks or months).
- Tumour architecture: follicular or diffuse.
- Functional cell type: either T cell or B cell.

Classification of NHLs based on the Kiel system		
Grade	**B cell**	**T cell**
low grade malignancy	follicular: • centrocytic • centroblastic–centrocytic diffuse: • lymphocytic: chronic lymphocytic and hairy cell leukaemia • lymphoplasmacytoid • plasmacytic: multiple myeloma • centrocytic • centroblastic–centrocytic	lymphocytic small cerebriform cell: • mycosis fungoides • Sézary's syndrome lymphoepithelioid angioimmunoblastic T zone pleomorphic small cell
high grade malignancy	diffuse: • centroblastic • immunoblastic • anaplastic • lymphoblastic • 'Burkitt-type': small, non-cleaved cell	pleomorphic medium or large cell (HTLV-1) immunoblastic anaplastic lymphoblastic

Fig. 14.16 Classification of NHLs based on the Kiel system.

- Specific cell type or size, e.g. centroblastic or immunoblastic, large or small cell.

A similar staging system to that used in HD may be used but is less clearly related than the histological type to the prognosis.

Treatment is by single or combination chemotherapy with which some show long-term remission if not cure. Bone marrow transplantation is under evaluation.

The prognosis depends on the type of lymphoma and varies widely from highly proliferative and rapidly fatal diseases (e.g. immunoblastic lymphoma) to indolent and well-tolerated malignancies with a mean survival of about 7 years (e.g. follicular centrocytic lymphoma).

Leukaemias

Leukaemias are neoplastic proliferations of white blood cell precursors in the bone marrow.

Classification of leukaemias

Leukaemias are classified into two broad groups according to the ability of the leukaemic cells to differentiate which also reflects the rate of disease progression.

- Acute: characterized by numerous immature 'blast' cells (leukocyte precursors), and rapid disease progression.
- Chronic: characterized by large numbers of precursor cells that are more differentiated than blast cells, and associated with slower disease progression.

These groups are then further classified into two main groups depending on neoplastic cell types:

- myeloid leukaemia (cells of granulocytic series).
- lymphocytic leukaemia (cells of the lymphoid series).

Aetiology of leukaemias—In the majority of cases, the cause of leukaemia is unknown. However, certain factors are known to initiate leukaemic transformation:

- Genetics: slight familial tendency (high concordance in monozygotic twins); chromosome abnormalities (both quantitative and qualitative) are present in about 50% of patients; increased incidence in Down syndrome.
- Ionizing radiation: excessive exposure in therapy, e.g. for ankylosing spondylitis, malignant disease; nuclear explosions/accidents as at Hiroshima and Chernobyl.

- Drugs: prolonged chemotherapy, e.g. with alkylating agents.
- Immune status: increased incidence in immunosuppressed individuals.
- Viruses, e.g. HTLV-I causes adult T cell leukaemia/lymphoma; HTLV-II is associated with hairy cell leukaemia.

Common features of leukaemias

The common features of leukaemias are bone marrow failure, gout and metastasis.

Bone marrow failure

Overproduction of leukocyte precursor cells causes the suppression of normal blood cell production, thus:

- Deficiency of red cell production leads to anaemia.
- Deficiency of platelet production (thrombocytopenia) leads to haemorrhage.
- Deficiency of normal leukocyte production (granulocytes and lymphocytes) leads to failure to control infection.

Gout

Increased cell turnover leads to increased uric acid synthesis which may result in gout.

Metastasis

There is infiltration of organs such as the liver, spleen, lymph nodes, meninges and gonads by the leukaemic cells.

Acute leukaemia

In acute leukaemia, blast cells (lymphoblasts or myeloblasts) fail to differentiate properly and proliferate in an uncontrolled manner.

There are two main types: acute lymphoblastic leukaemia (ALL) and acute myeloblastic leukaemia (AML).

See Fig. 14.17 for a table with the features of ALL and AML.

Clinical features of both AML and ALL are similar. They commonly present with symptoms of anaemia (e.g. tiredness, malaise) and their course is typified by a series of overwhelming infections and mucosal haemorrhage.

Onset is frequently rapid, and progression to death from anaemia, haemorrhage or infection occurs within weeks if no treatment is given.

The clinical course is less catastrophic in childhood ALL. Haematological investigations reveal:

- Anaemia: normocytic, normochromic.

- Leukocytosis, although leukopenia may be an occasional feature, despite massive marrow infiltration with blast cells.
- Neutropenia—overt infections.
- Thrombocytopenia—petechiae, purpura, epistaxis, bleeding gums, GI haemorrhage, cerebral haemorrhage.

Involvement of other organs:
- Skeleton (bone pain, especially in children): probably caused by osteolytic lesions.
- Lymphadenopathy.
- Hepatomegaly and splenomegaly: usually slight.
- Symptoms and signs secondary to CNS infiltration.

Management:
- Repeated courses of combination chemotherapy.
- Intensive blood transfusions.
- Antimicrobial agents.
- Bone marrow transplantation: encouraging results in younger patients but largely depends on availability of suitable donor.

For the prognosis see Fig. 14.17.

Chronic leukaemias
Chronic myeloid leukaemia
There is neoplastic proliferation of an abnormal myeloid clone of leukocyte precursors in the bone marrow.

Over 95% of cases are characterized by the presence of a karyotypic abnormality—the Philadelphia chromosome—within the haemopoietic stem cells. This involves reciprocal translocation of part of the long arm (q) of chromosome 22 with the long arm of chromosome 9. The Philadelphia chromosome-positive cases are referred to as chronic granulocytic leukaemia (CGL).

CML occurs in all age groups but most frequently between the ages of 40 and 60 years. The disease has a mild chronic phase characterized by anaemia and massive splenomegaly. However, in over 70% of cases, the disease enters a more aggressive phase due to the emergence and dominance of a more malignant clone of myeloid cells.

Clinical features of the aggressive phase are much more severe, and bear a close resemblance to those of acute leukaemia (usually AML) and are rapidly fatal.

Haematological investigation reveals leukocytosis and normocytic anaemia. Note that in contrast to acute leukaemias, neutropenia, lymphopenia and thrombocytopenia are not common in the chronic phase, and infection and bleeding are not typical.

There is often massive splenomegaly due to infiltration by CGL cells, and hepatomegaly is also frequently present.

Treatment is by:
- Chemotherapy.
- Interferon treatment.
- Bone marrow transplantation.

Features of acute lymphoblastic and acute myeloblastic leukaemia		
	Acute lymphoblastic leukaemia (ALL)	**Acute myeloblastic leukaemia (AML)**
epidemiology	mainly (>90%) affects children of <14 years with highest incidence at 3–4 years; second increase in incidence occurs around middle-age	occurs at all ages and is the commonest form of leukaemia in adults
proliferating cell type	neoplastic lymphoblasts (lymphocyte precursor cells)	neoplastic myeloblast (granulocyte/monocyte precursor cell)
degree of differentiation	blast cells show no differentiation	blast cells usually show some evidence of differentiation to granulocytes
prognosis	children aged 2–9 years: 50–75% cure rate; adults: 35% cure rate with chemotherapy; 50% with allogeneic bone marrow transplant	20–25% cure rate with standard chemotherapy; 50% with allogeneic bone marrow transplant

Fig. 14.17 Features of acute lymphoblastic and acute myeloblastic leukaemia.

Prognosis—CGL is a fatal disorder with a mean survival of about 4 years. However, a minority of patients do survive for 10 years or more.

Chronic lymphocytic leukaemia
This chronic lymphoproliferative disorder is characterized by the proliferation of an abnormal lymphoid clone of leukocyte precursors in the bone marrow.

This is the commonest leukaemia of adults comprising about 30% of all leukaemias, with males more than females by 2:1.

Clinical features—A slowly progressive disease of the elderly which follows a predictable course over a period of years summarized in Fig. 14.18. Features are similar to a low-grade lymphoma but with predominant blood and bone marrow involvement.

This disease is much less aggressive than other leukaemias.

Haematological changes are:
- Leukocytosis: small, non-functional lymphocytes of B cell origin.
- Anaemia and thrombocytopenia are late developments.
- Secondary autoimmune haemolytic anaemia develops in 10% of cases.

The lymph nodes, liver and spleen are characteristically involved, and normal architecture may become completely effaced by the infiltrating cells.

Survival for more than 10 years from diagnosis is common, and, as CLL is a disease of the elderly, death is often from an unrelated cause. However, anaemia, haemorrhage and infection may become life threatening in the later stages.

In younger subjects, a more aggressive course of CLL may develop with massive glandular enlargement and severe infections secondary to a compromised immunity.

Myelodysplastic syndromes
This group of acquired neoplastic disorders of the bone marrow is characterized by increasing bone marrow failure with quantitative and qualitative abnormalities of all three myeloid cell lines (red cell, granulocyte/monocyte and platelets) due to a defect of stem cells. They are also known as refractory anaemias.

In most cases, the disease arises *de novo* and the aetiology is likely to be as for the leukaemias. However,

in a significant proportion of cases, the disease is secondary to treatment with chemotherapy (with or without radiotherapy) for a previous neoplastic disease.

The hallmark of the disease is ineffective haemopoiesis resulting in pancytopenia despite a marrow of either normal or increased cellularity.

Bone marrow contains morphologically abnormal cells including ring sideroblasts and hypogranular white cells, often with abnormal chromosomes.

The disease has tendency to progress to acute leukaemia, and is therefore considered 'preleukaemic'.

Clinical features—More than half the patients are over 70 years old, and more than 75% are over 50; males are affected more often than females.

Symptoms are generally sequelae of cytopenia and include anaemia, infection, and haemorrhage. Disease progression is slow but there is a tendency for it to transform into acute myeloid leukaemia.

Diseases are subclassified depending on the presence of ring sideroblasts and the proportion of leukaemic-type blast cells in the bone marrow (Fig. 14.19).

Treatment is largely supportive, by blood transfusion and treatment of the infection.

Morbidity and deaths are largely attributable to the refractory cytopenias either directly (e.g. from haemorrhage) or indirectly (e.g. from transfusion-related haemosiderosis).

In a minority of patients deaths are related to leukaemic transformation.

Clinical features and staging of chronic lymphocytic leukaemia according to the RAI classification	
Stage	Feature(s)
0	lymphocytosis of blood and marrow
I	lymphocytosis and enlarged nodes
II	lymphocytosis and enlarged liver or spleen
III	haemoglobin <11 g/dl, with features of stages 0, I or II
IV	platelet count <100 × 10^9/l, with features of stages 0, I, II or III

Fig. 14.18 Clinical features and staging of chronic lymphocytic leukaemia according to the Rai classification.

Hairy cell leukaemia

This rare, B cell leukaemia is characterized by variable numbers of 'hairy' cells in the blood, bone marrow, liver and other organs. Hairy cells are so named because of their characteristic irregular outline caused by cytoplasmic projections or 'hairs'.

The disease has a peak incidence at 40–60 years old, males more so than females by 4:1.

It is characterized clinically by features of pancytopenia and splenomegaly.

The disorder typically runs a chronic course and remission is common with chemotherapy or interferon treatment. Splenectomy is also useful in management.

Myeloproliferative disorders

These are autonomous proliferations of one or more myeloid cells (erythroid, granulocytic, megakaryocytic) with differentiation to mature forms (Fig. 14.20).

Progression from one disorder to another within the group is common.

Polycythaemia rubra vera

This idiopathic condition is characterized by an above normal increase in red cell concentration, usually with concomitant increases in haemoglobin concentration and haematocrit.

The disorder has a prevalence of 1 per 100 000 in the UK and typically affects the middle-aged, males more so than females.

Progression of this disease is chronic but about 20% of cases evolve into myelofibrosis, and another 5–10% into acute leukaemia.

Onset is usually insidious and non-specific, e.g. malaise, fatigue, headache and dizziness. The principal symptoms are due to vascular engorgement, increased haematocrit, and thrombosis, with or without haemorrhage. Splenomegaly is common, and hepatomegaly is occasional.

Treatment is by venesection or myelosuppression with chemotherapy or use of radioactive ^{32}P. Treated patients have a mean survival of about 13 years.

Note that most cases of polycythaemia are not due to polycythaemia rubra vera but are secondary to conditions resulting in chronic hypoxia (p.319). Splenomegaly and pancytosis are not usually features of these conditions.

Myelofibrosis

This condition is characterized by a proliferation of fibroblasts in the bone marrow and gross marrow fibrosis, with a corresponding massive extramedullary haemopoiesis in the liver and spleen. It is also known as myelosclerosis.

The condition is a chronic disorder of late and middle age, and may arise *de novo* (with unknown aetiology), or as an end-stage of other myeloproliferative disorders, in which case the reactive fibrosis is thought to be stimulated by factors released from proliferating pathological megakaryocytes.

Classification of myelodysplastic syndromes (MDS)			
Type of MDS	**Peripheral blood**	**Bone marrow**	**Median survival (months)**
refractory anaemia (RA)	blasts <1%	blasts <5%	50
RA with ring sideroblasts (RARS)	blasts <1%	blasts <5% ring sideroblasts >15% of total erythroblasts	50
RA with excess blasts (RAEB)	blasts <5%	blasts 5–20%	10
RAEB in transformation (RAEB-t)	blasts >5%	blasts 20–30% or Auer rods present	5
chronic myelomonocytic leukaemia (CMML)	blasts <1% monocytes >1.0 × 10^9/l	blasts 5–20% promomonocytes	10

Fig. 14.19 Classification of myelodysplastic syndromes (MDS).

303

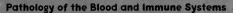
The disease is usually slowly progressive. However, in about 10% of patients transformation to acute leukaemia occurs.

Clinical features are:
- Blood film: typically leukoerythroblastic; erythropoiesis is ineffective leading to anaemia with marked anisocytosis and tear-drop poikilocytes.
- Splenomegaly is invariable.
- Hepatomegaly is common.
- Increased bone density due to sclerosis (hence the alternative name).

Symptoms are usually caused by anaemia and massive splenomegaly. Systemic symptoms (e.g. fever, weight loss, etc.) are usually late features.

Treatment is generally supportive, and with careful management median survival is about 5 years.

Primary (essential/idiopathic) thrombocythaemia
This condition is characterized by increased platelet production due to a clonal myeloproliferative disorder. It is most commonly seen in patients over 50 years of age. Its features are:
- Large, atypical platelets with increased platelet count, often $>1000 - 10^9/L$.
- Combined pathological haemorrhages and thromboembolic episodes.

- Iron-deficiency anaemia due to chronic blood loss is an occasional feature.
- Spleen may be enlarged but is usually normal or reduced in size because of thromboembolic infarction.

Treatment with chemotherapy and antiplatelet drugs (e.g. aspirin) is effective and median survival with treatment is 8–10 years.

Proliferation of plasma cells
Myeloma
Multiple myeloma
This diffuse, neoplastic, monoclonal proliferation of plasma cells throughout the red marrow typically affects the elderly, with almost all cases occurring after the age of 40. It is also known as myelomatosis.

Pathogenesis—Proliferating plasma cells produce a monoclonal immunoglobulin or light chain, referred to as the 'M component' (NB: The 'M' stands for myeloma not IgM).

The M component is usually IgG (>60%) but may be IgA (20%) or immunoglobulin light chain (κ being more frequent than λ).

(IgD and IgE are unusual, and IgM-producing plasma cells are a feature of a different type of plasma cell neoplasm: Waldenström's macroglobulinaemia).

Myeloproliferative disorders and their basic features			
Disorder	**Principal proliferations**	**Bone marrow morphology**	**Clinical features**
polycythaemia rubra vera	erythroblasts	increased cellularity, especially erythroid	erythrocytosis with increased Hb and PCV often neutrophilia and thrombocytosis pruritus (related to basophilia) thrombosis or haemorrhage splenomegaly
myelofibrosis	fibroblasts	increased deposition of collagen/reticulin; bone marrow difficult to aspirate	leukoerythroblastic blood picture anaemia with tear-drop poikilocytes hepatosplenomegaly
chronic granulocytic leukaemia	myeloblasts	increased cellularity, especially myeloid	leukoerythroblastic blood picture anaemia, neutrophilia, basophilia splenomegaly
essential thrombocythaemia	megakaryoblasts	increased megakaryocytes	thrombocytosis thrombosis or haemorrhage occasional splenomegaly

Fig. 14.20 Myeloproliferative disorders and their basic features. Hb = haemoglobin, PCV = packed cell volume.

The presence of a single type of immunoglobulin is reflected in the electrophoretic pattern which shows normal levels of α- and β-globulins but a dramatic increase in the levels of γ-globulins (Fig. 14.21).

Renal impairment

Whole immunoglobulins are too large to pass through the glomerular filter but in two-thirds of cases of IgG and IgA myelomas, monoclonal free light chains are also produced which are small enough to enter the urine, where they are called Bence Jones proteins.

During passage through the tubules, the protein precipitates as 'casts', causing damage to the tubular epithelial cells, with concomitant formation of surrounding giant cells—'Bence Jones or myeloma kidney'.

Light chains that pass through capillaries are incorporated into amyloid (systemic amyloidosis; p. 293) by mechanisms not yet fully elucidated, causing damage to many organs including the kidneys.

Raised blood uric acid (from increased cell turnover) worsens renal impairment, as does increased blood calcium from bone osteolysis.

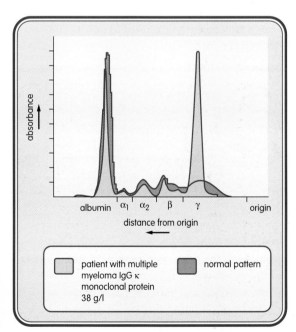

Fig. 14.21 Serum electrophoresis showing characteristic gamma band of multiple myeloma. (Adapted with permission from *Essential Haematology*, 3rd edn, by V. Hoffbrand and J. Pettit, Blackwell Science, 1993.)

Bone changes

These are as follows:

- Hypercellular marrow with large proportion of abnormal plasma cells, especially in the skull, ribs, vertebrae and pelvis.
- Osteolysis of medullary and cortical bone due to increased numbers of bone-resorbing osteoclasts: thought to be stimulated by activation factors (e.g. interleukins) produced by the malignant plasma cells.
- Osteolytic lesions are seen as 'punched out' defects in the bones, the skull showing this appearance particularly well.
- Generalized osteoporosis may result in pathological fractures or vertebral compression.

Haematological findings

These are as follows:

- Anaemia: usually normochromic, normocytic.
- Marked rouleaux formation (red cells pile together adhering by their rims forming cylinders).
- Raised blood viscosity (depending on type of immunoglobulin).
- Reduced concentration of unaffected immunoglobulins: 'immune paresis'.
- Abnormal plasma cells: occasionally seen in peripheral blood.
- Neutropenia and thrombocytopenia: common features in late stages.

Clinical features are:

- Bone pain (especially backache and pathological fractures).
- Features of anaemia: lethargy, weakness, dyspnoea, pallor, tachycardia.
- Repeated infections: related to deficient antibody production and, in advanced disease, to neutropenia.
- Abnormal bleeding tendency: M component may interfere with platelet function and coagulation factors, and thrombocytopenia occurs in advanced disease.
- Features of renal failure and/or hypercalcaemia.

Treatment involves chemotherapy and radiotherapy. Median survival is about 2 years with treatment.

Solitary myeloma

This rare disease is characterized by discrete solitary tumours of proliferating monoclonal plasma cells, usually in the bone.

Proliferation does not occur in parts of the skeleton beyond the primary lesion, and marrow aspirates distant from the primary tumour are usually normal.

The associated M component usually disappears following radiotherapy to the primary lesion. However, a minority of cases progress to multiple myeloma.

- Name the most common type of leukopenia. What are its causes and effects?
- Describe the morphological features and cellular composition of affected lymph nodes in Hodgkin's disease.
- Explain the classification basis of leukaemia.
- Describe the common clinical features of leukaemia.
- List the myeloproliferative disorders, and describe their basic features.
- Describe the pathogenesis of multiple myeloma.

DISORDERS OF THE SPLEEN AND THYMUS

Splenomegaly

The spleen serves as the site of filtration and phagocytosis of the following:

- Effete cells and cell debris, especially red cells.
- Micro-organisms.
- Abnormal or excess material derived from metabolic processes.

Splenomegaly (enlargement of the spleen) is a common physical sign, and may have many causes, the main types of which are summarized in Fig. 14.22.

A palpable spleen is at least twice its normal size, and is vulnerable to traumatic rupture, e.g. in glandular fever or malaria.

Effect of splenomegaly

Irrespective of the cause, enlargement of the spleen may result in the development of hypersplenism, i.e. a decrease in the circulating numbers of erythrocytes, leukocytes and platelets (pancytopenia), resulting from the destruction or pooling of these cells by the enlarged spleen.

Hypersplenism is often accompanied by a compensatory response: hyperplasia of the bone marrow.

Splenectomy leads to clinical and haematological improvement.

Congestive splenomegaly

This is enlargement of the spleen caused by any condition that leads to a persistent elevation of splenic venous blood pressure. Causes of raised splenic venous pressure are outlined in Fig. 14.23.

Morphological features—Sinusoids of spleen are initially distended with red cells. Fibrosis eventually occurs, and sinusoids then appear ectatic and empty.

The cut surface of the spleen has a purple-red colour with an inconspicuous white pulp, and is often flecked with firm, brown nodules (called Gamna–Gandy nodules) which represent areas of healed infarction.

Foci of extramedullary haemopoiesis are an occasional feature and are thought to be secondary to local hypoxia.

A quick revision of splenic venous anatomy is helpful in understanding the causes of raised splenic venous pressure (Fig. 14.23).

Splenic infarcts

Splenic infarction follows occlusion of the splenic artery or its branches and may be caused by:

- Emboli that arise in the heart: most commonly.
- Local thrombosis, e.g. in sickle cell diseases, myeloproliferative disorders and malignant infiltrates.

Infarcts may be single or multiple and are generally wedge shaped and pale.

Causes of splenomegaly	
Cause	**Comments**
infections	bacterial, e.g. typhoid, tuberculosis, brucellosis, infective endocarditis viral: infectious mononucleosis protozoal: malaria, leishmaniasis, trypanosomiasis, toxoplasmosis
congestion	due to persistent elevation of splenic venous blood pressure, the cause of which may be: • prehepatic: thrombosis of hepatic, splenic or portal vein • hepatic: long-standing portal hypertension associated with cirrhosis • posthepatic: raised venous pressure of inferior vena cava, e.g. due to right-sided heart failure, which is transmitted to the spleen via the portal system
storage diseases	heritable enzyme deficiencies, which result in storage of material in splenic macrophagic cells, e.g. Gaucher's disease, Niemann–Pick disease and Tay–Sachs disease
neoplasia	primary: rare secondary: • lymphomas: Hodgkin's disease and non-Hodgkin's lymphomas • leukaemias: especially chronic leukaemias • metastases: splenic metastases from solid tumours, e.g. carcinomas or sarcomas, are rare • extramedullary haemopoiesis, e.g. in myeloproliferative diseases and diseases with diffuse marrow replacement by tumour
haematological disorders	haematological anaemias, e.g. hereditary spherocytosis, β-thalassaemia, autoimmune haemolysis autoimmune thrombocytopenia: destruction of antibody-coated platelets in spleen results in accumulation of foamy histiocytes in sinuses
immune disorders	Felty's syndrome: follicular hyperplasia in spleen associated with hypersplenism and rheumatoid disease sarcoidosis: spleen infiltrated by granulomas amyloidosis: spleen infiltrated with amyloid

Fig. 14.22 Causes of splenomegaly.

Rupture of the spleen

Rupture of a normal spleen usually occurs following a considerable abdominal trauma, particularly as occurs in some automobile accidents.

Spontaneous rupture of an abnormal enlarged spleen may occur particularly in infectious mononucleosis, malaria and in splenic haemopoietic proliferations such as myelofibrosis.

A massive intraperitoneal haemorrhage usually follows splenic rupture, necessitating emergency splenectomy.

Disorders of the thymus

The thymus is composed of lymphoid cells and specialized epithelial cells, and is known as the 'primary' lymphoid organ. It is concerned with the development and processing of the long-lived T lymphocytes prior to their distribution to lymphoid tissues and to a circulating pool of T lymphocytes.

Thymic activity is maximal in fetal and childhood stages; regression is rapid after puberty.

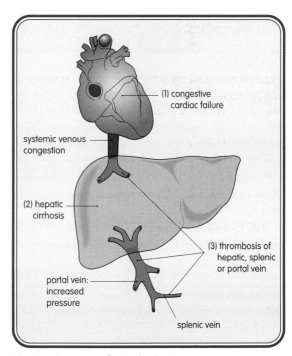

Fig. 14.23 Causes of raised splenic venous pressure.

Developmental disorders
Thymic hypoplasia and aplasia
These occur due to the developmental failure of either:
- Epithelial tissue: thymus is completely absent or is represented by a fibrous streak, e.g. DiGeorge syndrome (p. 291) and Nezelof's syndrome.
- Lymphoid tissue: severe combined immunodeficiency syndromes, ataxia telangiectasia and reticular dysgenesis.

Both types of developmental disorders result in T cell deficiency associated with a disordered, cell-mediated immune response.

Thymic cysts
These are cysts lined with thymic tissue and occur in the neck or anterior mediastinum. Usually congenital, they may be acquired due to degeneration within the thymus gland or within thymic neoplasms.

Thymic hyperplasia
This is a rare condition in which lymphoid follicles (germinal centres) composed of B cells develop in the thymic medulla. It is often accompanied by an increase in the size of the thymus and associated with autoimmune disease, especially myasthenia gravis; in some cases autoantibodies are thought to be produced by the lymphoid tissue.

Thymomas
These rare tumours are derived from thymic epithelial cells, which may be benign or malignant. Most arise within the thymus but ectopic thymomas occasionally arise in the soft tissues of the neck, the hilum of the lung, and other sites within the mediastinum or rarely the thyroid.

Histologically, thymomas are composed of uniform epithelial cells variably admixed with reactive lymphoid cells.

They are associated with a variety of disorders including myasthenia gravis and non-organ specific autoimmune diseases.

Benign thymomas
The majority (80–90%) of thymomas are benign, well-circumscribed, encapsulated, lobulated tumours. Most are asymptomatic but some present with local disease caused by the compression of adjacent mediastinal structures:

- Respiratory passages—dyspnoea and cough.
- Oesophagus—dysphagia.
- Great veins—cyanosis and suffusion of the face.

The remainder present with autoimmune disease. Complete surgical excision is curative.

Malignant thymomas
Around 10–20% of thymomas are malignant and invade the local tissues. There are two types:
- Type 1: histologically indistinguishable from benign thymomas but invade the local tissues, e.g. pericardium, lungs, pleura. Rarely spread outside the thorax.
- Type 2: rare malignant thymomas histologically distinct from benign and from type 1 thymomas, e.g. squamous cell carcinoma, oat cell carcinoma. Poor prognosis.

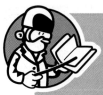

- List the causes of splenomegaly.
- Define hypersplenism.
- State the causes of splenic infarcts.
- Name four developmental disorders of the thymus.
- Describe the different types of thymoma.

DISORDERS OF RED BLOOD CELLS

Abnormalities of red cell size and shape
Many haematological and systemic disorders are associated with specific abnormalities of red cell size (anisocytosis) and/or abnormal red cell shape (poikilocytosis).

It is useful to know the red cell abnormalities associated with specific diseases as they are readily detected microscopically and are of diagnostic importance.

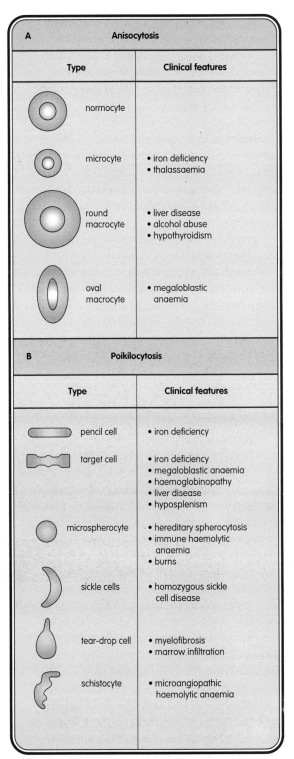

Fig. 14.24 Diagrammatic representation of (A) abnormalities in red cell size (anisocytosis) and (B) abnormalities in red cell shape (poikilocytosis). (Adapted with permissin from *General and Systematic Pathology*, 2nd edn, by J.C.E. Underwood, Churchill Livingstone, 1996.)

A diagrammatic representation of some of the variations in red cell size and shape, and the disorders that cause them is shown in Fig. 14.24.

Anaemia
Anaemia may be defined as a state in which the blood haemoglobin level is below the normal range for the patient's age and sex. The normal haemoglobin range is males 15.5 g/dl ± 2.5, females 14.0 g/dl ± 2.5. The causes of anaemia are shown in Fig. 14.25.

Blood loss
Acute blood loss
Following acute blood loss, a state of cardiovascular collapse may occur, and the shock syndrome is often the predominant feature.

On cessation of haemorrhage, the plasma volume begins to be restored, and anaemia becomes apparent.

Causes of anaemia	
Cause	**Clinical features**
increased red cell loss, lysis or pooling	blood loss haemolysis: • intrinsic abnormalities of red cells: hereditary: membrane defects, enzyme defects, haemoglobinopathies acquired: paroxysmal nocturnal haemoglobinuria • extrinsic abnormalities of red cells: antibody-mediated red cell destruction mechanical trauma to red cells hypersplenism
impaired red cell production	deficiency of haematinics: • megaloblastic anaemias: lack of B_{12} or folate • iron-deficiency anaemia dyserythropoiesis (production of defective cells): • anaemia of chronic disorders • myelodysplasia • sideroblastic anaemia hypoplasia of marrow (failure to produce cells): • aplastic anaemia • red cell aplasia invasion of marrow by malignant cells: • leukaemias • myeloproliferative diseases • non-haematological malignancies

Fig. 14.25 Causes of anaemia.

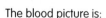

The blood picture is:
- Normocytic and normochromic anaemia.
- Polychromatic erythrocytes and reticulocytes, reflecting increased haemopoiesis.
- Transient leukocytosis and thrombocytosis.

Plasma proteins and other biochemical constituents are restored rapidly (in 2–3 days). Full red cell restoration may take up to 6 weeks.

Chronic blood loss

Chronic blood loss is the commonest cause of iron-deficiency anaemia. The main causes of chronic haemorrhage are:
- Diseases of the gastrointestinal tract: particularly peptic ulceration, carcinoma of the stomach and carcinoma of the colon.
- Menorrhagia.
- Lesions in the urinary tract.

Patients with unexplained iron-deficiency anaemia require careful screening for an occult cause of blood loss.

Haemolytic anaemias

In all haemolytic anaemias, the basic pathological change is a reduction in the life span of the red cells due an increased rate of destruction: haemolysis. The effects of increased haemolysis are:
- Anaemia: normocytic with increased reticulocytes in the blood.
- Erythroid hyperplasia of bone marrow.
- Splenomegaly.
- Unconjugated hyperbilirubinaemia, which may lead to development of pigment gallstones, jaundice, (kernicterus in neonates).
- Haemoglobinuria: leading to tubular damage in the kidney.

The aetiology of haemolytic anaemias can be broadly classified into:
- Intrinsic abnormalities of red cells: hereditary defects, acquired defects.
- Extrinsic abnormalities of red cells: antibody-mediated red cell destruction, mechanical trauma to red cells.

Hereditary defects of the red cell

Hereditary defects of the red cell can be classified into:

- Cell membrane defects: hereditary spherocytosis and hereditary elliptocytosis.
- Enzyme deficiencies: deficiency of glycolytic enzymes or hexose monophosphate shunt enzymes.
- Haemoglobinopathies: e.g. thalassaemias and sickle cell disease.

Hereditary spherocytosis and hereditary elliptocytosis

Hereditary spherocytosis is the commonest cause of hereditary haemolytic anaemia in the UK. It is an autosomal dominant condition caused by an abnormality of the cytoskeletal-associated membrane protein, spectrin.

The cells are spherical, of reduced deformability, and abnormally fragile.

Reduced deformability of the spherical red cells causes their retention in the splenic microcirculation where they undergo metabolic stress caused by a lack of glucose and acidosis. Increased fragility of metabolically stressed cells causes their spontaneous lysis or premature phagocytosis by the splenic macrophages.

Blood film shows:
- Increased microspherocytes, which are more deeply staining with loss of the central pallor of normal erythrocytes.
- Increased polychromatic cells and reticulocytes.

The general clinical features of chronic haemolysis are present. Splenectomy is performed to prevent haemolysis.

Hereditary elliptocytosis is similar to spherocytosis but the red cells are elliptical. This is caused by abnormalities of the cytoskeletal-associated membrane proteins ankyrin, spectrin, or band 42 protein.

This condition is not as severe as hereditary spherocytosis, and does not usually cause anaemia or jaundice.

Enzyme deficiencies

In erythrocytes, 90% of glucose is metabolized anaerobically to lactate via the Embden–Meyerhof glycolytic pathway (pathway is similar to regular glycolysis except that the end product is lactate not pyruvate); 10% of glucose is used in the hexose monophosphate shunt (also known as the pentose phosphate pathway) to increase the levels of NADPH to those required for the reduction of glutathione. Reduced glutathione is essential for maintaining Hb in the reduced (ferrous) state (Fig. 14.26).

Deficiencies of glycolytic enzymes

Pyruvate kinase deficiency is a rare, autosomal recessive defect which results in congenital chronic haemolytic anaemia. Red cells become rigid due to reduced ATP formation and are removed by the spleen.

Anaemia is generally mild, but blood film shows raised poikilocytosis and distorted 'prickle cells'.

Clinically, jaundice is usual and gallstones are frequent.

Many other enzymopathies of glycolytic enzymes exist but are extremely rare, e.g. deficiencies of hexokinase, glucose phosphate isomerase, and phosphofructokinase. The effects are similar to pyruvate kinase deficiency.

Deficiencies of hexose monophosphate shunt enzymes

The most common deficiencies are glucose-6-phosphate dehydrogenase (G6PD) deficiency, and glutathione synthetase deficiency.

G6PD deficiency is an X-linked recessive condition especially common among Black races. It results in a decreased ratio of NADPH/NADP, which leads to an impaired reduction of glutathione, and an increased susceptibility to oxidative stress.

Spontaneous anaemia is rare but haemolytic crises are frequently precipitated by infections, ingestion of fava (broad) beans or the administration of certain drugs (quinine, phenacetin, aspirin).

Blood film during haemolytic crises shows raised poikilocytosis with bite-shaped defects ('bite' cells) or surface blebs ('blister' cells), and Heinz bodies (red cells containing oxidized, denatured haemoglobin). The blood picture is normal between haemolytic episodes.

Female heterozygotes have the advantage of being resistant to falciparum malaria.

A deficiency of glutathione synthestase leads to defective synthesis of glutathione causing a similar syndrome to G6PD deficiency.

Haemoglobin abnormalities (haemoglobinopathies)

Haemoglobinopathies are caused by either:

- Decreased α- or β-globin synthesis: the α- and β-thalassaemias.
- Synthesis of abnormal haemoglobin: e.g. sickle cell disease, unstable haemoglobins.

Anaemias resulting from haemoglobinopathies are usually a combined result of both dyshaemopoiesis and haemolysis.

Thalassaemias

Normal adult haemoglobin (HbA) is composed of two α-globin chains and two β-globin chains ($\alpha_2\beta_2$). In thalassaemia, one or more of the genes responsible for synthesis of α- or β-globin chains is abnormal, resulting in α- or β-thalassaemia, depending on which chain is affected.

The disease is inherited and is common in the Mediterranean, the Middle and Far East, and South-East Asia, where carrier rates of 10–15% are found.

Fig. 14.26 Metabolic pathways of the red cell. (H_2O_2, hydrogen peroxide; GSH, GSSG, glutathione; NADP, NADPH, nicotinamide-adenine-dinucleotide phosphate; glucose-6-P = glucose-6-phossphate; fructose-6-P = fructose-6-phosphate).

(Figure 14.26 diagram)

hexose monophosphate shunt pathway

H_2O_2 → H_2O

glutathione peroxidase

GSH → GSSG

glutathione reductase

NADP → NADPH

Embden–Meyerhof glycoytic pathway

glucose

hexokinase

glucose-6-P

glucose-6-phosphate dehydrogenase

6-phospho gluconate

ribulose-5-phosphate

fructose-6-P

phosphoenol pyruvate

pyruvate kinase

pyruvate

lactate

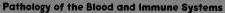

α-thalassaemia—Mainly caused by deletion (rather than mutation) of parts of the α-globin genes. Normal individuals have four copies of the α-globin gene, two copies on each chromosome 16. There are therefore four possible degrees of α-thalassaemia, depending on how many genes are abnormal (Fig. 14.27).

Haemolysis is less severe in α-thalassaemia than in β-thalassaemia.

β-thalassaemia—Caused by a mutation of the β-globin gene(s) leading to either reduced (β^+) or absent (β^0) synthesis of the β-globin chain. Normal individuals have two copies of each β-globin gene (one on each chromosome 11). There are therefore two possible degrees of β-thalassaemia:

- Thalassaemia minor: heterozygous trait associated with mild anaemia.
- Thalassaemia major: homozygous syndrome associated with severe haemolytic anaemia.

Sickle cell disease

This is caused by an abnormal form of haemoglobin, HbS ($a_2\beta^S_2$), caused by a point mutation (resulting in the substitution of valine for glutamate) in the gene coding for the β-globin chain.

The disease is common in west and central Africa, the Mediterranean and the Middle East. Carriage of the gene may confer some protection against falciparum malaria.

HbS polymerizes at low oxygen saturations, causing an abnormal rigidity and deformity of red cells, which assume a sickle shape (Fig. 14.28). As a result, deoxygenated red cells undergo aggregation (causing vascular occlusion of small vessels) and haemolysis (due to increased fragility).

Heterozygous versus homozygous state

Heterozygous condition—Sickle cell trait in which only 30% of the haemoglobin is HbS, resulting in no significant clinical abnormality.

Thalassaemia disorders			
Type of thalassaemia		**Globin chains present**	**Clinicopathological features**
β-thalassaemia	thalassaemia minor	heterozygous $\beta^0\beta$	moderate reduction in HbA
		heterozygous $\beta^+\beta$	compensatory increase in HbA_2 ($\alpha_2\delta_2$)
			mild anaemia with hypochromic cells
	thalassaemia major	homozygous $\beta^0\beta^0$	hypochromic microcytic anaemia
		homozygous $\beta^+\beta^+$	severe haemolysis with hepatosplenomegaly
		or occasionally $\beta^+\beta^0$	marrow hyperplasia causing skeletal deformities
			iron overload from repeated transfusions
α-thalassaemia	silent carrier	-α/αα	asymptomatic with normal haematology or slightly reduced MCV
	α-thalassaemia trait	--/αα or α-/α-	asymptomatic but mild haemolytic anaemia with some microcytic cells
	haemoglobin H disease	--/α-	excess β-chains form tetramers: HbH
			moderate haemolytic anaemia with hypochromia and microcytosis
			splenomegaly
	hydrops fetalis	--/--	death *in utero*

Fig. 14.27 Summary of the thalassaemia disorders.

Homozygous condition—Sickle cell disease in which more than 80% of the haemoglobin is HbS, the rest being HbF and HbA_2. It is associated with serious clinicopathological features.

Fig. 14.29 shows a table with the pathogenesis and clinical features of sickle cell disease.

'Crises' of sickle cell disease

In addition to the effects of aggregation and haemolysis, sickle cell disease is characterized by various 'crises' that occur after the age of 1 or 2 years, when HbF levels have fallen and the proportion of HbS has increased. These are of three main patterns:

- Sequestration crises: sudden pooling of red cells in the spleen may develop in the early years of the disease causing a rapid fall in haemoglobin concentration, which can lead to death.
- Infarctive crises: due to obstruction of the small blood vessels. Commonly affected tissues are bone (especially femoral head), the spleen (leading to splenic atrophy) and skin (leg ulcers).
- Aplastic crises: splenic infarction predisposes to infection leading to depression of red cell production and exacerbation of pre-existing anaemia.

Treatment is by the avoidance of factors known to precipitate crises, especially hypoxia. Blood transfusions are necessary during crises.

Mean survival figures are variable reflecting differing standards of medical care. However, death in infancy or childhood is usual in underdeveloped countries.

Unstable haemoglobins

Hereditary abnormalities in globin chains result in the decreased stability of the haemoglobin molecule with haemolytic anaemia of variable severity. Examples are haemoglobins Köln and Zurich.

Acquired defects of the red cell
Paroxysmal nocturnal haemoglobinuria

This rare disorder of young adults is caused by a clonal abnormality of erythrocytes, which renders them abnormally sensitive to lysis by complement. This may arise *de novo* or follow an episode of aplastic anaemia. Venous thrombosis is a frequent complication.

Haemosiderinuria is conspicuous in all cases. However, nocturnal haemolysis with or without haemoglobinuria is present in only about 25% of cases.

Antibody-mediated red cell destruction
Isoimmune

This antibody-mediated haemolysis of red cells is derived from another individual of the same species.

Incompatible ABO blood transfusion

The classic example red cell haemolysis, this is caused by iso-antibodies (Fig. 14.30).

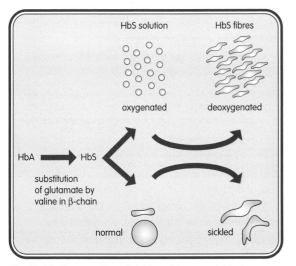

Fig. 14.28 Aggregation of sickle cell haemoglobin in conditions of low oxygen.

Pathogenesis and clinical features of sickle cell disease	
Pathogenesis	**Clinical features**
vascular occlusion	cerebral infarction retinopathy → blindness pulmonary infarction → acute respiratory distress cor pulmonale haematuria and polyuria splenic atrophy → hyposplenism → infections bone necrosis → osteomyelitis leg ulcers
chronic haemolysis	anaemia jaundice and gallstones haemochromatosis (due to iron overload in transfused patients)

Fig. 14.29 Pathogenesis and clinical features of sickle cell disease.

For example, if donor blood is group A (i.e. cells contain A antigen) and recipient blood is group O (cells do not possess A or B antigens but plasma contains both anti-A and anti-B antibodies), then anti-A antibodies of the recipient will cause agglutination and haemolysis of donor RBCs.

Clinical and pathological effects:
- Massive intravascular haemolysis leading to collapse, hypotension and pain in the lumbar region.
- Haemoglobinuria is common, and renal failure may ensue.
- Disseminated intravascular coagulation may be triggered by red cell lysis.

The effects may be precipitated with only a few millilitres of incompatible red cells.

Transfusion-induced haemolysis due to incompatibility of the rhesus system is generally milder since antibodies to the rhesus system are not complement fixing.

Haemolytic disease of the newborn (HDN)
This haemolysis of red blood cells in rhesus (Rh)-positive fetuses is caused by the placental passage of maternal anti-rhesus IgG antibodies from rhesus-negative mothers. It is particularly associated with D antigen of the rhesus blood group.

The pathogenesis is as follows:
- First pregnancy: Rh-positive fetus in Rh-negative mother with no antibodies—healthy baby. However, if fetal red blood cells enter maternal circulation during breach of placental barrier (e.g. at birth or miscarriage), then isoimmunization of mother will occur.
- Subsequent pregnancies: anti-Rh antibodies acquired by mother during previous pregnancy cause HDN in Rh-positive fetuses.

HDN is categorized into three groups according to severity.
1. Congenital haemolytic anaemia: mild anaemia and jaundice, usually self limiting.
2. Icterus gravis neonatum: rapidly developing severe anaemia and jaundice. May result in brain damage due to kernicterus, hepatosplenomegaly due to extramedullary haemopoiesis, or death from severe anoxia.
3. Hydrops fetalis: death *in utero* associated with severe anoxia and cardiac failure.

The incidence of HDN has been reduced due to the prophylactic removal of fetal cells entering the maternal circulation by the injection of anti-D before isoimmunization can occur.

Autoimmune haemolytic anaemia
This is the commonest type of haemolytic anaemia, caused by the immune destruction of red blood cells by the host's own antibodies. It may be idiopathic, secondary to other diseases or drug related.

It is divided into two main groups according to the temperature at which haemolytic reactions occur.

'Warm' antibody type
Autoantibody is IgG and most reactive at 37°C, leading to chronic anaemia with microspherocytes. Red cell destruction occurs in the spleen.

Clinical features are those of haemolytic anaemia: pallor, jaundice and splenomegaly (Fig. 14.31).

'Cold' antibody type
Autoantibody is IgM and most reactive at 4°C but can still bind complement and agglutinate red cells at 30°C, the temperature of peripheral tissues (hands, feet, nose and ears). There is destruction of red cells by Kupffer's cells of the liver.

Clinical features are of anaemia and of blueness and coldness of the fingers, toes, nose and ears, occasionally progressing to ischaemia and ulceration. Disorder is chronic and usually mild (Fig. 14.32).

Fig. 14.33 is a summary of antibody-mediated haemolytic anaemias.

ABO blood group system			
Genotype	Phenotype	Antibodies	Frequency of phenotype in UK
OO	O	anti-A, -B	most common
AA or AO	A	anti-B	common
BB or BO	B	anti-A	rare
AB	AB	none	rarest

Fig. 14.30 ABO blood group system.

Mechanical trauma to red cells

Mechanical damage to red cells may lead to reduced life span and haemolysis.

There are several groups of mechanical haemolysis, as follows.

Microangiopathic haemolytic anaemia

Haemolysis is caused by physical trauma to erythrocytes as they are forced through narrow areas in the vasculature. It is commonly present in:

- Disseminated intravascular coagulation: red blood cells are damaged on fibrin strands deposited in small blood vessels.
- Haemolytic uraemic syndrome.
- Thrombotic thrombocytopenic purpura (TTP).

Blood film shows the presence of schistocytes, helmet cells and crenated cells.

Macroangiopathic haemolytic anaemia

This is caused by physical trauma to erythrocytes as they are forced through prosthetic heart valves. Blood film is as above.

Splenic sequestration

Splenic sequestration of red cells causes their premature haemolysis resulting in hypersplenism (p. 306).

Malaria

Haemolysis is common in malaria; *Plasmodium* spp. enter the erythrocytes where they multiply and mature to

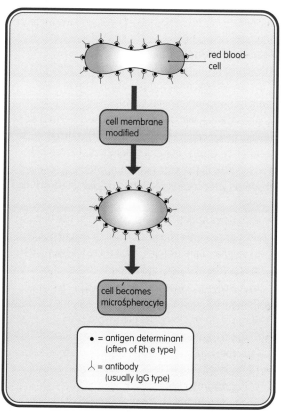

Fig. 14.31 'Warm' antibody type haemolysis. The red cell membrane is modified, and becomes a microspherocyte with consequences similar to hereditary spherocytosis: early sequestration in the spleen, etc. (Adapted with permission from *Pathology Illustrated*, 4th edn, by A. Govan, P. Macfarlane and R. Callander, Churchill Livingstone, 1995.)

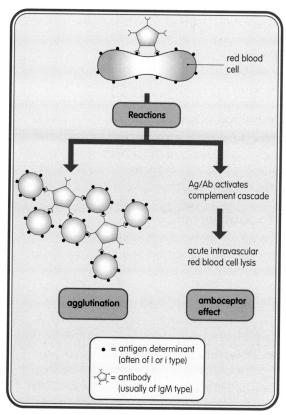

Fig. 14.32 'Cold' antibody type haemolysis. The antibody combines with red blood cells resulting in agglutination (clinically presenting as painful hands and feet) or the amboceptor effect (clinically presenting as paroxysmal cold haemoglobinuria—haemoglobinaemia and haemoglobinuria). (Adapted with permission from *Pathology Illustrated*, 4th edn, by A. Govan, P. Macfarlane and R. Callander, Churchill Livingstone, 1995.)

315

Summary of antibody-mediated haemolytic anaemias		
Isoimmune	**Autoimmune**	
	'warm' antibody type (autoantibody is IgG class)	**'cold' antibody type (autoantibody is IgM class)**
transfusion reactions haemolytic disease of the newborn	idiopathic (50%) secondary: • chronic lymphatic leukaemia • lymphoma related • systemic lupus erythematosus and other autoimmune disorders • viral infections • drug related, e.g. methyl-dopa, penicillin, quinidine	idiopathic secondary: • lymphoma related • infectious mononucleosis • mycoplasma pneumonia

Fig. 14.33 Summary of antibody-mediated haemolytic anaemias.

form schizonts, which eventually escape by rupturing the erythrocytes. Extreme splenomegaly is often present.

Chemical
Snake bites, spider bites, scorpion stings and chemicals are occasionally causes of haemolysis.

Hypersplenism
There is a decrease in the numbers of circulating of erythrocytes, leukocytes and platelets (pancytopenia) as a direct result of their destruction or pooling by an enlarged spleen (p. 306).

Haematinic deficiency
There is a deficiency of those dietary factors required for either haemoglobin synthesis or erythrocyte production.

Megaloblastic anaemia
This type of anaemia is the result of impaired DNA synthesis in marrow precursor cells and is caused by a deficiency of vitamin B_{12} or folic acid.

In the marrow, lack of B_{12} or folate causes the development of abnormally large red cell precursors (megaloblasts), which develop into abnormally large red cells (macrocytes).

Bone marrow becomes hypercellular with megaloblasts—macrocytic anaemia, neutropenia and thrombocytopenia. Defective cells are prematurely destroyed—haemolytic anaemia.

Note that the effects of B_{12} and folate deficiency occur in most organs of the body but are prominent where cell turnover is rapid, e.g. in the marrow and mucous membranes of the alimentary tract and genitalia.

Vitamin B_{12} (cobalamin)
The source is animal products, e.g. meat and eggs.

Requirements are 1 mg per day but up to several years' supply stored in the liver.

Absorption—Vitamin B_{12} is normally absorbed from the diet by binding to intrinsic factor (IF) which is secreted by gastric parietal cells. The B_{12}–IF complex binds to cells in the terminal ileum, where B_{12} is absorbed. The causes of vitamin B_{12} deficiency are as follows:
• Pernicious anaemia: most common cause of B_{12} deficiency, and in females more than males. Caused by autoimmune atrophic gastritis resulting in lack of production of IF and malabsorption of B_{12}. Corrected by injections of vitamin B_{12}.
• Congenital: lack of IF.
• Surgical gastrectomy: results in loss of IF.
• Surgical removal of the terminal ileum: loss of B_{12} absorption site.
• Disease of terminal ileum (e.g. Crohn's disease): loss of B_{12} absorption site.
• Bacterial overgrowth: compete for B_{12}.
• Malnutrition: rare but occasionally seen in veganism.

The effects of vitamin B_{12} deficiency are as follows:
• Megaloblastic anaemia, with associated neutropenia and thrombocytopenia.
• Lesions of the nervous system: myelin degeneration of posterior and lateral columns of spinal cord—subacute combined degeneration of the cord (see Chapter 6).

• Malabsorption: due to mucosal changes—weight loss.

Treatment is by correction of the underlying cause (if possible), and/or injections of vitamin B_{12}.

Folic acid

The source is vegetables, cereals, meat and eggs.

Requirements are 50 mg per day and only 50–100 days' supply stored mainly in the liver.

Absorption—Folic acid is normally absorbed from the diet in the jejunum. The causes of folate deficiency are as follows:

• Malnutrition, e.g. from anorexia, alcoholism, poverty, overcooking of food. This is the most common cause of deficiency.
• Malabsorption, e.g. coeliac disease, dermatitis herpetiformis, Crohn's disease.
• Increased requirements, e.g. pregnancy and lactation, haemolysis, malignancy, extensive psoriasis or dermatitis.
• Drugs may cause malabsorption (e.g. anticonvulsants) or may block utilization, e.g. methotrexate.

The effects of folate deficiency—Blood and bone marrow changes are identical to those in B_{12} deficiency. However, deficiency of folate is not associated with the neurological features of B_{12} deficiency (Fig. 14.34).

Treatment is by oral folic acid supplements, resulting in a complete reversal of the pathological features, even in malabsorption states.

Iron-deficiency anaemia

Iron deficiency is the most common cause of anaemia.

Iron is abundant in meat, vegetables, eggs and dairy foods.

Requirements are:
• In men and postmenopausal women: 1 mg per day.
• In menstruating women: 2 mg per day.
• In pregnancy: 3 mg per day.

Absorption is via the duodenum and upper jejunum in ferrous (Fe^{2+}) form.

The causes of iron deficiency are:
• Chronic blood loss: most common cause (e.g. diseases of the GI tract, menorrhagia, lesions of the urinary tract).
• Increased requirements, e.g. in childhood and pregnancy.
• Malabsorption due to gastrectomy, coeliac disease.
• Malnutrition.

The effects of iron deficiency in blood film are:
• Hypochromic microcytic erythrocytes.

Comparison of vitamin B_{12} and folate deficiency		
	Vitamin B_{12} deficiency	**Folate deficiency**
source	animal produce	most foods
requirements	1 µg/day (heat stable, body stores = several years)	minimally 50 µg/day (heat labile, body stores = months)
nutritional deficiency	uncommon (only in vegans)	common
time of onset	slow (years)	over several weeks
area of absorption	absorbed in terminal ileum and requires intrinsic factor	absorbed in jejunum (and duodenum)
disease causing deficiency	gastric or terminal ileal disease may cause deficiency	jejunal disease may cause deficiency
drug involvement	no	may be drug related (anticonvulsants or antimetabolites)
neurological involvement	neurological lesions frequent	no

Fig. 14.34 Comparison of vitamin B_{12} and folate deficiency.

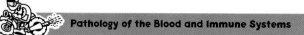

- Low numbers of reticulocytes for degree of anaemia.
- Poikilocytosis (especially 'pencil' cells).
- Anisocytosis.

Laboratory findings are as follows: reduced total serum iron, reduced serum ferritin and reduced transferrin saturation, but with a greatly increased total iron binding capacity.

Clinical features are:
- Anaemia: lethargy, dyspnoea, headache, palpitations.
- Angular cheilitis: fissures at angles of mouth.
- Atrophic glossitis (smooth tongue).
- Oesophageal webs.
- Hypochlorhydria.
- Koilonychia (spoon nails).
- Brittle nails.
- Pica (indiscriminate eating of non-nutritious substances such as grass, stones or clothing).

Treatment is of the underlying cause and iron supplements.

Dyserythropoiesis

This group of disorders is characterized by the production of defective red cells. The pathogenesis of associated dyserythropoiesis is poorly understood.

Anaemia of chronic disorders

Chronic disorders are a common cause of anaemia, being second only to iron-deficiency.

It may develop in patients with:
- Non-organ specific autoimmune diseases, e.g. rheumatoid disease and SLE.
- Chronic infective diseases, e.g. tuberculosis, malaria and schistosomiasis.
- Neoplasia: lymphoma and some carcinomas.

Blood film—Mainly normocytic and normochromic but a mild degree of microcytic, hypochromic anaemia.

Laboratory findings are a reduced serum iron and reduced serum iron-binding capacity, with an increased or normal serum ferritin (cf. iron-deficiency anaemia).

The disorder may be due to the failure of macrophages to transfer their iron stores to the bone marrow. Circulating red cells have a reduced life span, and the marrow shows a lack of response to erythropoietin.

Myelodysplasia

This acquired neoplastic disorder is caused by a defect of stem cells and characterized by progressive bone marrow failure with quantitative and qualitative abnormalities of all three myeloid cell lines (red cell, granulocyte/monocyte and platelets) (p. 302).

Sideroblastic anaemia

This anaemia caused by defective haem synthesis results in the accumulation of excess iron in the cytoplasm of red cell progenitor cells in the form of haemosiderin, forming cells termed ring sideroblasts.

There are two groups of the disease:
- Primary sideroblastic anaemia: myelodysplastic syndrome.
- Secondary sideroblastic anaemia: drug-, toxin-, and neoplasia-related.

Hypoplasia

This anaemia is due to the failure of red cell production by bone marrow.

Aplastic anaemia

A severe life-threatening disease caused by failing bone marrow stem cells, this is characterized by pancytopenia. The marrow is hypocellular and is replaced by fat.

It may be idiopathic or secondary to:
- Radiation.
- Antineoplastic chemotherapy.
- Drugs: chloramphenicol, gold, NSAIDs.
- Toxins: benzene.
- Viruses: papovavirus, HIV-1.
- Fanconi's anaemia.

Red cell aplasia

This anaemia is caused by the suppression of red cell progenitor cells. In contrast to aplastic anaemia, other blood cells are not affected. There are three main types:
- Self-limited red cell aplasia: occurs after parvovirus infection or exposure to certain toxins.
- Chronic acquired red cell aplasia: autoimmune and may be associated with thymomas (p. 308).
- Chronic constitutional red cell aplasia: due to hereditary defect in progenitor cells.

Marrow infiltration

Extensive infiltration of the bone marrow may cause the

obliteration of normal haemopoietic elements. It is caused by:

- Leukaemias.
- Myelofibrosis.
- Disseminated carcinomas.
- Disseminated lymphomas.

Patients develop leukoerythroblastic anaemia characterized by circulating erythroblasts and primitive white cells. Extramedullary haemopoiesis commonly develops.

Polycythaemia

Polycythaemia (erythrocytosis) is defined as a sustained increase in red cell numbers, usually with a corresponding increase in haemoglobin concentration and haematocrit.

Relative polycythaemia

This occurs when the haematocrit reading is raised due to a decrease in plasma volume, usually as a result of fluid loss. This is not 'true' polycythaemia.

Absolute polycythaemia

Primary

Primary polycythaemia occurs in a rare condition termed polycythaemia rubra vera, which is one of the myeloproliferative disorders (pp. 303–304).

Secondary

Most cases of polycythaemia are secondary to conditions resulting in:

- Chronic hypoxia (common)—'appropriate'

polycythaemia, e.g. high altitude, cyanotic heart disease, respiratory disease (such as chronic bronchitis, emphysema), smoking, haemoglobinopathy (resulting in defective release of O_2 to tissues).
- Renal tumours and ischaemia (rare)—'inappropriate' polycythaemia, e.g. renal carcinomas or cysts, renal artery stenosis.

Both chronic hypoxia and renal tumours/ischaemia result in increased erythropoietin production, which stimulates the bone marrow production of red cells.

See Fig. 14.35 for a comparison table of the main features of primary and secondary polycythaemia.

- Describe the classification of anaemia.
- Name the common haemoglobinopathies and describe their basic pathology.
- Compare the different types of antibody-mediated red cell destruction.
- State the causes of mechanical trauma to red cells.
- Describe the types of anaemia caused by haematinic deficiency.
- What are the causes of polycythaemia?

Fig. 14.35 Comparison of the main features of primary and secondary polycythaemia.

Comparison of main features of primary and secondary polycythaemia		
	Primary	**Secondary**
prevalence	rare	common
cause	unknown	hypoxia renal tumours/ischaemia
erythropoietin	normal or decreased	increased
blood film	↑ RBCs (may be hypochromic) ↑ leukocytes ↑ megakaryocytes	↑ RBCs (normochromic)
splenomegaly	common	none

DISORDERS OF HAEMOSTASIS

Definitions
Purpura
This skin rash results from bleeding into the skin from capillaries. It is caused either by defects in capillaries or by defects or deficiencies of blood platelets. Individual purple spots of the rash are called petechiae.

Ecchymosis
This bruise presents as a bluish-black mark on the skin resulting from the release of blood into the tissues either through injury or through the spontaneous leaking of blood from the vessels.

Haematoma
This accumulation of blood within the tissues clots to form a solid swelling.

Abnormalities of the vessel walls
This heterogeneous group of conditions is characterized by easy bruising and spontaneous bleeding from small vessels. The underlying lesions are of two main types:
- Abnormal perivascular connective tissue which leads to inadequate vessel support.
- Intrinsically abnormal or damaged vessel wall.

Haemorrhages are mainly in the skin, causing petechiae or ecchymoses, or both. In some disorders there is also bleeding from the mucous membranes.

Infections
Many bacterial and viral infections may cause purpura as a result of either vascular damage by the organism or immune complex formation, e.g. measles, dengue fever or meningococcal septicaemia.

Drug reactions
A variety of drugs may sometimes cause vasculitic reactions.

Scurvy and Ehlers–Danlos syndrome
Vitamin C is required for the hydroxylation of proline as a step in collagen synthesis. In both Ehlers–Danlos syndrome (an inherited disorder of collagen synthesis) and scurvy (vitamin C deficiency) capillaries are fragile due to defective collagen synthesis.

Perifollicular petechiae, bruising and mucosal haemorrhages are common.

Steroid purpura
Long-term steroid therapy or Cushing's syndrome results in purpura caused by defective vascular supportive tissue.

Henoch–Schönlein purpura
This immune complex (type III) hypersensitivity reaction is usually found in children, and often following an acute infection. It is characterized by red wheals and a purple rash on the buttocks and lower legs due to bleeding into the skin from inflamed capillaries and venules.

Arthritis, haematuria and GI symptoms may also occur.

It is a self-limiting condition but occasionally patients develop renal failure.

Osler–Weber–Rendu syndrome (hereditary haemorrhagic telangiectasia)
This rare, autosomal dominant disorder is characterized by multiple dilatations of small vessels (telangiectasia) that appear during childhood and become more numerous in adult life.

Telangiectasia develops in the skin, mucous membranes and internal organs and frequently bleeds spontaneously or following relatively mild trauma. Recurrent GI tract haemorrhages and epistaxis may cause chronic iron-deficiency anaemia.

Disordered platelet function
Reduced platelet count (thrombocytopenia)
Decreased production
This is the commonest cause of thrombocytopenia.

Generalized disease of bone marrow
Aplastic anaemia—This severe, life-threatening disease is caused by failing bone marrow stem cells and characterized by pancytopenia. The marrow is hypocellular and is replaced by fat (p.318).

Marrow infiltration—Extensive infiltration of bone marrow may cause the obliteration of normal haemopoietic elements.

Specific impairment of platelet production
Selective megakaryocyte depression may result from either drug toxicity (alcohol, cytotoxics) or viral infections (measles, HIV).

Ineffective megakaryopoiesis
This runs as follows:
- Megaloblastic anaemia (folate or B_{12} deficiency) is characterized by decreased numbers of platelets or increased numbers of megakaryocytes.
- Paroxysmal nocturnal haemoglobinuria: may cause ineffective megakaryopoiesis.

Decreased platelet survival
Immune destruction—autoimmune thrombocytopenic purpura
The destruction of antibody-coated platelets by the reticuloendothelial system, especially the spleen, results in spontaneous or post-traumatic haemorrhage at various sites:
- Skin: petechiae and ecchymoses.
- Mucous membranes, e.g. epistaxis, bleeding gums.
- Menorrhagia, haematuria, melaena.
- CNS: may be fatal.

This is often associated with anaemia (secondary to haemorrhage).
Clinical types are:
- Acute: often in children and usually self-limiting with spontaneous resolution. May be post infective, e.g. measles.
- Chronic: usually in adults, mainly idiopathic but occasionally symptomatic of CLL or lymphoma, or may occur in association with other autoimmune disease, e.g. rheumatoid arthritis, SLE.
- Drug induced, e.g. quinine, heparin, sulphonamides.

Non-immune destruction
This is mainly through thrombotic thrombocytopenic purpura (TTP) and haemolytic–uraemic syndrome (HUS).
HUS and TTP are thought to represent the same disease process but with different distributions of thrombotic lesions.
Thrombocytopenia occurs due to abnormal platelet activation and consumption. Platelets adhere to the endothelium of capillaries and precapillary arterioles where they undergo aggregation and release, with fibrin deposition, which results in microvascular occlusive platelet plugs and microangiopathic haemolytic anaemia (p.315).

Aetiology—The underlying cause of the disorder is obscure but the following pathogenetic factors have been implicated:
- Immune-mediated vessel damage.
- Platelet hyperaggregation due to deficiency of an IgG inhibitor of platelet-agglutinating factor in normal plasma.
- Diminished production of prostacyclin by vessel walls.
- Excess of high molecular weight multimers of von Willebrand's factor, which interact with platelet agglutinating factor, causing platelet adhesion to vascular endothelium.

In TTP, occlusive plugs lead to widespread ischaemic organ damage, especially of the brain and kidney, resulting in neurological abnormalities and progressive renal impairment. In HUS, organ damage is limited to the kidney.
Disseminated intravascular coagulation can also cause widespread consumption of platelets results in simultaneous thrombosis and haemorrhage (p.324).

Splenic sequestration
Thrombocytopenia is common in splenomegaly due to platelet 'pooling' by the spleen. Unlike red cells, platelets tolerate splenic stasis without injury and so platelet lifespan is unaffected.

Dilutional thrombocytopenia
Platelets are unstable at 4°C and so transfusion with massive amounts of stored blood may cause abnormal bleeding. The effect can be minimized by replacement with specific screened products, e.g. fresh frozen plasma and platelet concentrates.
See Fig. 14.36 for a summary of the causes of thrombocytopenia.

Defects of platelet function
Congenital
Defective adhesion (Bernard–Soulier syndrome)
This rare disease causes life-threatening haemorrhages. The platelets are deficient in glycoprotein receptors, which are essential for the binding of von Willebrand factor. The platelets are larger than normal and there is a defective adherence to exposed subendothelial connective tissues and defective platelet aggregation. There is also a variable degree of thrombocytopenia.

Causes of thrombocytopenia	
Cause	Clinical features
decreased platelet production	generalized disease of bone marrow: • aplastic anaemia, marrow infiltration specific impairment of platelet production: • drugs: alcohol, thiazides, cytotoxics • infections: measles, HIV ineffective megakaryopoiesis: • megaloblastic anaemia and paroxysmal nocturnal haemoglobinuria
decreased platelet survival	immune destruction: • autoimmune thrombocytopenic purpura non-immune destruction: • thrombotic thrombocytopenic purpura/ haemolytic–uraemic syndrome • disseminated intravascular coagulation
splenic sequestration	–
dilutional thrombocytopenia	–

Fig. 14.36 Causes of thrombocytopenia.

Defective aggregation—thromboaesthenia (Glanzmann's disease)
This failure of primary platelet aggregation is due to a deficiency of membrane receptors (glycoproteins IIb and IIIa) for fibrinogen binding.

Defective secretion (storage pool disease)
A common, mild defect of platelet function, this causes easy bruising and bleeding after trauma. It is caused by a deficiency of 'dense granules' within the platelets, which normally store ADP. The decreased storage pool of ADP prevents the secondary wave of platelet aggregation.

Acquired
Aspirin
Aspirin therapy is the commonest cause of defective platelet function, and produces an abnormal bleeding time.

Aspirin inhibits cyclooxygenase, causing an impairment in thromboxane A_2 synthesis, which is necessary for release reaction and aggregation. After a single dose the defect lasts 7–10 days.

Bleeding tendency is mild, with increased skin bruising and bleeding after surgery. The defect may contribute to the associated GI haemorrhage from acute mucosal erosions and may be life threatening.

Uraemia
In uraemia, defects may be caused by an abnormal arachidonate metabolism with reduced synthesis of thromboxane. Platelet interactions with subendothelium are abnormal and bleeding may be severe.

Clotting factor abnormalities
Hereditary factor abnormalities
Von Willebrand's disease
This is the commonest of the hereditary coagulation disorders. It is an autosomal dominant disorder of abnormal platelet adhesion associated with low factor VIII activity. The primary defect is a reduced synthesis of von Willebrand factor, which has two main functions:
• Promotes platelet adhesion.
• Carrier molecule for factor VIII, protecting it from premature destruction.

The disease is characterized by operative and post-traumatic haemorrhage, mucous membrane bleeding (e.g. epistaxes, menorrhagia) and excessive blood loss from superficial cuts and abrasions.

Bleeding episodes are treated with intermediate-purity factor VIII concentrates that contain both von Willebrand factor and factor VIII.

Haemophilia A (factor VIII deficiency)
A common hereditary disorder of blood coagulation, this is characterized by absence or low levels of plasma factor VIII.

Its inheritance is X-linked but 33% of patients have no family history and the disorder presumably result from spontaneous mutation; it affects 1 per 10 000 in the UK.

Blood clotting time is prolonged, and in severe disease, the blood is incoagulable.

The disease is characterized by frequent episodes of spontaneous haemorrhage into a major joint, especially knees, hips, elbows and shoulders. Without factor replacement therapy, bleeding continues until the intra-articular pressure rises sufficiently to prevent further haemorrhage.

Resolution of acute haemarthrosis occurs slowly with recurrent bleeds producing massive synovial hypertrophy, erosion of joint cartilage and bone, and changes of severe osteoarthritis.

Bleeding into muscles, retroperitoneal tissues, urinary tract and epistaxes also occurs.

Operative and post-traumatic haemorrhage is life threatening, both in severely and mildly affected patients.

Mild, moderate and severe forms of the disease are recognized depending on the residual clotting factor activity (Fig. 14.37).

Treatment—Control can be achieved by intravenous clotting factor replacement.

Factor IX deficiency

Inheritance, clinical features and treatment of factor IX deficiency are identical to those of haemophilia A. However, factor IX deficiency is less common, the incidence being only about one-fifth of that of haemophilia A. This is also known as haemophilia B and Christmas disease.

The features of the most common hereditary clotting factor deficiencies are summarised in Fig. 14.38.

Other deficiencies

Hereditary deficiencies of most of the other coagulation factors have also been described but are extremely rare.

Acquired factor abnormalities

Acquired disorders of coagulation are far more common than the inherited disorders, and multiple clotting factor deficiencies are usual.

Vitamin K deficiency

Vitamin K is essential for the γ-carboxylation and hence activation of factors II, VII, IX and X and proteins C and S. The deficiency is associated with decreased activity of these proteins leading to coagulopathies. This may present in the newborn or in later life.

Vitamin K is obtained from green vegetables and bacterial synthesis in the gut. It is a fat soluble vitamin and requires bile for its absorption.

Causes of vitamin K deficiency:
- Inadequate diet.
- Malabsorption, e.g. obstructive jaundice (reduced bile), coeliac disease.
- Drugs: warfarin (a vitamin K antagonist).

Neonates are particularly susceptible to vitamin K

Fig. 14.37 Classification of haemophilias.

Classification of haemophilias			
Category	Frequency	Coagulation factor activity (% of normal)	Clinical features
severe	40%	<1%	frequent spontaneous bleeding episodes from birth degenerative joint disease
moderate	10%	1–5%	post-traumatic bleeding occasional spontaneous episodes bruising
mild	50%	5–20%	post-traumatic bleeding may be subclinical

Common hereditary clotting factor abnormalities			
	Haemophilia A	Factor IX deficiency	Von Willebrand's disease
deficiency	factor VIII	factor IX	von Willebrand factor → factor VIII deficiency
inheritance	X-linked	X-linked	dominant
prevalence in UK	1 in 10 000	1 in 50 000	1 in 5000
main sites of haemorrhage	muscle, joints: post-trauma or postsurgery	muscle, joints: post-trauma or postsurgery	mucous membranes, post-trauma and operation

Fig. 14.38 Common hereditary clotting factor abnormalities.

deficiency due to their lack of gut bacteria and low concentrations of the vitamin in breast milk. The combined effect of vitamin K deficiency and low levels of clotting factors due to liver immaturity may produce life-threatening disease: haemorrhagic disease of the newborn.

Treatment is by vitamin K supplementation.

Liver disease

This is commonly associated with coagulation defects due to:

- Impaired absorption of vitamin K caused by biliary obstruction, producing decreased activation of factors II, VII, IX and X and proteins C and S.
- Reduced synthesis of clotting factors and of fibrinogen, and increased amounts of plasminogen activator in severe hepatocellular disease.
- Thrombocytopenia from hypersplenism associated with portal hypertension.
- Dysfibrinogenaemia: functional abnormality of fibrinogen found in many patients with liver disease.
- Qualitative platelet disorders.

Disseminated intravascular coagulation

This condition, characterized by increased coagulation, leads not only to widespread thrombosis but also to haemorrhage due to consumption of platelets and coagulation factors. Thus both thrombosis and haemorrhage are a feature of this disorder.

The disorder may cause a severe haemorrhagic syndrome with high mortality or may run a milder, more chronic course.

Aetiology—This is shown in Fig. 14.39.

Pathogenesis—The causes listed in Fig. 14.39 activate the coagulation system in small vessels throughout the body via:

- Release of procoagulant material into circulation, e.g. obstetric disorders, certain malignancies, liver disease, severe falciparum malaria and haemolytic transfusion reactions.
- Widespread endothelial damage, e.g. septicaemia, certain viral infections, severe burns or hypothermia.
- Platelet aggregation: some bacteria, viruses and immune complexes may have a direct effect on platelets.

The main effects of DIC are:

- Vascular occlusion results in organ dysfunction (from ischaemic damage) and microangiopathic haemolysis (p.315).
- Consumption of platelets, clotting factors and fibrinogen causes haemorrhage.
- Activation of fibrinolytic system results in increased fibrin degradation products, which themselves have anticoagulant effect causing haemorrhage.

Treatment is of the underlying cause, with clotting factor and platelet replacement.

Thrombosis

Thrombosis is the formation of a solid mass of blood constituents—thrombus—within the vascular system during life.

Thrombosis can affect both arteries and veins:

- Arterial thrombosis: most commonly superimposed on atheroma, and may result in tissue infarction distal to thrombus due to ischaemia.
- Venous thrombosis: most commonly due to stasis and may result in oedema due to impaired venous drainage.

Causes of disseminated intravascular coagulation	
Problem	**Cause**
infections	septicaemia, viral infections (purpura fulminans), malaria
malignancy	mucin-secreting adenocarcinomas, acute promyelocytic leukaemia
obstetric complications	amniotic fluid embolism, premature separation of placenta, eclampsia
hypersensitivity reactions	anaphylaxis, incompatible blood transfusion
widespread tissue damage	burns, major accidental trauma, major surgery, shock, intravascular haemolysis, dissecting aortic aneurysm
liver disease	

Fig. 14.44 Causes of disseminated intravascular coagulation.

A thrombus is different from a clot! A clot is defined as blood coagulated outside the vascular system, or within the vascular system after death.

Virchow's triad

Factors that predispose to thrombosis can be classified into three main groups, collectively known as Virchow's triad, namely hypercoagulability, endothelial injury, and abnormalities of blood flow.

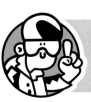

Questions about Virchow's triad are extremely common in examinations.

Hypercoagulability

Primary (hereditary)

Hereditary defects of hypercoagulability lead to a lifelong tendency to thrombosis (thrombophilia) and usually affect the venous system:

- Antithrombin III deficiency: autosomal dominant condition characterized by recurrent venous thromboses usually starting in early adult life. Primary defect is a deficiency of antithrombin III, which usually neutralizes thrombin and other activated clotting factors.
- Protein C deficiency: commonest form of hereditary thrombophilia. Autosomal dominant condition resulting in failure of neutralization of activated factors V and VIII. Protein S is a cofactor for protein C, thus protein S deficiencies produce a similar pathology.
- Abnormal factor Va: mutated factor Va, which is resistant to neutralization by protein C.
- Defective fibrinolysis: rare causes of thrombophilia resulting from defects of fibrinogen (dysfibrinogenaemia) or of plasminogen.

Secondary (acquired)

Defects are as follows:

- Malignancy: patients with carcinoma of the breast,

lung, prostate, pancreas or bowel have an increased risk of venous thrombosis.
- Blood disorders, e.g. increased viscosity (especially polycythaemia rubra vera), and thrombocytosis lead to an increased risk of venous thrombosis.
- Oestrogens: associated with raised plasma levels of various clotting factors leading to an increased risk of venous thrombosis.
- Antiphospholipid antibody leads to the interaction of the antibody with phospholipid-bound proteins involved in coagulation and causes prolongation of clotting times *in vitro*, with a paradoxical increased risk of venous and arterial thrombosis. Often found in patients with autoimmune disease, especially SLE.
- Cholesterol: partly genetic, partly acquired (diet/lifestyle), leads to an increased risk of arterial thrombosis.

Endothelial injury

Direct injury to the endothelium as seen in trauma and inflammation may lead to thrombosis. Damage to the endothelium also occurs in association with atheroma.

Alterations to blood flow

Alterations are:

- Stasis: allows platelets to come in contact with endothelium, and slow flow prevents blood from diluting activated coagulation components.
- Turbulence: may cause physical trauma to endothelial cells, and loss of laminar flow may bring platelets into contact with endothelium.

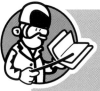

- Describe the various aetiologies of vessel wall abnormalities.
- List the causes of thrombocytopenia.
- What are the most common hereditary clotting factor abnormalities? Describe their basic features.
- List the causes of acquired clotting factor abnormalities.
- What are the components of Virchow's triad and how do they cause thrombosis?

15. Pathology of the Skin

TERMINOLOGY OF SKIN PATHOLOGY

The vocabulary of dermatology is quite distinct from that of other specialities. Learning the common dermatological terms is essential in order to correctly describe different skin disorders.

Macroscopic appearances

Macule
This localized, flat area of altered skin colour can be hyperpigmented as in a freckle, hypopigmented as in vitiligo, or erythematous as in a capillary haemangioma.

Papule
A small, raised, solid lesion of the skin, this is generally defined as being less than 5 mm in diameter.

Nodule
This is similar to a papule but greater than 5 mm in diameter. It may be solid or oedematous, and can involve any layer of the skin.

Plaque
An extended papule which forms a plateau-like elevation of skin, a plaque is usually more than 20 mm in diameter but rarely more than 5 mm in height.

Wheal
This is similar to a papule or plaque but transitory and compressible. It is caused by dermal oedema, red or white in colour and usually signifies urticaria.

Blister
This fluid-filled space within the skin is caused by the separation of cells and the leakage of plasma into the space.

Vesicle
This small blister (less than 5 mm in diameter) contains clear fluid within or below the epidermis.

Bulla
This is similar to a vesicle but larger than 5 mm in diameter.

Pustule
A small, pus-containing blister, a pustule commonly indicates infection, but not always (e.g. those seen in psoriasis are not infected).

Scale
This thickened horny layer of keratin forms readily detached fragments of skin. Scaling is caused by disturbances in the processes of keratinization, and usually indicates inflammation of the epidermis (Fig. 15.1A).

Lichenification
There is a thickening of the epidermis with exaggeration

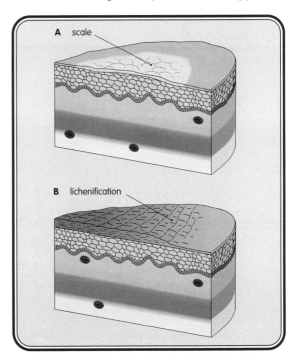

Fig. 15.1 Basic lesions of the skin showing scale and lichenification.

of the normal skin creases caused by abnormal scratching or rubbing of skin (Fig. 15.1B).

Excoriation
This is caused by the destruction or removal of the surface of the skin usually by scratching, but also by chemical application or other means.

Onycholysis
This is the separation of part or all of a nail from its bed. It may occur in psoriasis and in fungal infections of the skin and nail bed, and is more common in women.

Microscopic appearances
See Fig. 15.2 for a diagrammatical representation of normal skin and normal epidermis.

Hyperkeratosis
Thickening of the outer horny layer of skin (stratum corneum) occurs.

Parakeratosis
There is excessive keratin in which nuclear remnants persist (a histological sign of increased epidermal growth).

Acanthosis
The thickening of the epidermis is caused by an increased number of prickle cells in the stratum spinosum (prickle cell layer).

Dyskeratosis
There is an abnormal premature keratinization of cells in the prickle cell layer.

Acantholysis
The loss of cellular cohesion and separation of epidermal keratinocytes are due to the rupture of intercellular bridges. Bulla formation often results.

Spongiosis
Epidermal oedema causes partial separation of keratinocytes.

Vacuolization
This is the formation of intracellular, fluid-filled spaces (vacuoles).

Papillomatosis
In this condition many papillomas grow on an area of skin or mucous membranes.

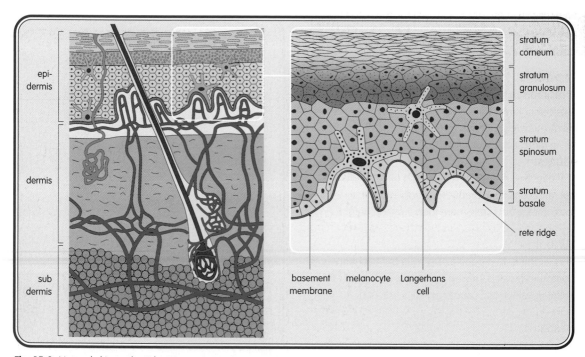

Fig. 15.2 Normal skin and epidermis.

Lentiginous
This describes skin whose increased pigmentation is a result of increased numbers of melanocytes.

Exocytosis
Migratory inflammatory cells appear in the epidermis.

Erosion
This is the loss of all or part of the epidermis which does not extend into the dermis, but which heals without scarring.

Ulceration
A full thickness defect (epidermis and dermis) of the skin forms.

- **What is the dermatological terminology used to describe the macroscopic and microscopic appearance of skin?**

INFLAMMATION AND SKIN ERUPTIONS

Psoriasis

Definition
Psoriasis is a chronic, non-infectious, inflammatory disease of the skin characterized by erythematous plaques covered with thick, silvery scales.

It affects about 2% of the population in the UK and can start at any age, but the peak onset is in the second and third decades.

The aetiology of psoriasis is unclear; however, about 35% of patients show a family history.

Environmental factors are thought to trigger the disease in genetically susceptible individuals.

Pathogenesis:

- Epidermal cell proliferation rate is increased 20-fold or more.
- Epidermal turnover time is greatly reduced.
- Keratinocytes are normal but the stem cell number is increased.

Characteristic histological features are:

- Long, rete ridges separated by a markedly oedematous papillary dermis in which there are large numbers of dilated capillaries.
- Scale: composed of flakes of thickened surface keratin, which contains remnants of nuclei (parakeratosis).
- Neutrophil polymorphs migrate through the epidermis and may be trapped beneath the thickened horny layer.

Precipitating factors—A number of factors have been identified which can precipitate psoriasis:

- Köbner's phenomenon: trauma to skin (e.g. scratch, surgical scar, or burn).
- Infection: streptococcal sore throat may precipitate guttate psoriasis.
- Drugs: β-blockers, lithium, and antimalarials can precipitate or worsen psoriasis.

Psoriasis most commonly affects the knees, elbows, trunk and scalp (Fig. 15.3).

Several types of psoriasis exist which are of variable appearance and behaviour (as described below).

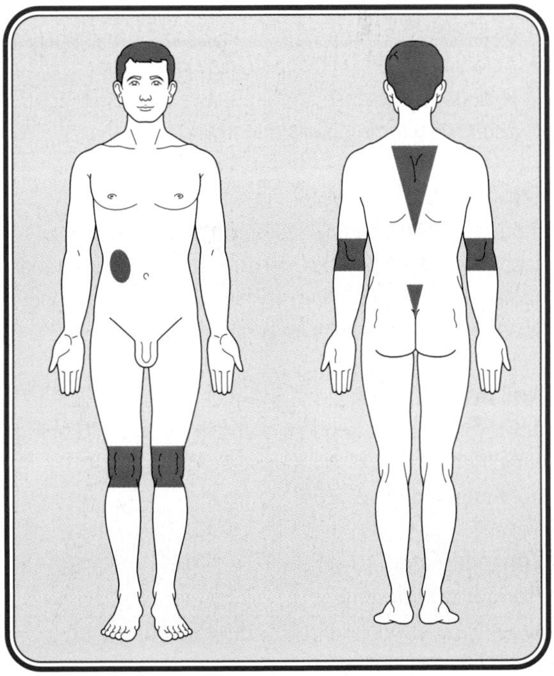

Fig. 15.3 Common sites of psoriasis.

Plaque

This is the commonest form of psoriasis, characterized by disc-shaped, erythematous plaques (up to several cm in diameter) covered with waxy white scales, which, if detached, reveal small areas of punctate bleeding. Distribution follows the pattern illustrated in Fig. 15.3.

Guttate

Acute, symmetrical, 'drop-like' lesions (about 1 cm in diameter are seen), usually on the trunk and limbs. It is common in adolescents and young adults and may follow a streptococcal throat infection.

Flexural

Smooth, erythematous plaques, often glazed, commonly affect axillae, submammary areas and the natal cleft. It is found mostly in the elderly.

Localized forms

There are four varieties:

- Scalp psoriasis: commonly confused with dandruff but is better demarcated and more thickly scaled.
- Palmoplantar pustulosis: yellow-brown sterile pustules on the palms or soles. Most common in middle-aged females and associated with smoking.
- Napkin psoriasis: psoriasis-like lesions of the nappy area of infants, some of whom later develop true psoriasis.
- Acrodermatitis of Hallopeau (also known as Hallopeau's disease): rare, persistent form of psoriasis affecting digits and nails.

Generalized pustular

Though rare, this can be life threatening, requiring hospital admission. Small sterile pustules (collections of neutrophils) develop on an erythematous background. Onset is often acute with fever and malaise.

Nail involvement

Nail involvement is frequent, with pitting and thickening of the nail which may be followed by onycholysis. Treatment is often difficult.

Complications

Psoriatic arthropathy

About 5% of psoriasis patients develop arthropathy, which takes one of four forms:

- Distal arthritis: the commonest form. Affects the distal interphalangeal joints of the hands and feet, causing 'sausage-like' swelling of the digits.
- Rheumatoid-like arthritis: polyarthropathy similar to rheumatoid disease, but less symmetrical and with negative test for rheumatoid factor.
- Mutilans arthritis: progressive deformity of the hands and feet caused by erosion of the small bones. Often associated with severe psoriasis.
- Ankylosing spondylitis/sacroiliitis: in HLA-B27-positive patients.

Erythroderma

This rare complication of psoriasis (and other disorders) is characterized by a generalized reddening, flaking and thickening of all, or nearly all, of the skin surface. It is accompanied and often preceded by pyrexia, malaise and shivering. Associated systemic effects are potentially fatal, and inpatient treatment is required.

Fig. 15.4 provides a table of the management of psoriasis.

Eczema and contact dermatitis

Definitions

Eczema and dermatitis are non-infective inflammatory conditions of the skin. They are not diseases, but are reactive conditions occurring in response to certain stimuli, many of which are unknown. They can be acute or chronic.

Dermatitis and eczema essentially describe the same reactive condition, i.e. they are histopathologically identical, and are often used interchangeably. However, eczema is used to describe the reaction that occurs in response to an endogenous stimulus, whereas dermatitis is used to describe the reaction that occurs in response to an exogenous stimulus.

Acute and chronic forms of eczema and dermatitis

Acute eczema/dermatitis

Acute eczema/dermatitis is characterized by:

- Erythema: caused by chronic inflammatory cell infiltrate (lymphocytes) around dilated vessels in the upper dermis.
- Spongiotic, fluid-filled vesicles: caused by epidermal oedema (leakage of fluid from the dilated vessels) with separation of keratinocytes (spongiosis).
- Erythematous lesions are itchy (histamine release) and vesicles may weep and crust.

Chronic eczema/dermatitis

Scratching of the itchy, acute-stage lesions causes secondary changes which result in the chronic form of the condition. It is characterized by:

- Thickening of the prickle cell layer (acanthosis).
- Thickening of the stratum corneum (hyperkeratosis).
- Elongation of the rete ridges and dermal collagenization.
- Dilation of dermal vessels and infiltration of the dermis with inflammatory cells.

Characteristic thickening, which occurs as a result of scratching, is termed lichenification (see above).

Atopic eczema

This chronic form of eczema is often associated with a strong family history of other atopic diseases such as asthma and hayfever. Uncontrollable itching is common, and the condition follows a remitting/relapsing course.

Although 10–15% of the population are atopic, only about 5% of these individuals will develop atopic eczema.

The aetiology of atopic eczema and other atopic diseases is not well understood; however, the strong family history associated with these conditions suggests at least a partial genetic cause for the disease.

The pathogenesis is as follows:

- Individuals prone to atopy have higher circulating levels of IgE antibodies than non-atopic individuals
- On exposure to certain allergens, IgE-mediated, type I hypersensitivity reactions are triggered, causing large scale, mast cell degranulation with the release of histamine and other inflammatory mediators.
- In the skin, this type of hypersensitivity reaction results in the histological changes of acute eczema, which on scratching becomes chronic eczema.

Management of psoriasis	
Topical therapy (first line treatment for mild to moderate psoriasis)	
tar preparations	suitable for plaque or guttate psoriasis; inhibit DNA synthesis; safe but messy
dithranol	antimitotic preparation; irritant to normal skin; applied specifically to plaques of psoriasis
topical corticosteroids	treatment of choice for face, genitalia and flexures, and useful for stubborn plaques on the hands, feet and scalp; risk of side effects
keratolytics	e.g. 5% salicylic acid; useful for hyperkeratotic psoriasis of the palms and soles
Systemic therapy (for severe or life threatening psoriasis)	
photochemotherapy	PUVA (psoralen + ultraviolet-A): photoactivation of psoralen with UV-A causes crosslinking of DNA resulting in inhibition of cell division; treatment is effective, but with long-term risk of skin cancer
retinoids	vitamin A derivatives effective in treatment of pustular psoriasis and in the thinning of hyperkeratotic plaques; often used in combination with topical therapies or PUVA; side effects including teratogenicity are common
methotrexate	folate antagonist with anti-inflammatory and immune modulatory effects; side effects include hepatotoxicity and teratogenicity

Fig. 15.4 Management of psoriasis.

Atopic eczema presents at an early age, with 60% presenting before one year and 90% by five years.

The appearance of atopic eczema varies between different age groups (Fig. 15.5):

- Infancy: babies develop the typical acute form of eczema on the face and hands, often with secondary infection.
- Childhood: progression from acute to chronic condition. Usually involves the antecubital and popliteal fossae, neck, wrists and ankles.
- Adults: chronic condition with lichenified (and sometimes nodular) lesions. The hands are most commonly affected but a few adults also develop the chronic, severe form of generalized atopic eczema, which is often precipitated by stressful situations.

The complications are:

- Bacterial infection: typically with *S. aureus*.
- Viral infection: increased susceptibility to the development of viral warts, molluscum contagiosum, and to secondary infection with herpes simplex (eczema herpeticum).
- Growth retardation: may occur in children with severe eczema. The cause is unknown.

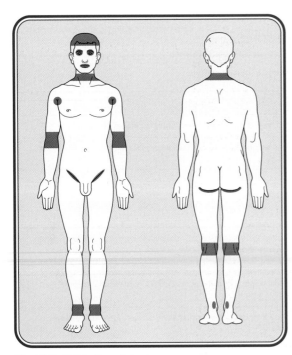

Fig. 15.5 Distribution of atopic eczema.

- Cataracts: rare; may occur in young adults in association with severe atopic eczema.

The treatment for atopic eczema is shown in Fig. 15.6.

Contact dermatitis

Contact dermatitis is a form of dermatitis precipitated by exogenous agents (Fig. 15.7). It can be classified into:

- Irritant contact dermatitis: the most common form. Caused by contact of the skin with water, abrasives, acids, alkalis, solvents or detergents.
- Allergic contact dermatitis: caused by a type IV hypersensitivity reaction to allergens such as nickel.

Lesions are localized to the site of contact, and are commonest on the hands and face.

Management is by identification and reduction in contact of the offending allergen/irritant, e.g. by protective gloves, and by topical therapy, e.g. steroids.

Other forms

Seborrhoeic dermatitis

This is a common, chronic inflammatory condition in which the skin is reddened and covered by thick, waxy or white scale. The eruption often occurs in the sebaceous gland areas of the scalp and face, although other areas may also be involved.

The aetiology is unknown but genetic factors and overgrowth of the yeast commensal *Pityrosporum ovale* have been implicated.

There are four common patterns in the clinical presentation (as shown in Fig. 15.8):

- Scalp and facial involvement: affects the side of the nose, scalp margin, eyebrows and ears and excessive dandruff is usually present. Most common in young males.
- Petaloid: affects presternal area.
- *Pityrosporum folliculitis*: erythematous follicular eruption with papules or pustules typically affecting the back.
- Flexural: involvement of the axillae, groins and submammary areas, often secondarily colonized by *Candida albicans*.

The management is as follows:

- Medicated shampoos for scalp lesions.
- Topical antifungals for facial, truncal and flexural involvement.
- Topical hydrocortisone.

Discoid (nummular) eczema

A condition of unknown aetiology, this is characterized by 'coin-shaped', symmetrical, eczematous lesions which typically affect the limbs of middle-aged or elderly men. Secondary bacterial infection is common.

Venous (stasis) eczema

This typically affects the legs of middle-aged or elderly women, and is associated with underlying venous disease. It may present with haemosiderin pigmentation around the ankles or with fibrosis of the dermis and subcutaneous tissue and ulceration.

It is also known as gravitational eczema.

Treatment of atopic eczema		
Therapy	**Treatment**	**Comments**
topical therapy	emollients	moisturize dry skin and decrease itching
	topical steroids	anti-inflammatory effects
	topical antibiotics	useful for infected eczema
	coal tar bandage	useful for lichenified or excoriated eczema
systemic therapy	oral antihistamine	sedative form taken at night is useful to reduce desire to scratch
	oral antibiotics	used for infected exacerbations
	evening primrose oil: linoleic and γ-linolenic acid	beneficial in small proportion of patients with moderate/severe eczema
	PUVA	used for very resistant eczema only
dietary manipulation	–	useful for food allergies or resistant eczema

Fig. 15.6 Treatment of atopic eczema.

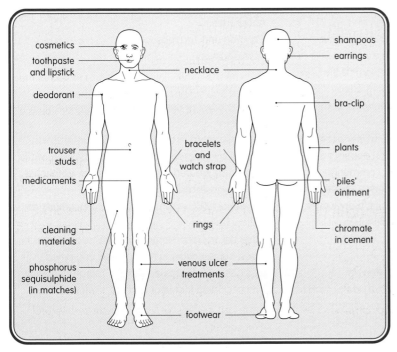

Fig. 15.7 Distribution and causes of contact dermatitis.

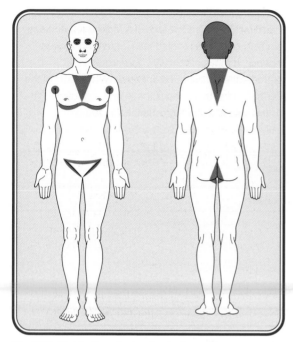

Fig. 15.8 Distribution of seborrhoeic dermatitis.

- Describe the histological changes that occur in psoriasis.
- Name the different types of psoriasis, and describe their distribution.
- Describe the histological changes that occur in eczema/dermatitis.
- Name the different types of eczema and describe their distribution.

Hand dermatitis and pompholyx

This common, acute or chronic eczema may appear as a vesicular eruption known as pompholyx—with 'sago-like' vesicles on the sides of the fingers and on the palms.

Pompholyx is caused by the formation of eczematous vesicles which cannot rupture the thick, horny layer of the skin on the hands. The vesicles therefore persist and cause intense itching until the skin eventually peels. Onset is usually in young adults, especially in warm weather, and is often recurrent.

Asteatotic eczema (eczema craquelé; winter eczema)

This dry eczema with cracking of the skin appears as a fine, 'crazy-paving' pattern of fissuring, commonly affecting the limbs and trunk of the elderly. Causes are the overwashing of patients in institutions, a dry winter climate, hypothyroidism or the use of diuretics.

Lichen striatus

A rare, self-limiting linear eczema of unknown aetiology, this typically affects the limbs of adolescents.

INFECTIONS AND INFESTATIONS

Bacterial infections

Normal skin microflora

The skin is colonized by numerous micro-organisms known as microflora or commensals (see Chapter 4), which may number as many as 0.5 million per cm^2. Some examples are:

- *Staphylococcus epidermidis*.
- *S. aureus*.
- Diphtheroids.
- Streptococci.
- *Pseudomonas aeruginosa*.
- Anaerobes.
- *Candida* and *Torulopsis*.
- *Pityrosporum*.

Overgrowth of normal flora

Some diseases are caused by an overgrowth of normal flora:

- Erythrasma: dry, scaly, reddish-brown eruption caused by corynebacteria. Usually asymptomatic but can be treated with topical or oral antibiotics.
- Trichomycosis axillaris: overgrowth of corynebacteria, which form yellow concretions on axillary hair.
- Pitted keratolysis: overgrowth of micrococci, which digest keratin causing malodorous and pitted erosions with depressed discoloured areas. Occurs with occluding footwear and sweaty feet.

Staphylococcal infections

Impetigo

This highly contagious superficial skin infection is caused by either streptococci, staphylococci or both. The clinical features of impetigo are as follows:
- Relatively rare in the UK.
- Generally occurs in children and spreads rapidly through populations, e.g. in schools.
- Characterized by the development of large, thin-walled bullae, often on the face, which leave areas of yellow crusted exudate.
- Commonly confused with herpes simplex or fungal infections.

The management of impetigo is by the removal of crusts with saline soaks and the application of topical antibiotics; widespread infection can be treated with systemic antibiotics.

Ecthyma

This is a full-thickness infection of epidermis by *Staphylococcus aureus*.

The clinical features of ecthyma are as follows:
- Characterized by circumscribed, ulcerated and crusted infected lesions which eventually heal with scarring.
- Occurs most commonly on the legs, usually as a result of an insect bite or neglected minor injury.
- May also be seen in drug addicts due to use of contaminated needles.

The management of ecthyma is by systemic and topical antibiotics.

Folliculitis

This infection of multiple hair follicles is usually caused by *Staphylococcus aureus*.

The clinical features of folliculitis are:
- Characterized by the production of tiny pustules located in the necks of hair follicles (superficial folliculitis).
- In men, it commonly affects the beard area (sycosis barbae).
- In women, it commonly affect the legs after hair removal by shaving or waxing.

A furuncle (boil) is a deep infection of a follicle resulting in an expanding collection of pus, which destroys the follicle and extends into the surrounding dermis.

A carbuncle is a deep abscess formed in a group of follicles with multiple drainage channels forming a painful suppurating mass; it may cause systemic symptoms.

The management of folliculitis is through systemic and topical antibiotics.

Carbuncles often need surgical drainage.

Staphylococcal scalded skin syndrome

An acute toxic illness usually of infants, this is characterized by the shedding of sheets of skin, and is caused by the potent exotoxin produced by a specific strain of *S. aureus*.

The clinical presentation is as follows:
- Extensive disruption of the epidermis, with widespread confluent blistering and denuded erythematous areas resembling scalding of the skin.
- Condition may follow impetigo.

Management—It is a serious condition requiring hospital admission and systemic antibiotic treatment.

Streptococcal infections

Erysipelas

This acute, erythematous, spreading infection of the dermis is caused by *Streptococcus pyogenes*.

The clinical presentation is as follows:
- Usually affects the face or the lower leg and appears as a painful red swelling.
- Lesion is usually well demarcated and is often oedematous and tender.
- Often preceded by fever and flu-like symptoms.
- Streptococci usually gain entry to the skin via a fissure, e.g. behind the ear or between the toes.

Severe infection requires parenteral antibiotic treatment, usually penicillin. Less severe cases can be treated with oral antibiotics.

Necrotizing fasciitis

A deep-spreading infection of the fat, fascia and muscle, this is caused by *Streptococcus pyogenes*.

The condition presents as an ill-defined erythema typically affecting the leg, and associated with a high fever. Infected tissues become rapidly necrotic.

It usually occurs in otherwise healthy subjects after minor trauma.

Management is by extensive emergency surgical debridement (removal of dead tissue); systemic antibiotics are essential.

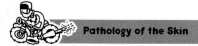
Mycobacterial infections

TB has become uncommon in the UK but it is still occasionally seen in the elderly and in Asian immigrants.

Cutaneous manifestations of TB:

- Lupus vulgaris: the commonest *M. tuberculosis* skin infection in the UK. Usually occurs following reactivation of pre-existing disease, and presents as a slowly progressive chronic skin lesion characterized by reddish-brown plaques. Typically affects the head or neck.
- Scrofuloderma: cutaneous involvement resulting from spread of infection from underlying lymph node. Fistulae and scarring may occur.
- Warty tuberculosis: warty plaque that occurs on inoculation of the skin in an individual with immunity from previous infection. Typically affects the hands, knees or buttocks. Rare in Western countries but is the commonest form of cutaneous TB in the Third World.

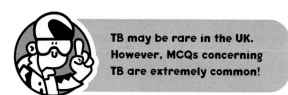

TB may be rare in the UK. However, MCQs concerning TB are extremely common!

All types are characterized by giant cell granulomatous inflammation in the dermis leading to the destruction of dermal collagen and skin appendages. Scarring is common and sometimes destruction of deeper tissues such as cartilage occurs.

Treatment is with a 6–9 month course of antibiotics.

Spirochaetal infections

Syphilis

Syphilis is a chronic infectious disease caused by the spirochaete *Treponema pallidum* and is usually transmitted by sexual intercourse. It typically involves three stages: primary, secondary and tertiary.

Skin lesions may be seen in all stages, but predominant skin manifestations present during the secondary stage.

Secondary syphilis

This is an inflammatory response in the skin and mucous membranes to the disseminated spirochaete.

The clinical presentation is as follows:

- Presents about 4–12 weeks after the onset of primary chancre (primary stage).
- Characterized by a non-itchy, pink or copper-coloured papular eruption on the trunk, limbs, palms and soles, and is often accompanied by lymphadenopathy and general malaise.
- Other signs are moist warty papules (condyloma lata) in the anogenital area, buccal erosions and diffuse patchy alopecia.
- Untreated, the eruption resolves in 1–3 months.

Management is by intramuscular penicillin and contact tracing of sexual partners and assessment for other venereal diseases.

Non-venereal treponemal infections

Rare in the UK but endemic in tropical and subtropical areas, these are transmitted by direct contact:

- Yaws—Central Africa, Central America and South East Asia (*Treponema pertenue*)
- Pinta—Central America (*T. carateum*).
- Endemic syphilis (bejel)—Middle East (*T. pallidum*).

Lyme disease

This cutaneous and systemic infection is caused by the spirochaete *Borrelia burgdorferi* and spread by certain ticks. The majority of cases develop a slowly extending erythematous rash at the site of the tick bite. Intermittent systemic symptoms include fever, malaise, headache, neck stiffness, and muscle and joint pain.

Other bacterial infections

Anthrax

This rare infection is caused by *Bacillus anthracis* associated with farm animals, particularly cattle.

A haemorrhagic bulla forms at the site of inoculation, and may be followed by vasculitis and a necrotizing, haemorrhagic inflammation of the skin.

The disease has a variable clinical course but death can occur if it is not rapidly diagnosed and treated.

Gram-negative infections

Gram-negative bacilli, such as *Pseudomonas aeruginosa,* can readily infect burns, ulcers or other moist skin lesions. They can also cause folliculitis and cellulitis (infection of subcutaneous tissues).

Fig. 15.9 provides a summary of bacterial skin infections.

Viral infections
Viral warts (verrucae)

These common, benign, hyperkeratotic, papillomatous growths on the skin are caused by infection with human papillomavirus (HPV).

Keratinocytes in the stratum granulosum (granular layer) beneath the wart are often vacuolated due to the viral infection. They clinically present as described below.

Common warts

Firm, dome-shaped, horny papules (1–10 mm across), usually multiple, these are found mainly on the hands, but may also affect the feet, face and genitalia.

Plantar warts

These occur on the soles of the feet and are often covered by callus (hyperkeratosis). Pressure causes inward growth, which results in tenderness.

Plane warts

Flat, skin-coloured papules usually found on the face, these are usually multiple and resist treatment but eventually resolve spontaneously.

Genital warts

These affect the genitalia and the perianal region. The warts may be small or may coalesce into large, cauliflower-like, warty growths called condylomata acuminata. Affected women have an increased risk of developing cervical cancer.

Management—Hand and foot warts frequently disappear spontaneously. Resistant varieties are treated with topical 'wart paints' (salicylic acid, lactic acid, gluteraldehyde, etc.) or with cryotherapy. Genital warts generally require cryotherapy or curettage and cautery with a local anaesthetic.

Molluscum contagiosum

This presents as discrete, multiple, pale papules with a central depression caused by a DNA poxvirus.

Clinical presentation—It mainly affects children or young adults. The most commonly affected areas are the face, neck and trunk.

The virus is transmitted by contact, including sexual transmission, or on towels.

Untreated, the papules disappear in 6–9 months.

The treatment is by curettage, cryotherapy or by expressing the content of papule (which contains a cheesy material) under local anaesthetic.

Herpes simplex

A common, acute vesicular eruption of the skin or mucous membranes, this is caused by infection with herpes simplex virus (HSV).

Pathologically:
- HSV blisters are highly contagious and are transmitted through direct contact.
- Virus penetrates the epidermis or mucous membrane and replicates with the epithelial cells.
- Following primary infection, the virus enters a latent stage within infected cells.
- Reactivation can occur at any time, even years after initial infection.
- Recurrence is thought to be precipitated by respiratory infection, sunlight or local trauma.

Clinical presentation—There are two types of HSV: Types 1 and 2.

HSV type 1

Primary infection usually occurs in childhood and causes the common cold sore, present on or around

Summary of bacterial skin infections	
Causative bacteria	**Associated skin disease**
commensal overgrowth	erythrasma, trichomycosis axillaris, pitted keratolysis
staphylococci	impetigo, ecthyma, folliculitis, scalded skin syndrome
streptococci	erysipelas, impetigo, necrotizing fasciitis
mycobacteria	TB (lupus vulgaris, scrofuloderma, warty tuberculosis), leprosy
spirochaetes	secondary syphilis, yaws/bejel/pinta, Lyme disease
others	anthrax, Gram-negative infections

Fig. 15.9 Summary of bacterial skin infections.

the lips. Epithelial infection may be accompanied by fever, malaise or local lymphadenopathy and lasts for about two weeks.

HSV type 2

This is mainly associated with genital herpes and is sexually transmitted.

However, both type 1 and 2 viruses can cause both genital herpes and cold sores, depending on the site of the initial infection.

Complications are:

- Secondary bacterial infection: usually staphylococcal.
- Eczema herpeticum: atopic eczema may be complicated by herpes simplex infection. Potentially fatal.
- Disseminated herpes simplex: occasionally occurs in the newborn or in immunosuppressed patients.
- Chronic herpes simplex: common in patients with HIV infection.
- Herpes encephalitis: serious complication of HSV infection.
- Erythema multiforme: immune-mediated disease characterized by erythematous lesions on the hands and feet.

Management is by topical acyclovir (used for mild facial or genital herpes simplex) and oral acyclovir (prescribed for severe episodes of HSV infection).

Herpes zoster (shingles)

This acute, vesicular eruption occurs in a dermatomal distribution and is caused by the reactivation of latent varicella zoster virus.

Following an attack of chickenpox, the virus remains dormant in the dorsal root ganglion of the spinal cord. On reactivation (the causes of which are unknown), the virus migrates down the sensory nerve to affect one or more dermatomes on the skin. The clinical presentation is as follows:

- Usually presents as densely grouped vesicles and erythema on one dermatome.
- Thoracic dermatomes are most commonly affected, except in the elderly where the ophthalmic division of the trigeminal nerve is particularly common.
- Vesicles become pustular and form crusts which separate in 2–3 weeks to leave scarring.
- Vesicular blisters contain virus which when shed may

cause chickenpox in contacts with no previous exposure.

- Associated with pain, tenderness or paraesthesia in the dermatome, which may also precede the eruption by 3–5 days.
- Local lymphadenopathy is common.

Complications are:

- Secondary bacterial infections.
- Ophthalmic scarring: corneal ulcers and scarring may occur following shingles of the ophthalmic division of the trigeminal nerve.
- Motor palsy: rare; viral involvement may spread from the posterior horn of the spinal cord to the anterior horn to infect motor nerves resulting in palsies or paralysis of individual muscles or muscle groups.
- Disseminated herpes zoster: may occur in the immunosuppressed leading to potentially fatal varicella pneumonia or encephalitis.
- Postherpetic neuralgia: occurs in one-third of those over 60 years old, but infrequent in patients under 40 years old. Pain usually subsides within 12 months.

Management of mild shingles is by symptomatic treatment with rest, analgesia and calamine lotion.

Severe cases are treated with oral acyclovir which, if taken within 48 hours of onset, decreases the duration and the intensity of the disease and may prevent postherpetic neuralgia.

Fungal infections

Dermatophyte infections

Dermatophytes are filamentous (hyphal) fungi which reproduce by spore formation. They commonly inhabit keratin of the skin, hair and nails producing superficial mycoses (Fig. 15.10).

Dermatophytes are collectively termed 'ringworm' but comprise three genera:

- *Microsporum*, e.g. *M. canis*.
- *Trichophyton*, e.g. *T. rubrum* and *T. interdigitale*.
- *Epidermophyton*, e.g. *E. floccosum*.

Management is by topical therapy for minor fungal infections, with systemic therapy for widespread involvement or disease of the nails or scalp. Humid and sweaty conditions, including occlusive footwear, should be minimized.

Candida albicans infections

Candida albicans is a yeast-type fungus and is a commensal of the vagina and alimentary canal. It commonly produces opportunistic infections which may be predisposed to by humidity, obesity, diabetes and oral antibiotic therapy.

Clinical presentation—In infection, hyphal forms of *C. albicans* are seen, and the infection is termed candidosis (or candidiasis).

Candidosis may present as described below.

Genital

This is especially common in the vagina ('thrush') where white-yellowish plaques on the inflamed mucous membranes produce itching/discomfort, and sometimes a white vaginal discharge. It can be spread by sexual intercourse; males develop similar changes on the penis.

Oral

White plaques adhere on the tongue or inside the cheeks.

Intertrigo

A superficial inflammation of two skin surfaces that are in contact (e.g. between the thighs or under the breasts) is often aggravated by *C. albicans* infection. Interdigital clefts are commonly affected in wetworkers.

Paronychia

The nail-fold becomes inflamed and swollen, the cuticle is lost, and the nail may be ridged transversely. It is often seen in wetworkers.

Systemic

This occurs in the immunosuppressed, producing red nodules on the skin with small, satellite pustules.

Mucocutaneous candidosis

This is a rare (and sometimes inherited) disorder of immune deficiency. It causes chronic *C. albicans* intertrigo and nail and mouth infections.

Management is by:

- Topical therapy: for body folds, oral and genital *Candida*.
- Systemic therapy: short course useful for recurrent or persistent candidosis (reduces bowel carriage), long-term treatment for mucocutaneous candidiasis.

Infestations

Insect bites

These are a cutaneous inflammatory reaction to insect

Dermatophyte infections and their clinical effects		
Affected area	**Commonest organism**	**Clinical presentation**
tinea corporis (trunk and limbs)	*Trichophyton verrucosum, Microsporum canis, T. rubrum*	single or multiple ring lesions with scaling and erythema, especially at the edges
tinea pedis (athlete's foot)	*T. rubrum, T. interdigitale, Epidermophyton floccosum*	redness, erosion and scaling which is often interdigital, but diffuse involvement of skin also occurs common in young men; increased predisposition by communal washing, swimming baths, occlusive footwear, and hot weather
tinea capitis (scalp/hair)	*M. canis, M. audouinii, T. tonsurans, T. schoenleinii*	hair loss and scaling usually affects children
tinea cruris (groin)	*T. rubrum, E. floccosum, T. interdigitale*	red, scaly rash with brown patches; more common in men and often seen in athletes ('jock itch')
tinea mannum (hand)	*T. rubrum*	unilateral diffuse powdery scaling of the palm
tinea unguium (nails)	*T. rubrum, T. interdigitale*	thick, crumbling nails more commonly affecting toenails incidence of onychomycosis increases with age

Fig. 15.10 Dermatophyte infections and their clinical effects.

parts or to injected foreign substances. Common culprits include garden insects (gnats, etc.), insects of household pets (fleas, mites), and bedbugs (inactive within furniture during the day but emerge at night).

Bites are usually grouped on a limb, and lesions vary from itchy wheals to quite large bullae depending on the insect and the type of immune response elicited.

Secondary bacterial infection of excoriated insect bites is common.

It can be managed by the elimination of the cause if within the household, and with topical hydrocortisone or calamine lotion.

Pediculosis (lice)

Lice are blood-sucking insects which, using their well-adapted legs and claws, attach to, and lay eggs (nits) in, hair and clothing of humans. There are two types:

- Pubic louse: sexually transmitted and mostly found in young adults (colloquially known as 'crabs').
- Body louse: associated with poor social conditions. Spread is by infested bedding or clothing. A variant, the head louse, is quite common in school children and is spread by head to head contact.

Clinical presentation—Intense itching caused by bites results in excoriation and commonly in secondary bacterial infection.

Lice are found in the seams of clothes, and their eggs can often be seen on hair shafts.

Scabies

Scabies are caused by the burrowing of the female mite *Sarcoptes scabei* through the stratum corneum where she lays her eggs. After a few days the eggs hatch into larvae which moult and mature in the epidermis. The new mites mate in the stratum corneum; the male dies, and the fertilized female burrows and continues the cycle.

Clinical presentation—Very itchy, raised lesions, often red and scaling, typically arise on the sides of fingers, palms, nipples and genitalia.

Linear tracks (the burrows), about 1 cm long, can often be seen, and the mite itself is occasionally visible as a white dot at the end of the burrow.

Itching causes excoriation which frequently results in secondary bacterial infection. Untreated, the condition becomes chronic.

Management—Scabies is transmitted by direct transfer, and therefore all contacts require treatment.

Treatment is with topical scabicides applied to the whole body.

Tropical skin infections and infestations

Leprosy

This chronic granulomatous disease is caused by *Mycobacterium leprae.*

Leprosy is rare in the UK but occurs in tropical and subtropical areas with about 10 million patients worldwide.

Transmission is by the inhalation of nasal droplets, after which the incubation period may be many years.

The clinicopathological features of leprosy (a.k.a. Hansen's disease) are dependent on the degree of hypersensitivity response (delayed type IV) instigated against the infection by the host.

The spectrum of disease ranges from tuberculoid (strong, cell-mediated immunity) to lepromatous (weak, cell-mediated immunity) forms.

Clinical presentation—*M. leprae* has a predilection for nerves (see Chapter 6) and the skin. Fig. 15.11 shows the skin involvement in the lepromatous and tuberculoid forms of leprosy.

Management is by triple therapy antibiotic treatment continued for at least two years.

Leishmaniasis

A common disease in the tropics and subtropics caused by the protozoan *Leishmania*, this is transmitted by sand flies. Three forms of the disease exist, caused by different species of *Leishmania* (Fig. 15.12).

Management—Cutaneous leishmaniasis often heals spontaneously. However, other forms require pentavalent antimony compound intravenously for 10–21 days.

Filariasis

This tropical disease is caused by the nematode worms *Wuchereria bancrofti* and *Brugia malayi*. The worms, which are transmitted by various mosquitoes, cause inflammation and eventual blockage of the lymph vessels. The net result is gross oedema of the surrounding tissues—elephantiasis—especially of the legs or scrotum.

Larva migrans

Also known as 'creeping eruption', this is caused by the larvae of nematode hookworms. Larvae burrow through the skin, leaving intensely itchy tracks in their wake. Treatment is with topical thiabedazole, although the larvae eventually die spontaneously after a few weeks, as they cannot complete their life cycle in humans.

Deep mycoses

These systemic diseases are caused by fungal invasion. They include:
- Blastomycosis—wart-like ulcers on the face, neck and limbs.
- Histoplasmosis—lung disease plus granulomata of the skin.
- Mycetoma—chronic granulomata on the foot.
- Sporotrichosis—chronic skin infection.

Onchocerciasis

This is endemic disease of Africa and Central America caused by the nematode worm, *Onchocerca volvulus*, which is transmitted to humans by a gnat. The worms cause an itchy papular eruption on the skin, which progresses to form fibrous nodules with lichenification and pigmentary change. Microfilariae also invade the eye and result in total or partial blindness (called 'river blindness' in Africa).

Skin involvement in lepromatous and tuberculoid forms of leprosy	
Lepromatous form	**Tuberculoid form**
minimal immune response (occurs in patients with low cellular immunity)	vigorous T cell mediated (delayed) hypersensitivity
bacteraemia occurs to peripheral sites	bacteraemia rare
many skin lesions with symmetrical distribution	few skin lesions with asymmetrical distribution
macules, papules, plaques and nodules	raised, red plaques with hypopigmented centre sensation is often impaired within the plaque
typically involves arms, legs, buttocks and face	often affects the face
progression causes a thickened, furrowed appearance of face (leonine facies) with eyebrow loss	progression is slow; combined effect of extensive destruction of tissue by immune response and repeated trauma to desensitized areas results in severe disfigurement, especially to hands and feet
untreated, this form is lethal due to the impaired immune response	eventually heals spontaneously

Fig. 15.11 Skin involvement in lepromatous and tuberculoid forms of leprosy.

Different types of leishmaniasis			
Type of leishmaniasis	**Endemic areas**	**Protozoan**	**Clinical presentation**
visceral (kala azar)	Asia, Africa and South America	*Leishmania donovani*	affects lymphatic system, spleen and bone marrow, causing splenomegaly, hepatomegaly, anaemia and disability; patchy pigmentation may occur on face, hands and abdomen
cutaneous	Mediterranean coast, Middle East and Asia	*L. tropica*	characterized by 'oriental sore', a red–brown nodule that appears at site of inoculation and which either ulcerates or spreads slowly to form crusty plaque
mucocutaneous	Central and South America	*L. braziliensis*	characterized by a skin lesion similar to that of oriental sore but is followed by necrotic ulcers which cause deformity of nose, lips and palate

Fig. 15.12 Different types of leishmaniasis.

- **Name the bacterial groups that commonly cause skin disease.**
- **Describe the skin conditions caused by each category of bacteria.**
- **Outline the clinical presentation of four common viral skin diseases.**
- **Name the body sites that can be infected by dermatophytes.**
- **Describe the main tropical skin infections and infestations.**

DISORDERS OF SPECIFIC SKIN STRUCTURES

Sweat and the sebaceous structures

Acne vulgaris

This inflammatory disorder of the pilosebaceous glands is characterized by comedones (blackheads and whiteheads), papules, pustules, cysts and scars. It is extremely common in adolescents, the peak age for clinical acne being 18 years.

Aetiopathogenesis—The cause of acne is uncertain, but the androgen-sensitive sebaceous glands show a hyperresponsiveness to testosterone that results in the following sequence of events:

- Increased sebum excretion.
- Hyperkeratosis of pilosebaceous ducts.
- Blockage of pilosebaceous units with excess keratin and sebum causing comedo formation.
- Colonization of ducts with *Propionibacterium acnes*.
- Release of inflammatory mediators.

Fig. 15.13 gives a diagrammatical representation of the pathogenesis of acne.

Clinical presentation—Comedones (sing. comedo) are of two types:

- Open as in blackheads: dilated pores with dark plugs of keratin and sebum.
- Closed as in whiteheads: small cream-coloured, dome-shaped papules.

The colonization of ducts with *P. acnes* causes the evolution of comedones into inflammatory papules, pustules or cysts, which often form scars on healing. This may persist until the early 20s and may even continue into the fifth decade in a few patients, especially in women.

There is a predilection for areas that have many sebaceous glands—the face, shoulders, back and upper chest.

Management of acne is shown in Fig. 15.14.

Rosacea

This chronic inflammatory disease of the face is characterized by erythema, telangiectasia and pustules.

The aetiology of rosacea is unknown.

Telangiectatic dilatation of the upper dermal vessels is common and causes erythema. Fragments of the mite *Demodex folliculorum* are commonly found in follicles, but its role in the pathogenesis is unclear.

Follicular pustules often develop in the markedly dilated hair follicles.

Rupture of the follicles leads to the development of a florid, lumpy form of rosacea, the result of a giant cell granulomatous reaction in response to follicular content release.

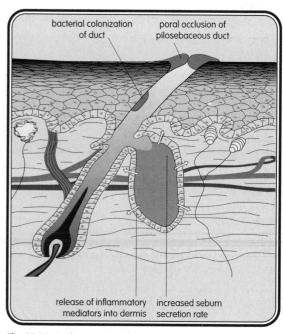

Fig. 15.13 Pathogenesis of acne.

Management of acne vulgaris		
Type	**Treatment**	**Comment**
topical treatment (mild acne)	benzoyl peroxide	reduces numbers of *Proprionibacterium acnes* but may cause irritation
	tretinoin	reduces number of non-inflamed lesions but may cause irritation
	antibiotics	used in treatment of mild or moderate acne
systemic treatment (moderate or severe acne)	antibiotics	e.g. tetracyclines or erythromycin for a minimum of 4 months
	antiandrogens	usually combined with an oestrogen and prescribed to females over a period of 6–12 months; suppresses sebum production and is also a contraceptive
	retinoids	isotretinoin: reduces sebum excretion, inhibits *P. acnes* and is anti-inflammatory; 4–6 month course; very effective but side effects common

Fig. 15.14 Management of acne vulgaris.

Clinical presentation—It typically affects the middle-aged or elderly, with a slightly higher incidence in women. It may persist for years, and is often complicated by:
- Rhinophyma: hyperplasia of sebaceous glands and connective tissue of the nose.
- Eye involvement: blepharitis (inflammation of the eyelids) and conjunctivitis.

The condition is exacerbated by sunlight and topical steroids.

Management is by oral antibiotic treatment, e.g. tetracycline or erythromycin. Plastic surgery is required for rhinophyma.

Hair disorders
Alopecia
This is commonly classified into three main types: diffuse non-scarring, localized non-scarring, and scarring (cicatricial).

Diffuse non-scarring
There is a diffuse reduction in hair density. The patient usually notices excessive numbers of hairs on the pillow, brush or comb.

The causes of diffuse non-scarring alopecia are:
- Male pattern/androgenic alopecia: inherited, androgen-dependent hair loss. Extremely common in men, but also occurs in women, becoming more pronounced after the menopause.
- Endocrine related: hypo- and hyperthyroidism, pituitary or adrenal underactivity. Androgen-secreting tumours in women can produce male pattern baldness.
- Nutrition related: iron or zinc deficiency, malnutrition —especially kwashiorkor (protein deficiency).
- Telogen effluvium: hair follicles, which are usually out of phase, can, under certain circumstances, become synchronized into the resting phase (telogen) and then be shed in unison three months later. The causes of synchronization are high fever, childbirth, surgery, drugs or stress.
- Drug induced, e.g. with cytotoxics, heparin, warfarin, carbimazole, colchicine and vitamin A.

Localized non-scarring
There is patchy hair loss. The causes are:
- Alopecia areata: common condition associated with autoimmune disorders in which growth phase of hair is prematurely arrested.

It typically presents in the second or third decade with bald patches on the scalp, but the eyebrows and beard can also be affected, and nails may show pitting.

The course is unpredictable, varying from the progressive enlargement of bald patches to the regrowth of hair (more common).

A poor prognosis is indicated if the onset is prepubertal, associated with atopy, or shows extensive involvement.

Rarely, complete scalp alopecia (totalis) or loss of all bodily hair (universalis) occurs.

- Infections, e.g. with scalp ringworm or secondary syphilis.
- Trauma/traction.

Scarring (cicatricial) alopecia
This is caused by scarring of the scalp with the destruction of hair follicles.

The causes of scarring are:
- Irradiation/burns (chemical or thermal).
- Infection, e.g. shingles of the ophthalmic division of the trigeminal nerve, kerion, or tertiary syphilis.
- Lichen planus/lupus erythematosus: erythema, scaling and follicular changes may result in scarring.
- Pseudopelade: end stage of an idiopathic or unidentified destructive inflammatory process in the scalp.

Excess hair
Hirsutism
This is the growth of coarse, pigmented hair with an androgenic distribution in a female.

Fig. 15.15 shows the aetiology of hirsutism.

Hypertrichosis
Excessive growth of hair in a non-androgenic distribution is less common than hirsutism. It can be:
- Localized, e.g. on melanocytic naevi or following topical steroid usage.
- Generalized: fine terminal hair appears on the face, limbs and trunk. Mostly drug induced, but can also be caused by anorexia nervosa (or malnutrition), porphyria, cutanea tarda or underlying malignancy.

Others
Hairshaft defects
These are rare, usually inherited, brittle hair conditions.

Dandruff
This is caused by excessive exfoliation of fine scales from an otherwise normal scalp.

Tinea capitis
Infection of the scalp with dermatophyte (p.338); may cause scarring alopecia.

Nail disorders
Congenital disease
Congenital conditions are as follows:

- Racket nails: commonest congenital nail defect characterized by broad, short, thumb nails.
- Nail–patella syndrome: nails (and patellae) are absent or rudimentary.
- Pachyonychia congenita: thickened, discoloured nails present from birth.

Trauma
Traumatic conditions are as follows:
- Subungual haematoma: bleeding under the nail following trapping of a finger- or toenail.
- Splinter haemorrhages: almost always occur with infective endocarditis, but may also be trauma induced.
- Ingrowing toenails: usually caused by ill-fitting shoes.
- Onychogryphosis: big toenails become thickened and horn-like, usually in response to trauma.
- Brittle nails: usually due to repeated exposure to detergents and water.

Nail involvement in the dermatoses
These are:
- Alopecia areata: pitting and roughness of nail surface.
- Psoriasis: pitting, nail thickening, onycholysis, brown patches, subungual hyperkeratosis.
- Eczema: pitting and transverse ridging.

Infections
Infections are:
- Tinea unguium: fungal infection of the nails (Fig. 15.16).
- Chronic paronychia: *C. albicans* infection of the nails, common in wetworkers (p.339).
- Acute paronychia: typically, a bacterial infection of the nails usually caused by staphylococci.

Aetiology of hirsutism	
idiopathic	most common form; probably due to increased hypersensitivity of end-organ to androgens
iatrogenic	e.g. androgens, progestogens
virilizing tumours	e.g. ovarian or adrenal tumours
endocrine disorders	congenital adrenal hyperplasia, Cushing's syndrome, acromegaly

Fig. 15.15 Aetiology of hirsutism.

Nail changes and their possible causes		
Nail change	**Description**	**Possible causes**
Beau's lines	transverse ridges	severe illnesses that affect nail growth, e.g. pneumonia or myocardial infarction
brittle nails	easily broken nails	repeated exposure to water/detergent, iron deficiency, hypothyroidism, ischaemia of digits
colour change	black transverse bands blue blue-green brown brown patches brown longitudinal streak red-brown streaks (splinter haemorrhages) white spots white (leuconychia) yellow yellow nail syndrome	cytotoxic drugs haematoma, cyanosis, antimalarials *Pseudomonas* infection fungal infection, cigarette stains, chlorpromazine, gold, Addison's disease psoriasis melanocytic naevus, malignant melanoma, Addison's disease infective endocarditis, trauma trauma to nail matrix (not calcium deficiency) hypoalbuminaemia psoriasis, tinea unguium, jaundice, tetracycline defective lymphatic drainage
clubbing	swelling of nail with loss of angle between nail fold and nail plate normal clubbed	respiratory: pulmonary tuberculosis, bronchiectasis, empyema, lung cancer fibrosing alveolitis cardiovascular: infective endocarditis, congenital heart disease other less common diseases, e.g. asbestosis, Crohn's disease, ulcerative colitis, cirrhosis
koilonychia	concave (spoon-shaped) nails	iron deficiency anaemia repeated exposure to detergents
nail fold telangiectasia	reddened nail folds caused by dilated capillaries	inflammatory connective tissue disorders including SLE, systemic sclerosis and dermatomyositis
onycholysis	separation of part or all of nail from its bed	psoriasis, tinea unguium, trauma, thyrotoxicosis, tetracyclines
pitting	small holes in nail bed	psoriasis, eczema, alopecia areata, lichen planus
ridging	transverse	Beau's lines, eczema, psoriasis, chronic paronychia
	longitudinal	secondary to trauma

Fig. 15.16 Nail changes and their possible causes.

Tumours of the nails
The tumours are:
- Viral warts: common around the nail-fold.
- Periungual fibroma: associated with tuberous sclerosis (see Chapter 6).
- Myxoid cysts: mucous cysts adjacent to the nail-fold which probably arise from folds of synovium.
- Malignant melanoma: subungual malignant melanoma which produces a pigmented longitudinal streak in a nail, and may cause its destruction.

Nail changes in systemic disease
Fig. 15.16 gives examples of nail changes and their possible causes.

Systemic disorders often cause specific nail changes. A thorough examination of the nails can often be helpful in the diagnosis of a disease.

- Describe the pathogenesis of acne and its distribution on the body.
- State the three main categories of alopecia and their causes.
- Compare the clinical presentation of acne and rosacea.
- What are the causes of excess hair?
- Name four types of nail tumour.

DISORDERS OF PIGMENTATION

Hypopigmentation
Vitiligo
This common disorder is characterized by the appearance of symmetrical white or pale macules on the skin which are caused by the patchy loss of pigmentation.

Aetiopathogenesis—Autoimmune disease of melanocytes is often associated with other autoimmune diseases such as pernicious anaemia, thyroid disease and Addison's disease.

The aetiology is unknown but about 30% of patients have a family history.

Clinical presentation—It affects about 1% of all races but is more conspicuous in dark-skinned races.

Onset is usually between 10 and 30 years, and may be precipitated by injury or sunburn.

It commonly affects the hands, wrists, knees, neck and areas around orifices (e.g. mouth), and has an unpredictable course ranging from progression to repigmentation (rarely).

Vitiligo is managed with camouflage cosmetics and sunscreens (to reduce contrast between pigmented and non-pigmented skin). Topical steroids occasionally induce repigmentation in darker skins. PUVA (psoralen and UV-A) is occasionally beneficial.

Albinism
This is a rare (1 in 20 000) autosomal recessive disease characterized by the lack of pigmentation in the skin, hair and eyes. Melanocyte numbers are normal but melanin production fails due to deficient or defective enzyme, tyrosinase.

The skin is white or pink, the hair is white and pigmentation is lacking in the eye. It is associated with poor sight, photophobia and nystagmus. Albinos have an increased risk of skin tumours on exposure to UV light.

Prenatal diagnosis is possible.

Phenylketonuria
This autosomal recessive inborn error of metabolism is caused by a deficiency of phenylalanine hydroxylase, which normally converts phenylalanine to tyrosine, thus:

$$\text{phenylalanine} \xrightarrow{\text{phenylalanine hydroxylase}} \text{tyrosine}$$

Patients also have fair hair and skin due to impaired melanin synthesis (tyrosine is a precursor of melanin). The concentration of phenylalanine and its metabolites is increased and causes damage to the neonatal brain. Untreated, mental retardation and choreoathetosis develop, although a low phenylalanine diet can prevent neurological damage.

The prevalence is 1 per 10 000 and it is detected by routine screening tests.

A summary of the causes of hypopigmentation is given in Fig. 15.17.

Hyperpigmentation
Freckles and lentigines
Freckles

Freckles and lentigines are common topics in MCQs.

Freckles are small, light brown macules which darken on exposure to sunlight. They contain normal numbers of melanocytes, but melanin production is increased. They are common in childhood, especially in fair skinned children. No treatment is required.

Lentigines

Lentigines (also known as lentigos) are similar in appearance to freckles but are more scattered and do not darken in the sun. They contain increased numbers of melanocytes and may develop in childhood but are more common in a sun-exposed, elderly skin. They respond to cryotherapy.

Chloasma (melasma)

This photosensitivity reaction in pregnant women (or in women taking oral contraceptives) causes the appearance of symmetrical, ill-defined brown patches on the face. These are caused by oestrogen-induced melanocyte stimulation.

Sunscreens and cosmetic camouflage can help mask the brown patches, which usually improve spontaneously.

Drug-induced pigmentation

This can be caused by stimulation of melanogenesis or by drug deposition in the skin. Drugs commonly responsible include amiodarone, bleomycin, psoralens, chlorpromazine and minocycline.

Other causes
Addison's disease

This is characterized by hypoadrenalism with overproduction of ACTH by the pituitary. ACTH stimulates melanogenesis resulting in hyperpigmentation of mucosae and flexures.

Addisonian-like pigmentation is also seen in Cushing's syndrome, hyperthyroidism and acromegaly.

Peutz–Jeghers syndrome

This rare, autosomal dominant disorder is characterized by perioral lentigines and intestinal polyps.

Fig. 15.18 provides a summary of the causes of hyperpigmentation.

Summary of causes of hypopigmentation		
	Cause	Example
generalized hypopigmentation	genetic	albinism and phenylketonuria
patchy hypopigmentation	endocrine	hypopituitarism (↓ ACTH and ↓ MSH)
	infective	leprosy, yaws, pityriasis versicolor
	postinflammatory	cryotherapy, eczema, psoriasis, morphoea, pityriasis alba
	chemical	substituted phenols, hydroquinone
	other	vitiligo, lichen sclerosus, halo naevus

Fig. 15.17 Summary of causes of hypopigmentation.

- List the causes of generalized hypopigmentation.
- List the causes of patchy hypopigmentation.
- Compare the pathogenesis of albinism and phenylketonuria.
- Describe the differences between freckles and lentigines.
- Categorize the causes of hyperpigmentation.

Summary of causes of hyperpigmentation	
Cause	**Problem**
genetic	inherited: freckles, neurofibromatosis (café au lait spots), Peutz–Jeghers syndrome acquired: lentigines
endocrine	chloasma, Addison's disease, Cushing's syndrome, hyperthyroidism and acromegaly
metabolic	biliary cirrhosis (jaundice), haemochromatosis (iron deposition), porphyria
nutritional	carotenaemia (orange discoloration), malnutrition/malabsorption, pellagra
postinflammatory	eczema, lichen planus, systemic sclerosis
drugs	e.g. oestrogens, amiodarone, bleomycin, psoralens, chlorpromazine and minocycline
other	acanthosis nigricans, malignant melanoma, naevi, argyria (deposition of silver), chronic renal failure

Fig. 15.18 Summary of causes of hyperpigmentation.

BLISTERING DISORDERS

Blisters are fluid-filled spaces within the skin caused by the separation of two layers of tissue and the leakage of plasma into the space. The type of blister formed (Fig. 15.19) depends on the level of separation, and can be:
- Subcorneal: bullous impetigo or pustular psoriasis.
- Intra-epidermal: acute eczema, herpes simplex/zoster, pemphigus, friction blisters.
- Subepidermal: pemphigoid, dermatitis herpetiformis, cold and thermal injury.

Pemphigus

This rare but potentially fatal group of autoimmune disorders is marked by successive outbreaks of blisters on the skin and in the mouth.

Aetiopathogenesis—Patients have circulating IgG autoantibodies which bind to intercellular junctions in the epidermis. Binding of IgG activates complement, and adjacent keratinocytes are induced to release proteolytic enzymes. Cellular adhesion is lost (acantholysis), and an intra-epidermal separation occurs.

This is also associated with other organ-specific autoimmune disorders such as myasthenia gravis.

Clinical presentation—The commonest form is pemphigus vulgaris which typically affects middle-aged people. Oral erosions precede cutaneous blistering in 50% of cases. Flaccid, superficial blisters develop over the scalp, face, back, chest and flexures.

If left untreated, the blistering is progressive and ultimately fatal (due to the loss of electrolytes and protein). It is managed with systemic steroids and other immunosuppressive agents.

Bullous pemphigoid

This is a chronic, itchy blistering disorder of the elderly.

Aetiopathogenesis—An autoimmune disorder in which IgG antibodies are deposited at the basement membrane.

Inflammatory cells attracted by complement activation release proteolytic enzymes resulting in subepidermal bullae formation.

Clinical presentation—Large, tense blisters commonly appear on the limbs, trunk and flexures, but are occasionally localized to one site, often the lower leg. Oral lesions occur in only 10% of cases. An urticarial eruption may precede the onset of blistering.

The disease is self limiting in about 50% of cases and is managed with systemic steroids and other immunosuppressants.

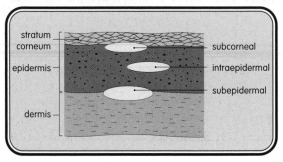

Fig. 15.19 Location of blisters within the skin.

Dermatitis herpetiformis

This presents as a rare eruption of symmetrical itchy blisters on the extensor surfaces.

Aetiopathogenesis—The aetiology is unknown but associated with coeliac disease (gluten hypersensitivity). It is characterized by granular IgA at the dermal papillae of normal-looking skin, and villus atrophy of the small intestine.

It usually presents in the third or fourth decade with males more often affected than females by 2:1. There are groups of small, intensely itchy vesicles on the knees, elbows, scalp, buttocks and shoulders.

Blistering diseases are rare but important as they can be severe, and are potentially fatal.
Pemphigus vulgaris is the most life threatening type of blistering disorder.

○ **What are the main characteristics of pemphigus vulgaris?**
○ **Compare the aetiopathogenesis of pemphigus and pemphigoid.**
○ **Describe the aetiopathogenesis and clinical presentation of dermatitis herpetiformis.**

Despite villus atrophy in most patients, symptoms of GI disturbances are uncommon. It should be managed with a gluten-free diet with or without dapsone.

A summary of blistering disorders is given in Fig. 15.20.

TUMOURS OF THE SKIN

Benign tumours of the skin
Epidermal tumours
Seborrhoeic wart

This common, benign tumour of basal keratinocytes typically occurs on the trunk, face and arms of the elderly. The aetiology of these tumours is unknown. They are also known as seborrhoeic keratosis and basal cell papilloma:

- Warts are often greasy looking (hence seborrhoeic) but are not associated with seborrhoea nor with sebaceous glands.
- Usually multiple, and vary in size from a few mm to several cm.
- Progress from lightly pigmented, small papules to darkly pigmented, warty nodules.
- Often have a 'pasted on' appearance with well-defined edges.

Microscopically, all lesions show basal cell proliferation, hyperkeratosis, and a variable degree of pigmentation.

Actinic keratosis

This presents as a roughened, scaly brownish-to-red lesions usually less than 1 cm across which bleed when

Summary of blistering disorders			
Disorder	**Type of bullae**	**Autoimmunity**	**Clinical features**
pemphigus vulgaris	intra-epidermal	IgG deposited on intercellular junctions	flaccid, superficial bullae more common in middle-aged high mortality
bullous pemphigoid	subepidermal	IgG deposited on basement membrane	large, tense bullae more common in elderly self-limiting in about 50% of cases
dermatitis herpetiformis	subepidermal	IgA deposited on dermal papillae	small, itchy vesicles usually presents in 3rd or 4th decade; males > females associated with coeliac disease

Fig. 15.20 Summary of blistering disorders.

rubbed. They typically arise on sun-exposed areas, especially the face, scalp and hands, of the middle-aged and elderly.

Histologically, they show hyperkeratosis and parakeratosis, abnormal keratinocytes with loss of maturation and a mild to moderate degree of pleomorphism and mitotic figures.

The lesions are considered as premalignant, with 20% of them evolving into squamous cell carcinoma.

Actinic keratosis is also known as solar keratosis or senile keratosis.

Skin tags

These common, benign, pedunculated polyps a few mm in length, typically affect the elderly or middle-aged, and have a predilection for the neck, axillae, groin and eyelids. They consist of a fibrovascular core with an epidermal covering.

Their aetiology is unknown but they are often found in obese individuals.

Cysts

These benign, keratin-filled, firm, skin-coloured cysts are normally 1–3 cm in diameter.

Common types are epidermal cysts (derived from the epidermis) and pilar cysts (derived from the outer root sheath of the hair follicle). These are often incorrectly grouped together as sebaceous cysts.

Milia

These small, white, keratin cysts, normally 1–2 mm in diameter, often affect the eyelids and the upper cheeks. They are common in children, but can appear at any age. (Milia is the plural of milium.)

Dermal tumours
Dermatofibroma (histiocytoma)

This firm, reddish-brown nodule of about 5–10 mm in diameter is common in young adults, females more than males, and usually appears on the lower legs.

Histologically, it consists of intertwining bands of collagen fibres formed by proliferating fibroblasts, with reactive hyperplasia and hyperpigmentation of overlying epidermis. It can be mistaken for a melanocytic naevus or malignant melanoma.

Pyogenic granuloma

A benign, rapidly-growing, bright-red nodule arising mainly on the fingers or face, this typically develops at a site of trauma, e.g. a thorn prick, and is more common in young adults and children. It is neither pyogenic nor granulomatous, but is a well-circumscribed dermal lesion of proliferating capillaries and inflammation which closely resembles a haemangioma.

Excision and histological examination are required to rule out malignant melanoma.

Keloid

This is an excessive proliferation of connective tissue occurring in previously injured skin, but extending beyond the margin of the original injury. Characteristics are:

- Firm, smooth, erythematous nodules occurring mainly over the upper back, chest or ear lobes.
- More common in Black people.
- Highest incidence in second to fourth decades.

Treatment is by steroid injection into the keloid.

Campbell De Morgan's spot (cherry angioma)

Small, bright red papules (about 1–2 mm diameter) composed of benign capillary proliferations commonly arise on the trunk in elderly or middle-aged patients.

Lipoma

A soft, subcutaneous tumour of mature adipocytes, is often multiple, and mostly found on the trunk, neck and upper extremities.

Chondrodermatitis nodularis

This small painful nodule on the upper rim of the pinna occurs usually in elderly men. It is caused by inflammation of the underlying cartilage, and is not a neoplasm. Excision is curative.

Fig. 15.21 provides a summary of benign skin tumours.

Naevi
Definition

Naevi are benign, coloured lesions on the skin formed from a proliferation of one or more of the normal constituent cells of the skin. Though often congenital (birthmarks), they may be acquired.

Melanocytic naevi

Consist of benign collections or nests of melanocytic

cells, and are the commonest type of naevus (also known as 'moles'). They present in most Caucasians, but are less prevalent in those with Down syndrome and in Black people.

The aetiology of naevi development is unknown but it seems to be an inherited trait in many families:

- About 1% of naevi are congenital.
- Majority develop during childhood or adolescence; numbers reach a peak at puberty and have a tendency to decline during adult life.
- A few new naevi develop during the third and fourth decade, especially if provoked by excessive sun exposure or pregnancy.

Naevi can be classified according to the position of the naevus cells within the skin as follows:

- Junctional naevi: flat macules consisting of rounded nests of melanocytes in the lower epidermis at the dermo-epidermal junction.

Summary of benign skin tumours	
Tumour type	**Example**
benign epidermal tumours	viral wart actinic keratosis seborrhoeic wart milia cysts skin tags
benign dermal tumours	dermatofibroma melanocytic naevus cherry angioma pyogenic granuloma keloid lipoma chondrodermatitis nodularis

Fig. 15.21 Summary of benign skin tumours.

- Compound naevi: papules or nodules with an irregular surface which consist of junctional nests of melanocytes combined with an intradermal mass of melanocytic cells.
- Intradermal naevi: dome-shaped papules/nodules composed entirely of melanocytic cell clusters within the upper dermis (no junctional component present).

These different types of naevi are thought to arise by progression from junctional to intradermal (Fig. 15.22). Other variants are:

- Congenital naevi: usually over 1 cm in diameter, and may be protuberant or hairy, and have a risk of malignant change.
- Blue naevi: steely blue intradermal naevus, usually solitary, and most commonly found on the extremities.
- Halo naevi: white halo of depigmentation surrounds naevi. Represents involution of naevus by immune destruction. Mainly seen in children and adolescents.
- Becker's naevi: rare, unilateral lesion on upper back or chest. Initially hyperpigmented and later becomes hairy. More common in adolescent males.
- Familial dysplastic naevus syndrome: familial condition characterized by large numbers of atypical and 'dysplastic' naevi. Affected individuals have a greatly increased risk of developing malignant melanoma.

The majority of naevi are entirely benign, but malignant changes can occur. Junctional components of junctional or compound naevi carry the highest risk for malignancy. Invasion is preceded by nuclear pleomorphism with increased mitoses and cellular atypia. Clinically, malignant naevi appear larger than

Fig. 15.22 Types of melanocytic naevi.

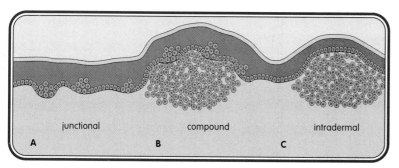

normal, and have an irregular edge, surface and pigmentation.

The management is as follows:
- Increase public awareness about significance of change in pigmented lesions.
- Problematical naevi or naevi with an increased risk of malignant change are excised and sent for histological examination.

Vascular naevi

These common naevi, usually congenital or developed soon after birth, are composed of small dermal blood vessels. There are four main types:
- Salmon patch: commonest type (present in about 50% of neonates), typically on neck or eyelids. Usually fade quickly.
- Port wine stain naevus: irregular red/purple macule which often affects one side of the face.
- Capillary haemangioma (strawberry naevus): red nodular lesion which develops during the first few weeks of life, reaches its maximum size in the first 12 months, and then involutes. Most cases have regressed by 5–7 years.
- Cavernous haemangioma: similar to strawberry naevus but composed of larger and deeper channels and presents as a nodular swelling. Regression is not as complete.

The treatment is by camouflage cosmetics or laser treatments for port wine stains. Strawberry naevi are usually left to involute.

Epidermal naevi

These warty, pigmented and often elongated naevi are usually congenital or develop in early childhood. Most are a few cm long but can be extensive.

Treatment is by excision but recurrence is common.

Connective tissue naevi

Rare, skin-coloured papules composed of coarse collagen bundles in the dermis, these are common in tuberous sclerosis.

Fig. 15.23 provides a summary of naevi.

Malignant melanoma

This malignant tumour of melanocytes usually arises in the skin. Incidence in the UK is 10 per 100 000 per year,

but is rising steadily. Females are more often affected than males by 2:1.

It occurs in all races, but is more common in caucasoids, with an incidence that is proportional to geographical latitude, suggesting an effect of UV radiation. The commonest site in males is on the back but in females it is the lower leg.

THe aetiology is unknown but repeated exposure to UV radiation is thought to play a part.

Major risk factors for the development of malignant melanoma (with decreasing risk) are:
- Familial dysplastic naevus syndrome.
- Multiple melanocytic naevi (50 naevi over 2 mm in diameter).
- Congenital naevus.
- Previous malignant melanoma.
- Immunosuppression.
- Fair skin.

Classification

Four main types of malignant melanoma are recognized:

Superficial spreading malignant melanoma

A flat tumour with variable pigmentation and irregular edges, this is the commonest type, accounting for 50% of all UK cases. There is a female preponderance, and it is commonest on the lower leg.

Lentigo malignant melanoma

A nodular lesion arising in a pre-existing lentigo maligna,

Summary of naevi	
Type of naevus	**Comments**
melanocytic	very common, usually multiple, pigmented and benign consist of nests of melanocytic cells classified into junctional, compound and intradermal types are congenital, blue, halo, Becker's and dysplastic
vascular	common, usually congenital, composed of small dermal blood vessels types are salmon patch, port wine stain, capillary haemangioma ('strawberry'), cavernous haemangioma
epidermal	warty, pigmented and often linear
connective tissue	rare, skin-coloured, collagenous naevi

Fig. 15.23 Summary of naevi.

typically occurs in sun-damaged skin of the face in elderly patients. It comprises about 15% of UK cases.

(The lentigo maligna is similar to a benign lentigine—p.347—but is generally larger, at over 2 cm, and has atypical melanocytes.)

Acral lentiginous malignant melanoma
This resembles the lentigo malignant melanoma but affects the palms, soles and nail-beds (subungual melanoma). It comprises 10% of UK cases but is the commonest form of malignant melanoma in oriental people. It is often diagnosed late and consequently has poor survival figures.

Nodular malignant melanoma
A pigmented nodule which may grow rapidly and ulcerate, this accounts for 25% of UK melanomas and is more common in males, typically arising on the trunk.

Staging and prognosis of malignant melanoma
Local invasion of the malignant melanoma is assessed using the Breslow method (Fig. 15.24). The Breslow

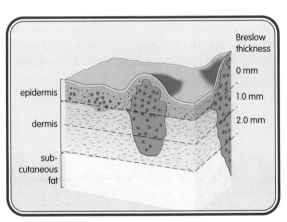

Fig. 15.24 Staging of malignant melanomas.

thickness is the measured thickness in mm (on a histological section) from the granular layer of the epidermis to the deepest identifiable melanoma cell.

The Breslow thickness is directly related to the risk of metastasis (Fig. 15.25). Tumours are divided into one of three prognostic groups depending on their Breslow thickness.

Diagnosis—One or more of following changes observed or reported in a naevus or pigmented lesion may suggest malignant melanoma:
- Size: usually increased.
- Shape: irregular outline.
- Colour: irregular pigmentation.
- Inflammation: at the edge of lesion.
- Crusting: oozing or bleeding lesion.
- Itchiness: a common symptom.

The differential diagnosis of malignant melanoma includes:
- Benign lentigine.
- Benign melanocytic naevi.
- Dermatofibroma.
- Haemangioma.
- Pigmented basal cell carcinoma.
- Seborrhoeic wart.

Management is by surgical excision with regular follow-up to detect recurrence which may be:
- Local: at edge of excised site.
- Lymphatic: in regional lymph nodes or in lymphatics between tumour and nodes.
- In distant sites: due to haematogenous spread.

Malignant epidermal tumours
Basal cell carcinoma (rodent ulcer)
A malignant tumour that arises from the basal keratinocytes of the epidermis. This is the commonest form of skin cancer, typically seen on the face in elderly or middle-aged subjects, with a male preponderance.

Fig. 15.25 Five-year survival rates for malignant melanomas of different Breslow thickness.

Five-year survival rates for malignant melanomas of different Breslow thickness		
Prognosis	Breslow thickness (mm)	5-year survival rate (%)
good	<1.0	93
intermediate	1–3.5	67
poor	>3.5	31

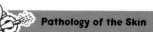

Tumours are locally very invasive but almost never metastasize.

Risk factors for the development of basal cell carcinoma include:

- Repeated UV exposure: tumours are more common in light-skinned races, with increasing incidence towards the Equator.
- X-ray irradiation.
- Chronic scarring.
- Genetic predisposition.

Tumours are typically composed of basophilic cells that invade the dermis as well-defined lobules and islands of cells.

Clinical presentation—They typically occur on sun-exposed sites, commonly around the nose, inner canthus of the eyelids and the temple.

Tumours grow slowly but relentlessly and may destroy underlying cartilage, bone and soft tissue structures.

There are three main types of basal cell carcinoma:

- Nodular: commonest form. Skin-coloured nodule which may show numerous telangiectatic vessels and a glistening pearly edge. Often has central ulceration with an adherent crust.
- Superficial (or multicentric): flat, red plaque often with an irregular rim-like edge, and light pigmentation. Often multiple, and occasionally seen on the trunk.
- Morphoeic: flat, thickened, whitish yellowish plaque with indistinct edges. These may have focal areas of ulceration.

Management—Complete excision is usually the best treatment but is not always possible. Radiotherapy is often used for non-excisable tumours. Recurrence is about 5% at 5 years for most methods of treatment.

Squamous cell carcinoma

This malignant tumour is derived from keratinocytes of the upper layers of the epidermis, and typically seen on the face in elderly or middle-aged subjects, with a male preponderance. Tumours are locally invasive and may also metastasize.

Its aetiology is related to:

- Chronic sunlight exposure.
- Chemical carcinogens (e.g. tar, arsenic and machine oil).
- X-ray radiation.
- Chronic ulceration and scarring.

- Smoking (lip lesions).
- Common wart virus with immunosuppression.
- Genetic (e.g. xeroderma pigmentosum).

Histologically, tumours consist of disorganized keratinocytes with typical malignant cytology, which destroy the dermo-epidermal junction and form invading strands into the dermis. Foci of keratinization are seen within the tumour.

The clinical presentation is:

- Dome-shaped nodules which usually arise in sun-exposed sites such as the face, neck, forearm or hand.
- Nodules typically develop into roughened keratotic areas, ulcers or horns.
- Often difficult to distinguish from keratoacanthomas.
- Less aggressive form may arise within actinic keratosis (pp. 349–350) as a small papule which progresses to ulcerate and then crust over.
- More aggressive forms may arise at the edge of chronic skin ulcers (rare).

Management—The treatment of choice is surgical excision. Radiotherapy can be used for carcinomas of the face or scalp in the elderly.

Intra-epidermal carcinoma (Bowen's disease)

This carcinoma *in situ* typically occurs on the lower leg in elderly women. Its predisposition is associated with previous exposure to arsenicals. It is characterized by:

There are only two skin neoplasms in which metastasis is a common feature:

- Malignant melanoma tumour of melanocytes, which metastasizes early.
- Squamous cell carcinoma tumour of upper epidermal keratinocytes, which metastasizes late.

Both are epidermal in origin.

- Slowly extending, pink or lightly pigmented, scaly plaques up to several cm in size.
- Atypical keratinocytes throughout whole thickness of the epidermis with prominent nuclear pleomorphism, and large numbers of mitoses.

Carcinomas usually remain *in situ* for many years but have the capacity to transform into squamous cell carcinomas.

Other tumours of the skin
Keratoacanthoma
This benign, self-limiting tumour typically arises on the face of elderly people. It grows very rapidly, changing from a small, red papule to a large, domed nodule with raised edges and a central mass of keratin within a few weeks. It resembles a squamous cell carcinoma, but does not invade deeply and never metastasizes.

The majority spontaneously regress within a few months.

Mycosis fungoides (cutaneous T cell lymphoma)
This rare, slowly progressive (years) tumour of CD4⁺ (T helper) lymphocytes evolves in the skin. There are four stages:
- Premycotic phase: erythematous eczematoid lesions. May persist for 10 or more years.
- Infiltrative phase: plaques develop, typically affecting the trunk. This stage may last for years.
- Fungoid phase: tumour nodules or ulcers develop within the plaques. Has a mean survival time of 2.5 years.
- Systemic disease: involvement of lymph nodes or internal organs.

Dermatofibrosarcoma
This is a locally invasive dermal tumour of proliferating myofibroblasts with low grade malignancy. It is similar in appearance to dermatofibromas but more aggressive in nature, and characterized by protuberant nodules on the epidermis. It has a tendency to recur following excision.

Kaposi's sarcoma
This malignant disorder is characterized by bluish-brown plaques or nodules formed from a proliferation of small blood vessels and spindle cells in the dermis.

Intradermal haemorrhage with haemosiderin deposition occurs within the nodules.

It commonly occurs in association with AIDS but is also endemic in certain African regions with cytomegalovirus. The lesions may be single or multiple, and have a tendency to metastasize.

- **Name the benign tumours of the epidermis and dermis.**
- **Describe the classification of melanocytic naevi.**
- **State the main risk factors for the development of malignant melanoma.**
- **What are the four clinical types of malignant melanoma?**
- **Describe the malignant tumours of the epidermis.**

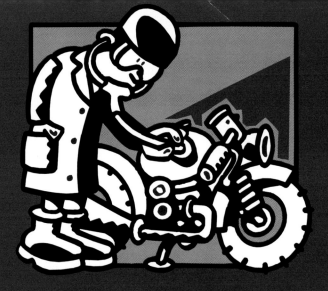

SELF-ASSESSMENT

Indicate whether each answer is true or false.

1. The following definitions are correct:

(a) Dysplasia is a change from one type of differentiated tissue to another.
(b) Anaplasia is an almost complete lack of differentiation.
(c) Carcinoma is a malignant tumour of epithelial derivation.
(d) Metaplasia is the disordered development of cells with loss of organization.
(e) Carcinoma *in situ* is a carcinoma with stromal invasion.

2. The following definitions are correct:

(a) Adenoma is a malignant tumour of glandular epithelium.
(b) Sarcoma is a benign tumour of connective tissue.
(c) Liposarcoma is a malignant tumour of adipose tissue.
(d) Chondroma is a benign tumour of cartilage.
(e) Lymphoma is a benign tumour of lymphoid cells.

3. Common features of benign tumours include:

(a) Invasion of surrounding stromal tissue.
(b) Cells of uniform size and appearance.
(c) Many mitotic figures.
(d) Ill-defined borders.
(e) Close resemblance to the original tissue.

4. In acute inflammation:

(a) The predominant cell type is the neutrophil polymorph.
(b) The inflammation is usually initiated by cell-mediated immunity.
(c) The duration may be for months.
(d) Plasma cells are frequently present.
(e) Lymphocytes are present at the start of the process.

5. The following are cytokines:

(a) Interleukins.
(b) Interferons.
(c) Bradykinin.
(d) Arachidonic acid.
(e) Tumour necrosis factor.

6. The following inflammatory processes often contain granulomas:

(a) Tuberculosis.
(b) Sarcoidosis.
(c) Ulcerative colitis.
(d) Leprosy.
(e) Ruptured silicone breast implant.

7. The following definitions are true:

(a) Virulence is the degree of pathogenicity of an organism.
(b) Commensal micro-organisms are those that are normally absent from the body and which cause disease.
(c) Opportunistic infections are those occurring in a fully immunocompetent host.
(d) Colonization is the habitation of external body surfaces by harmless micro-organisms.
(e) Infection is the invasion of a host by harmful micro-organisms.

8. A gene:

(a) Is composed of exons and introns.
(b) Is transcribed into DNA before splicing.
(c) Codes for a single polypeptide chain.
(d) On autosomal chromosomes is usually paired with a similar gene.
(e) Is regulated by promoters.

9. Anencephaly:

(a) Is commoner in male than female fetuses.
(b) Occurs in 1 in 100 live births.
(c) Is invariably fatal.
(d) Often results in spontaneous abortion.
(e) Has an absent cranial vault.

10. Extradural haemorrhage:

(a) Occurs between the dura and outer surface of the arachnoid membrane.
(b) Is not usually associated with a skull fracture.
(c) Is due to bleeding from the cortical bridging veins.
(d) May be associated with a post-traumatic lucid period.
(e) Requires urgent surgical intervention.

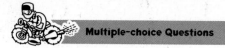

11. Ventricular septal defect:

(a) Usually produces a left-to-right shunt of blood.
(b) Produces cyanosis.
(c) Produces a pansystolic murmur.
(d) May be of a membranous or muscular location.
(e) Is the commonest congenital cardiac abnormality.

12. Benign hypertension is characterized by:

(a) Fibrinoid necrosis of arterioles.
(b) Hypertrophy of the muscular media of the arteries.
(c) Fibroelastic thickening of the initima.
(d) Hyaline deposition in arteriole walls.
(e) Sudden and severe increase in blood pressure.

13. Mitral valve incompetence may be caused by:

(a) Right ventricular dilatation.
(b) Infective endocarditis.
(c) Rheumatic fever.
(d) Papillary muscle rupture.
(e) Senile calcification.

14. Rheumatic fever:

(a) Is due to staphylococcal infection.
(b) Is due to a type IV hypersensitivity reaction.
(c) Is characterized by Aschoff nodules in the myocardium.
(d) Is becoming more common in Europe.
(e) May produce erythema marginatum.

15. Infective endocarditis:

(a) Usually occurs on structurally normal valves.
(b) Usually occurs on the mitral valve in IV drug abusers.
(c) May be caused by *Streptococcus viridans*.
(d) May be caused by *Candida* species.
(e) May cause mycotic aneurysms.

16. The following conditions predispose to the formation of aortic aneurysms:

(a) Atherosclerosis.
(b) Marfan's syndrome.
(c) Ehlers–Danlos syndrome.
(d) Syphilis.
(e) Osteopetrosis.

17. Carcinoma of the larynx:

(a) Is usually sited in the subglottic region.
(b) Has a positive association with cigarette smoking.
(c) Commonly spreads by the haematogenous route.
(d) Is usually of squamous cell differentiation.
(e) Usually presents after the age of 40 years.

18. Pulmonary emphysema:

(a) Is more common in females than males.
(b) Has a positive association with cigarette smoking.
(c) Has a positive association with a_1-antitrypsin deficiency.
(d) Has a positive association with chronic bronchitis.
(e) May produce pneumothoraces.

19. Bronchial asthma:

(a) May be caused by a type II hypersensitivity reaction.
(b) Is associated with hypotrophy of bronchial smooth muscle.
(c) May be precipitated by aspirin ingestion.
(d) May be precipitated by ozone.
(e) Is associated with bronchial mucosal oedema.

20. Cystic fibrosis:

(a) Is associated with infections with *Pseudomonas*.
(b) Is the commonest autosomal dominant condition in Europe.
(c) Is due to defective transport of chloride ions.
(d) May cause malabsorption.
(e) Is due to a mutation in a gene on chromosome 7.

21. Pulmonary tuberculosis:

(a) Is most commonly due to *Mycobacterium avium intracellulare*.
(b) Is caused by direct cytopathic effects of the infecting organism.
(c) Has a positive association with silicosis.
(d) Is a common cause of death in AIDS.
(e) Is characterized histologically by granulomas.

22. Lung carcinoma:

(a) Is most commonly of adenomatous differentiation.
(b) Has a positive association with cigarette smoking.
(c) Has a positive association with asbestos exposure.
(d) Has rarely metastasized at the time of presentation.
(e) Is the most common cause of death from neoplasia in the UK.

23. Coalworker's pneumoconiosis:

(a) May produce a restrictive pattern of pulmonary function.
(b) When associated with rheumatoid arthritis is named Caplan's syndrome.
(c) Is characterized by aggregates of pigment-laden macrophages in the lungs.
(d) Is associated with focal emphysema.
(e) Is classified as an industrial lung disease.

24. Asbestos exposure:

(a) Usually produces lung disease within 5 years of exposure.
(b) Has a positive association with mesothelioma.
(c) Of serpentine form is associated most strongly with pulmonary disease.
(d) May cause fibrotic lung disease.
(e) Is associated with lung carcinoma.

25. Pulmonary embolism:

(a) Has a positive association with heparin administration.
(b) Is usually caused by thromboembolism from the leg veins.
(c) Usually causes pulmonary infarction.
(d) Causes pulmonary hypertension.
(e) May be caused by tumour emboli.

26. Squamous cell carcinoma of the oral cavity:

(a) Occurs most commonly on the lips.
(b) Is commoner in women than men.
(c) Has a positive association with cigarette smoking.
(d) Has a positive association with moderate alcohol intake.
(e) Has a 5 year survival of about 50%.

27. Carcinoma of the oesophagus:

(a) Has a positive association with Barrett's metaplasia.
(b) May present with dysphagia.
(c) Has a 5% 5 year survival rate after treatment.
(d) Has a positive association with cigarette smoking.
(e) Has a positive association with tylosis.

28. *Helicobacter pylori*:

(a) Produces urease.
(b) Cannot be cultured in the laboratory.
(c) Causes antral gastritis.
(d) Is associated with antibodies to parietal cells.
(e) May be diagnosed by the urea breath test.

29. Gastric carcinoma:

(a) Is usually of squamous cell type.
(b) Is commoner in females than males.
(c) Occurs most commonly in the body of the stomach.
(d) Is commoner in Japan than Europe.
(e) Has a positive association with *Helicobacter pylori* infection.

30. Portal hypertension:

(a) May be caused by hepatic cirrhosis.
(b) May be caused by portal vein thrombosis.
(c) May be caused by hepatic vein thrombosis.
(d) Is not associated with ascites.
(e) Is associated with oesophageal varices.

31. Hepatitis A:

(a) Is caused by a DNA virus.
(b) Often causes chronic liver disease.
(c) Is transmitted by tattooing and IV drug abuse.
(d) May be prevented by vaccination.
(e) Is commoner in Europe than in the tropics.

32. Hepatocellular carcinoma:

(a) Is the commonest malignant hepatic tumour.
(b) Has a positive association with hepatitis A.
(c) Is commoner in males than females.
(d) Has a median survival of 3 years following diagnosis.
(e) Arises from bile duct epithelium.

33. Carcinoma of the pancreas:

(a) Has a positive association with excess alcohol ingestion.
(b) Is commoner in women than men.
(c) Is usually surgically resectable.
(d) Is an adenocarcinoma.
(e) Usually occurs in subjects older than 60 years.

34. Crohn's disease:

(a) Has a positive association with erythema nodosum.
(b) Has a negative association with cigarette smoking.
(c) May occur anywhere from the mouth to anus.
(d) Is characterized histologically by non-caseating granulomas.
(e) Has a positive association with uveitis.

35. Ulcerative colitis:

(a) Is characterized by transmural inflammation.
(b) Has a positive association with cigarette smoking.
(c) Is characterized by granulomatous inflammation.
(d) Is commonly complicated by fistulae.
(e) Is characterized by continuous disease distribution in the colon.

36. Colorectal carcinoma:

(a) Has a high incidence in Africa.
(b) Has a positive association with familial adenomatous polyposis.
(c) Is usually of squamous differentiation.
(d) Is staged by Dukes' system.
(e) Is incurable if it has metastasized to the liver.

37. Renal cell carcinoma:

(a) Is commoner in females than males.
(b) Is associated with von Hippel–Lindau syndrome.
(c) Rarely spreads by the haematogenous route.
(d) Has a positive association with cigarette smoking.
(e) Is usually of adenomatous differentiation.

38. Carcinoma of the uterine cervix:

(a) Is usually of adenomatous differentiation.
(b) Is often preceded by cervical intraepithelial neoplasia (CIN).
(c) Has a positive association with some serotypes of HPV.
(d) Has a positive association with cigarette smoking.
(e) Has a positive association with HIV infection.

39. The following are causes of primary hyperthyroidism:

(a) Graves' disease.
(b) Hashimoto's thyroiditis.
(c) Excess production of TSH.
(d) Multinodular goitre.
(e) Thyroid adenoma.

40. The following are causes of Cushing's syndrome:

(a) Addison's disease.
(b) ACTH administration.
(c) Prednisolone administration.
(d) Phaeochromocytomas.
(e) Adrenal cortical adenomas.

41. The human immunodeficiency virus (HIV)-1:

(a) Is a DNA virus.
(b) Requires reverse transcriptase from the host cell to replicate.
(c) Binds to CD4 lymphocytes.
(d) Is associated with *Pneumocytis carinii* infection.
(e) Is associated with *Mycobacterium avium intracellulare* infection.

42. Amyloid:

(a) Is an α helix protein.
(b) May be made of immunoglobulin light chains.
(c) May cause renal failure.
(d) Is found in cerebral plaques in Alzheimer's disease.
(e) Is associated with haemodialysis.

43. Neutropenia:

(a) In Caucasians is defined as a neutrophil count of less than 2.5 ± 10^9.
(b) May occur after phenylbutazone administration.
(c) Occurs in untreated chronic myeloid leukaemia.
(d) Occurs in Felty's syndrome.
(e) Occurs in folate deficiency.

44. Hodgkin's disease:

(a) Is characterized histologically by Reed–Sternberg cells.
(b) Is commoner in females than males.
(c) Is staged using the Rye classification.
(d) Has a better prognosis if B symptoms are present.
(e) Of the mixed cellularity type has the most favourable prognosis.

45. Chronic lymphocytic leukaemia:

(a) Is characterized cytogenetically by the Philadelphia chromosome.
(b) Is the commonest leukaemia in adults.
(c) Has a median survival of 9 months.
(d) Is commoner in males than females.
(e) May affect lymph nodes.

46. Sickle cell disease:

(a) Is caused by a point mutation in the DNA coding for the α-globin chain.
(b) Is commoner in Europe than Africa.
(c) Is associated with gallstones.
(d) Is associated with hypersplenism.
(e) May confer some resistance to malarial infection.

47. The following definitions are correct:

(a) Nodule is a raised lesion less than 5 mm across.
(b) Vesicle is a blister less than 5 mm across.
(c) Macular describes a raised lesion of altered skin colour.
(d) Pustule is a blister containing clear fluid.
(e) Spongiosis means epidermal oedema.

48. Psoriasis:

(a) Is an infective condition.
(b) Is characterized by a reduced turnover of epithelial cells.
(c) May be precipitated by lithium administration.
(d) Commonly affects skin over the elbows.
(e) Is associated with pitting of the nails.

49. Acne vulgaris:

(a) Is due to an increased sensitivity to oestrogen.
(b) Is associated with *Propionibacterium acnes* colonization.
(c) Has a predilection for the face.
(d) May be treated with erythromycin.
(e) Is associated with decreased sebum excretion.

50. Malignant melanoma:

(a) Arises from epidermal keratinocytes.
(b) Is associated with intermittent intense UV light exposure.
(c) Has an increased incidence in familial dysplastic naevus syndrome.
(d) With a depth of invasion of 3.5 mm has a good prognosis.
(e) May arise within lentigo maligna.

Short-answer Questions

1. What is inflammation? Compare the basic characteristics of acute and chronic inflammation.

2. Define 'syringomyelia'. List the causes and effects of this condition.

3. What is the most common congenital abnormality of the heart? Outline the pathology.

4. Define 'atherosclerosis' and describe the pathogenesis of atheromas.

5. What is Alzheimer's disease? Describe the histological hallmarks.

6. What is hypertension? Describe the features of benign and malignant hypertension.

7. Outline the aetiology and pathogenesis of chronic bronchitis.

8. Describe the pathogenesis of extrinsic (atopic) asthma.

9. Write short notes on lung cancer.

10. Outline the different respiratory diseases that may be caused by exposure to asbestos.

11. Define 'reflux oesophagitis' and list the predisposing factors and complications.

12. Describe the pathogenesis of autoimmune gastritis.

13. Define 'cirrhosis' and list the causes.

14. What is jaundice and what are the causes?

15. Describe the aetiology and pathogenesis of coeliac disease.

16. List three risk factors for colorectal carcinoma, and compare the pathological features of left- and right-sided colonic lesions.

17. Define 'osteoarthritis' and list the most commonly affected joints and four characteristic features that can be detected on X-ray.

18. What is amyloidosis? Describe the features of reactive systemic amyloidosis.

19. Define 'thyrotoxicosis' and outline the causes.

20. What is Cushing's syndrome? Describe the aetiology and clinical features.

Essay Questions

1. Describe the pathogenesis and complications of myocardial infarction.

2. Write an essay on the GI causes of anaemia.

3. Describe the pathology of breast carcinoma and the pathological factors that can predict its prognosis.

4. Write an essay on the effects of cigarette smoking on the respiratory system.

5. Describe the pathology of lesions causing haematuria.

6. Discuss the pathology of cerebrovascular disease.

7. Write an essay on rheumatoid disease.

8. Write an essay on the complications of diabetes mellitus.

9. Compare and contrast the pathology of ulcerative colitis and Crohn's disease.

10. Describe the pathology of malignant melanoma.

MCQ Answers

1. (a)F, (b)T, (c)T, (d)F, (e)F
2. (a)F, (b)F, (c)T, (d)T, (e)F
3. (a)F, (b)T, (c)F, (d)F, (e)T
4. (a)T, (b)F, (c)F, (d)F, (e)F
5. (a)T, (b)T, (c)F, (d)F, (e)T
6. (a)T, (b)T, (c)F, (d)T, (e)T
7. (a)T, (b)F, (c)F, (d)T, (e)T
8. (a)T, (b)F, (c)T, (d)T, (e)T
9. (a)F, (b)F, (c)T, (d)T, (e)T
10. (a)F, (b)F, (c)F, (d)T, (e)T
11. (a)T, (b)F, (c)T, (d)T, (e)T
12. (a)F, (b)T, (c)T, (d)T, (e)F
13. (a)F, (b)T, (c)T, (d)T, (e)F
14. (a)F, (b)F, (c)T, (d)F, (e)T
15. (a)F, (b)F, (c)T, (d)T, (e)T
16. (a)T, (b)T, (c)T, (d)T, (e)F
17. (a)F, (b)T, (c)F, (d)T, (e)T
18. (a)F, (b)T, (c)T, (d)T, (e)T
19. (a)F, (b)F, (c)T, (d)T, (e)T
20. (a)T, (b)F, (c)T, (d)T, (e)T
21. (a)F, (b)F, (c)T, (d)T, (e)T
22. (a)F, (b)T, (c)T, (d)F, (e)T
23. (a)T, (b)T, (c)T, (d)T, (e)T
24. (a)F, (b)T, (c)F, (d)T, (e)T
25. (a)F, (b)T, (c)F, (d)T, (e)T

26. (a)T, (b)F, (c)T, (d)F, (e)T
27. (a)T, (b)T, (c)T, (d)T, (e)T
28. (a)T, (b)F, (c)T, (d)F, (e)T
29. (a)F, (b)F, (c)F, (d)T, (e)T
30. (a)T, (b)T, (c)T, (d)F, (e)T
31. (a)F, (b)F, (c)F, (d)T, (e)F
32. (a)F, (b)F, (c)T, (d)F, (e)F
33. (a)T, (b)F, (c)F, (d)T, (e)T
34. (a)T, (b)F, (c)T, (d)T, (e)T
35. (a)F, (b)F, (c)F, (d)F, (e)T
36. (a)F, (b)T, (c)F, (d)T, (e)F
37. (a)F, (b)T, (c)F, (d)T, (e)T
38. (a)F, (b)T, (c)T, (d)T, (e)T
39. (a)T, (b)F, (c)F, (d)T, (e)T
40. (a)F, (b)T, (c)T, (d)F, (e)T
41. (a)F, (b)T, (c)T, (d)T, (e)T
42. (a)F, (b)T, (c)T, (d)T, (e)T
43. (a)T, (b)T, (c)F, (d)T, (e)T
44. (a)T, (b)F, (c)F, (d)F, (e)F
45. (a)T, (b)T, (c)F, (d)T, (e)T
46. (a)F, (b)F, (c)T, (d)F, (e)T
47. (a)F, (b)T, (c)F, (d)F, (e)T
48. (a)F, (b)F, (c)T, (d)T, (e)T
49. (a)F, (b)T, (c)T, (d)T, (e)F
50. (a)F, (b)T, (c)T, (d)F, (e)T

1. Inflammation is the response of living tissues to cellular injury. It serves to localize or eliminate the causative agent, limit tissue injury, and restore tissue to normality.

    Acute inflammation is the initial, rapid response of a tissue to injury. The reaction is accompanied by a prominent vascular response, and the predominant cell type is the neutrophil polymorph (innate immunity). The duration of the response varies from a few hours to a few weeks.

    Chronic inflammation is the persisting, slow response of a tissue to injury. It does not involve a prominent vascular response, and the predominant cell types are lymphocytes, plasma cells and macrophages (cell-mediated immunity). The duration of the response may be weeks, month or even years.

2. Syringomyelia is a rare condition in which a cyst lined by gliosis develops within the spinal cord, most commonly in the cervical region.

    The causes of syringomyelia are:
    *   Congenital (minority): often associated with maldevelopment of the cord or of the craniocervical junction.
    *   Acquired (majority): secondary to trauma, ischaemia or tumours of the spinal cord.

    The effects of syringomyelia are:
    *   Disassociated sensory loss, i.e. loss of the pain and temperature senses but with preservation of the position and vibration senses due to damage to the nerve fibres crossing the cord in the spinothalamic tract.
    *   Muscle weakness and atrophy in the upper limbs due to compression of the anterior horn cells.

3. Ventricular septal defects (VSDs) are the commonest cardiac abnormality, accounting for approximately 25% of all cases of congenital heart disease, and occurring in 1 in 500 live births. VSDs result in the shunting of blood from the left ventricle to the right (due to increased pressures on the left). The extent of shunting depends on the site and size of defects.

    The sites of VSDs are:
    *   Membranous portion: small defects.
    *   Muscular portion: larger defects.
    *   Junction of membranous and muscular portions (most common): small defects.

    Depending on the size of the defect, VSDs may present as cardiac failure in infants or as a murmur in older children or adults. Physical signs include a pansystolic murmur (caused by flow from the high pressure left ventricle to the low pressure right ventricle during systole), tachypnoea, and indrawing of the lower ribs on inspiration.

4. Atherosclerosis is a degenerative disease of large- and medium-sized arteries, characterized by the focal accumulation of lipid-rich material within the intima, with associated cellular reactions. The net result is a thickening and hardening of the arterial walls, which predisposes to ischaemia, vessel rupture, aneurysms, and thrombosis. These consequences of atherosclerosis account for half of all deaths in the Western world.

    Atherosclerotic lesions are known as atheromas. The most widely accepted theory proposes that their pathogenesis involves the following sequence of events:
    1. Chronic, low-grade endothelial injury results in the entry of cholesterol-rich, low-density lipoproteins (LDLs) into the intima; migration of macrophages into the intima; and platelet adhesion to the damaged endothelium.
    2. Intimal macrophages phagocytose lipid, forming barely visible pale bulges or 'fatty streaks'.
    3. Adhering platelets release platelet-derived growth factor (PDGF); there is a proliferation of intimal smooth muscle cells (myointimal cells).
    4. Myointimal cells deposit excess collagen and elastin in the intima forming 'lipid plaques', which are raised, yellow lesions consisting of free lipid (released by macrophages) and collagen.
    5. Increased collagen deposition eventually results in the formation of dense fibrous plaques—'fibrolipid plaques'—which cause pressure atrophy of the underlying media and elastic lamina, with weakening of the arterial wall.

5. Alzheimer's disease is a degenerative disorder characterized by marked atrophy of the cerebral cortex, especially of the frontal lobes.

    There are three histological hallmarks:
    *   Senile plaques: extracellular core of amyloid protein surrounded by dystrophic neurites.
    *   Neuropil threads: distorted, twisted dendritic processes of cortical axons found around amyloid plaques.
    *   Neurofibrillary tangles: intracellular tangles of insoluble cytoskeletal proteins (paired helical filaments) within cerebral neurons.

6. Chronic bronchitis is defined as a persistent productive cough for at least three consecutive months in at least two consecutive years.

    Aetiology—Cigarette smoking is thought to be the most important causative agent. Other causes include air polluting irritants such as sulphur dioxide or recurrent respiratory infections.

    Pathogenesis—Constant irritation of the bronchioles leads to chronic inflammation (bronchiolitis) with hypertrophy and hyperplasia of the mucous glands. Increased mucus secretion by the glands gives rise to the extensive mucus plugging responsible for the obstructive features of the disease. Sputum is typically sterile but is often complicated by infections of *Haemophilus influenzae* or *Streptococcus pneumoniae*.

7. Hypertension is defined as a sustained rise in systemic blood pressure above 160 mmHg systolic and/or above 95 mmHg diastolic. Hypertension is important as it is a treatable cause of cardiac failure and a major risk factor for the development of atherosclerosis.

   Benign hypertension is a common condition characterized by a stable elevation of blood pressure over many years. The disease affects at least 5% of the UK population, typically beginning at around 45 years old but prolonged into the sixth and seventh decades; males are affected more than females.
   Morphologically, there is a gradual thickening of the muscular media, elastic lamina and intima of the arteries with hyaline deposition in the arteriole walls (hyaline arteriolosclerosis).

   Malignant (accelerated) hypertension is a rare condition characterized by a dramatic elevation of blood pressure over a period of a few months to one or two years. The disease mainly affects young adults (25–35 years), females as much as males, and the majority of cases are secondary to renal disease. Acute destructive changes occur in the walls of the small arteries, namely necrosis of the vessel wall and infiltration of necrotic media by fibrin (fibrinoid necrosis). Destructive changes lead to the cessation of blood flow though the small vessels with multiple foci of tissue necrosis, e.g. in the glomeruli of the kidney, or abdominal viscera.

8. Pathogenesis of extrinsic asthma can be divided into three phases, correlating to the three clinical stages of the disorder:
   - Early (15–20 minutes): allergen binds to IgE antibodies on the surface of mast cells resulting in mast cell degranulation. Release of preformed histamine from the mast cell granules results in rapid onset bronchoconstriction.
   - Late (4–6 hours): inflammatory mediators released by mast cells during the early phase cause activation of macrophages and chemotaxis of polymorphs and eosinophils into the bronchial mucosa. These cells release further inflammatory mediators causing a secondary wave of bronchoconstriction after recovery from the early phase.
   - Prolonged hyper-reactivity (days): combined effect of damaged epithelial cells and persistence of inflammatory cells within the bronchial wall results in an exaggerated response of airways on further re-exposure to the allergen or other bronchoconstrictor trigger factors over ensuing days.

9. Incidence—Most common cancer in the UK, affecting 30 000 every year.
   Age—Peak incidence between 40 and 70 years.
   Sex—Males more than females, but with an increasing incidence in women.

Geography—The UK has a higher incidence than anywhere else in the world.
   Risk factors—Cigarette smoking.
   Occupational factors—Exposure to radioactive material, asbestos, nickel, chromium, iron oxides, and coal gas plants.
   Environmental factors—Radon (a natural radioactive gas in certain geographical areas).
   Macroscopic appearance—Tumours may be central (majority, all types) or peripheral (mainly adenocarcinomas).
   Microscopic appearance—Squamous cell carcinoma (50%), small ('oat') cell (20%), adenocarcinoma (20%), large cell anaplastic carcinoma (10%).
   Spread can be:
- Local: surrounding the lungs, pleura and adjacent mediastinal structures.
- Lymphatic: ipsilateral and contralateral peribronchial and hilar lymph nodes.
- Transcoelomic: across the pleural cavity.
- Haematogenous spread: brain, bone, liver and adrenal glands.

Prognosis—Related to type (worse with small cell) and stage (some squamous cell and adenocarcinomas may be surgically resectable) but, overall, 5 year survival is 5%.

10. Inhalation of asbestos, a fibrous silicate mineral, is associated with a number of pulmonary and pleural diseases. There is usually a latent period of about 15–30 years before clinical symptoms become evident.
    Asbestosis occurs within the interstitial fibrosis of the lungs resulting in a restrictive pattern of disease. Fibrosis is maximal at the lung bases, and asbestos bodies may be seen histologically.
    Lung cancer—There is a significantly increased risk of lung cancer in those exposed to asbestos, and the risk is greatly increased by smoking.
    Pleural plaques are asymptomatic discrete areas of asbestos-related pleural thickening usually identified on routine chest radiograph.
    Diffuse pleural fibrosis refers to diffuse areas of pleural thickening, causing a progressive restrictive defect of the lungs.
    Mesothelioma is a malignant tumour of the pleura. Over 90% of cases of mesothelioma are associated with asbestos exposure. Prognosis is poor.

11. Reflux oesophagitis is defined as inflammation of the oesophagus due to reflux of gastric acid from the stomach.
    The predisposing factors are:
- Factors that increase intra-abdominal pressure, e.g. over-eating, pregnancy, and poor posture.
- Factors that render the lower oesophageal sphincter incompetent, e.g. hiatus hernia, smoking or alcohol ingestion.

Complications are peptic ulceration of the lower oesophagus, stricture formation and Barrett's oesophagus, i.e. metaplasia of the lower oesophageal mucosa from squamous to glandular epithelium.

12. Autoimmune gastritis is an organ-specific autoimmune disease characterized by inflammation of the gastric mucosa, which is often associated with pernicious anaemia.

     Pathogenesis—Autoantibodies found in the serum are directed against gastric parietal cells and intrinsic factor (protein required for the absorption of dietary vitamin B_{12}). As a result, patients exhibit varying degrees of hypochlorhydria (decreased production of gastric acid) and have a macrocytic anaemia resulting from malabsorption of vitamin B_{12}. The association of autoimmune gastritis with macrocytic anaemia is known as pernicious anaemia. Histologically, there is glandular atrophy with a chronic inflammatory infiltrate. Also, the surface epithelium may show intestinal metaplasia, which is a premalignant condition.

13. Cirrhosis is defined as an irreversible process in which normal liver architecture is diffusely replaced by nodules of regenerated liver cells separated by bands of collagenous fibrosis. It is not in itself a diagnosis but represents the endstage of many diseases.
     The causes of cirrhosis are:
     - Common: idiopathic, alcoholic liver disease, chronic viral hepatitis (B or C).
     - Less common: autoimmune hepatitis, primary biliary cirrhosis, chronic biliary obstruction, cystic fibrosis, veno-occlusive disease, Budd–Chiari syndrome.
     - Rare: haemochromatosis, Wilson's disease, α_1-antitrypsin disease, glycogenosis, tyrosinaemia, drugs.

14. Clinical jaundice is defined as a yellowing of the skin or sclerae as a result of excess bilirubin in the blood. Levels of bilirubin must be above 50 mmol/L to manifest as yellow discoloration. Biochemical jaundice is defined as any increase in plasma bilirubin level above the normal (18–24 mmol/L).
     The aetiology of jaundice can be classified into pre-, intra- and posthepatic causes:
     - Prehepatic: haemolysis.
     - Intrahepatic: hepatocellular damage (e.g. alcoholic liver disease or viral hepatitis), small bile duct obstruction (e.g. primary biliary cirrhosis), hereditary enzyme defects (e.g. Gilbert's disease), pregnancy, drugs.
     - Posthepatic: large bile duct obstruction, e.g. gallstones, strictures, extrahepatic biliary atresia or pancreatic carcinoma.

15. Coeliac disease is a condition of malabsorption resulting from villous atrophy of the small intestine caused by abnormal sensitivity to gluten, a protein in wheat flour.
     Autoantibodies to the protein gliadin, a component of gluten, result in inflammation of the small intestinal mucosa with loss of villous architecture.
     Morphologically, the condition is characterized by a mosaic-like pattern of crypt openings with increased crypt depth and epithelial cell hyperplasia. Associations include HLA-B8 and dermatitis herpetiformis.

16. Risk factors for the development of colorectal carcinoma include the presence of multiple sporadic adenomatous polyps, ulcerative colitis and familial adenomatous polyposis.
     Right-sided carcinomas tend to have a polypoid growth pattern and often present later than left-sided lesions because of the easier passage of the softer faecal material in the ascending colon. Clinical features include weight loss, anaemia and right-sided abdominal mass.
     Left-sided carcinomas tend to have either annular or ulcerating growth patterns and present earlier due to mechanical obstruction to the passage of faeces. Clinical features include a change in bowel habit, rectal bleeding and obstruction.

17. Osteoarthritis is a degenerative disease of articular cartilage, associated with secondary changes in the underlying bone, resulting in pain and impaired function of the affected joint.
     The most commonly affected joints are the large weight-bearing joints of the hip, knee and vertebrae, or smaller joints that are constantly exposed to wear and tear such as in the hands.
     The four characteristic changes that can be recognized on X-ray are:
     - Narrowed joint space, due to loss of cartilage.
     - Increased bone density immediately adjacent to the joint space (sclerosis).
     - Irregularities of the bone surface, due to the presence of osteophytes.
     - Cystic appearance just beneath the sclerotic area.

18. Amyloidosis is the deposition of an abnormal extracellular fibrillar protein (amyloid) in the body's tissues.
     Reactive systemic amyloidosis describes the deposition of AA-type amyloid in different organs, especially the liver, spleen and kidney. AA amyloid is derived from serum amyloid A, an acute phase reactant protein synthesized in the liver in response to chronic inflammatory disorders such as chronic infections or rheumatoid arthritis.
     This condition results in hepatosplenomegaly and/or renal vein thrombosis, and nephrotic syndrome.

19. Thyrotoxicosis (a synonym for hyperthyroidism) is a clinical syndrome caused by excessive amounts of circulating thyroid hormones, typically both thyroxine and tri-iodothyronine.
     The signs and symptoms of thyrotoxicosis are the consequence of an increased metabolic rate and include tachycardia, palpitations, sweating, tremor, anxiety, increased appetite, loss of weight, fatigue and heat intolerance.
     Hyperthyroidism can be classified on the basis of aetiology into primary and secondary hyperthyroidism.
     Primary hyperthyroidism (increased thyroid hormones, decreased TSH): the hypersecretion of thyroid hormones which are not secondary to increased levels of TSH:
     - Graves' disease (exophthalmic goitre): this is

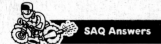

the commonest cause of thyrotoxicosis. It is an autoimmune disorder resulting in the overstimulation of the thyroid by autoantibodies.

- Toxic multinodular goitre (Plummer's disease).
- Toxic adenoma: solitary thyroid nodule producing excess hormone with the remainder of the thyroid gland being suppressed.
- Ingestion of large doses of thyroid hormone (thyrotoxicosis factitia).

Secondary hyperthyroidism (increased thyroid hormones, increased TSH): the overstimulation of the thyroid gland caused by excess TSH produced by a tumour in the pituitary or elsewhere (which is rare).

20. Cushing's syndrome is a condition resulting from prolonged inappropriate elevation of corticosteroid levels. The condition can by caused by:

- Excess ACTH, e.g. iatrogenic ACTH, pituitary hypersecretion of ACTH (Cushing's disease) or ectopic secretion of ACTH by malignant tumour of the lungs or elsewhere:
- Adrenal cortical tumours, either benign or malignant.
- Prolonged corticosteroid therapy.

The symptoms and signs include central obesity (buffalo torso) and moon face, reddening of the face and neck, hirsutism, hypertension, osteoporosis, diabetes and muscle wasting and weakness.

Index

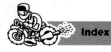

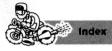

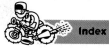

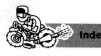

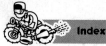